# Sensible Musculoskeletal Radiology

# Sensible Musculoskeletal Radiology:
## Case-Based Exercises in Clinical Decision Support

Edited by

Felix S. Chew, MD, MBA, FACR
Professor of Radiology
University of Washington

Hyojeong Lee, MD
Associate Professor of Radiology
University of Washington

Bare Bones Books
2021

First Printing: 2021

ISBN-13: 978-1721044337

ISBN-10: 1721044337

Bare Bones Books
9130 Fox Cove Ln NE
Bainbridge Island, WA 98110

barebonesbooks@yahoo.com

# Contents

# Preface

This book is intended to help physicians understand the nuances of ordering the most appropriate radiological exams for their patients, based primarily on the academic practice at the University of Washington and the evidence-based knowledge embedded in the American College of Radiology Appropriateness Criteria®. There is a wealth of published literature on the radiology of musculoskeletal diseases, but the results of idealized imaging in academic medical centers that is often described in the literature may not be obtainable in actual practice.

Radiologists have a unique perspective on the appropriateness of radiological exams because they see the results of imaging exams in much larger numbers than any individual referring clinician. It is from this perspective that we have written this book.

The book is divided into several parts by clinical presentation. Each part is further organized into chapters by anatomy. After the Introduction, each chapter is comprised of a number of individual cases that pose variations of a more general clinical problem. Following the concise presentation of a patient, the reader may choose among different imaging options for the presented patient. A sensible recommendation is made, and the specific clinical situation is then generalized, illustrated, and discussed, so that the reader can analogize to future cases in their real-world clinical practice.

Ordering radiology exams has become more difficult as the number imaging options has been expanding more rapidly than the administrative infrastructure. For example, many different radiological exams share identical Current Procedural Terminology (CPT) codes because of similarities in technology or historical factors. Ordering screens on electronic health records (EHR) may be slow to accept updates to radiology services being offered, increasing the level of difficulty for clinicians who wish to order a specific exam, and for radiologists who are trying to understand a generic order. Clinical decision support has the potential to improve patient access to diagnostic imaging by streamlining the ordering process for patients and healthcare providers. In this book, we provide exercises for clinicians to learn the nuances of how to order appropriate radiologic examinations for their patients.

Felix S. Chew
Hyojeong Lee

# Contributors

Laura Bancroft, MD
Professor, Radiology
University of Central Florida
Orlando, FL

Majid Chalian, MD
Assistant Professor, Radiology
University of Washington
Seattle, WA

Felix S. Chew, MD, MBA, FACR
Professor, Radiology
University of Washington
Seattle, WA

Carolyn Clark, MD
University of Washington
Seattle, WA

Tanner Clark, MD
University of Washington
Seattle, WA

Amanda M Crawford, MD
Assistant Professor, Radiology and Imaging Sciences
University of Utah
Salt Lake City, UT

Edward Derrick, MD
Department of Radiology
University of Central Florida
Orlando, FL

Jennifer Favinger, MD
Kaiser Permanente Washington
Seattle, WA

Erin M. Flaherty, MD
Tacoma, WA

Ryan P. Joyce, MD
Assistant Professor, Radiology
University of Washington
Seattle, WA

Kimia Kani, MD
Assistant Professor, Radiology
University of Maryland
Baltimore, MD

Vijaya Kosaraju, MD
Assistant Professor, Radiology
University Hospitals
Cleveland, OH

Hyojeong Lee, MD
Associate Professor, Radiology
University of Washington
Seattle, WA

Megan K. Mills, MD
Assistant Professor, Radiology and Imaging Sciences
University of Utah
Salt Lake City, UT

Jonelle Petscavage-Thomas, MD
Professor, Radiology
Penn State University
Hershey, PA

Jack A. Porrino, MD
Associate Professor, Radiology
Yale University
New Haven, CT

Michael L. Richardson, MD, FAUR
Professor, Radiology
University of Washington
Seattle, WA

Eira S. Roth, MD
Dallas, TX

Kurt F. Scherer, MD
Assistant Professor, Radiology
University of Central Florida
Orlando, FL

Maryam Soltanolkotabi, MD
Assistant Professor, Radiology and Imaging Sciences
University of Utah
Salt Lake City, UT

Lindsay Stratchko, DO
Department of Radiology
Penn State University
Hershey, PA

Eric A. Walker, MD, FACR
(1) Professor, Radiology
Penn State University
Hershey, PA
(2) Adjunct Assistant Professor, Radiology
Uniformed Services University of the Health Sciences
Bethesda, MD

# Part I. Introduction

# Chapter 1. The Sensible Approach

Felix S. Chew, MD

A sensible, pragmatic approach to ordering the most appropriate imaging test of musculoskeletal disorders should lead to the correct diagnosis in an efficient manner and not require the use of complicated diagnostic trees developed at academic medical centers. The patient populations may differ significantly from one practice to another, as may the availability of imaging technology, the expertise of local radiologists, and the expectations of patients, referring providers, and payors.

Healthcare facilities and systems have common features. Radiography (x-ray) is generally found in nearly every healthcare facility; CT and MRI are generally found in radiology departments or imaging centers. Radiography has relatively low cost, CT has higher cost, and MRI has even higher cost. Radiography is easily available, CT is available the same day, MRI may take a few days. MRI has higher cost but is nonetheless easily available to most of the U.S. population. Ultrasound (US) is commonly available, not only in radiology departments, but also in primary and specialty care clinics. There is a broad range of expertise among sonographers. Nuclear imaging requires more infrastructure support than other modalities to ensure the safe use of radioactive materials. Radiology options are summarized in Table 1.

| Table 1. Radiology Options | | |
|---|---|---|
| Modality Options | Contrast Options | Nuclear Options |
| Radiography (XR) | WO Contrast | Tc-99m Bone Scan |
| CT | W Contrast | Tc-99m SPECT |
| MRI | WO/W Contrast | 18-FDG PET/CT |
| US | Arthrography | Leukocyte Scan |
| Nuclear | Angiography | Gallium Scan |
| Interventional Procedures (injection, aspiration, biopsy) | | |

# Modality Options

Imaging modalities applicable to the musculoskeletal system work in the same way regardless of anatomic site. Musculoskeletal anatomy, physiology, biomechanics, pathophysiology, and pathology are the same regardless of specific location. Thus, imaging principles that apply to one anatomic region can be appropriately applied to another.

Radiography (XR)

Radiography uses x-rays to project shadows onto flat panel detectors, producing a two-dimensional representation of a three-dimensional structure. Proper positioning of the patient and correct exposure to x-rays are key determinants of radiographic quality. In most circumstances, multiple projections (also called views) are necessary for a radiographic study to be considered adequate. A poor quality or an abbreviated radiographic exam will provide less accurate diagnostic information than a good quality radiographic exam with the full number of views.

Fluoroscopy is a radiographic technology that can provide continuous real-time imaging. Its primary use in contemporary practice is for imaging guidance during invasive procedures.

Computed Tomography (CT)

CT uses computer algorithms to reconstruct slices of anatomy from data generated by an x-ray source and an array of detectors that rotate around the patient. CT scanners may differ in the number of x-ray sources and arrays of detectors; more of each generally translates into faster scans with higher spatial resolution. CT images are typically presented in axial, coronal, and sagittal planes. For CT of extremities, the imaging planes should be oriented relative to the anatomy itself, often requiring the manual selection of post-processing planes by the technologist that correspond to the actual position of the body part in the scanner. Three dimensional (3D) reconstructions may also be generated by the technologist or radiologist, and generally require interaction with the CT data on a workstation. Radiology departments vary in their policies regarding the retention of raw CT data, some keeping it for only a few hours. In general, the higher the level of radiation during the scan, the better the image quality. Current CT scanners are capable of generating images with exquisite bony detail (and high radiation doses), but because of concerns about unnecessary radiation, scanning protocols try to limit radiation (and consequently image quality) to just that which is medically necessary.

Metal objects included in the scan, such as orthopedic hardware or foreign objects such as bullets or shrapnel, cause artifacts that degrade the quality of the image. Software algorithms that reduce metal artifacts may partially correct for this image degradation. The greater the quantity of metal and the higher its density, the worse the resulting artifacts. Other than the increased radiation dose that may be used to mitigate metal artifacts, metal does not present a safety hazard inside or in proximity to CT scanners.

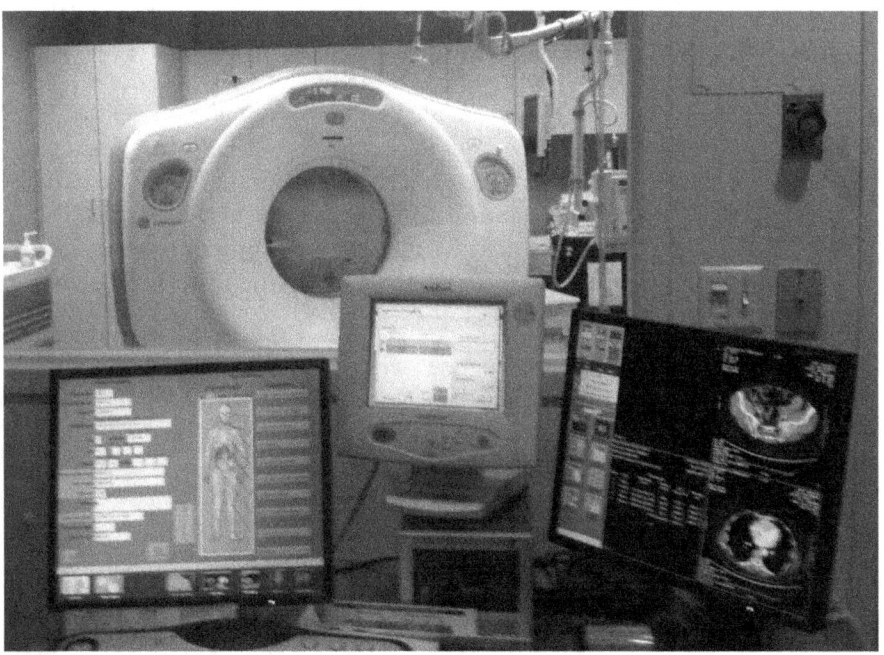

CT scanner from the operator's perspective.

Magnetic Resonance Imaging (MRI)

MRI uses magnetic fields and pulses of radiofrequency energy to generate signals that a computer reconstructs into cross-sectional images. The physical basis of the images is generally related to the density and mobility of hydrogen protons within the anatomic region of interest, and the appearance of the images depends on the technical parameters. No x-rays or ionizing radiation is involved. A particular series of energy pulses and signal collections is called a pulse sequence. When looking at MRI, white pixels are referred to as being bright or having high or intense signal (hyperintense) and dark pixels are referred to as being dark or having low signal (hypointense). Pixels of in-between intensity are referred to as having intermediate signal. A typical musculoskeletal MRI examination consists of images in two or three anatomic planes using two or more different pulse sequences.

An oversimplification for musculoskeletal MRI that many radiologists would nonetheless accept as practical would be to recognize two primary types of images that can be referred to as T1 MRI (T1-weighted MRI) and T2 FS MRI (T2-weighted fat-suppressed MRI). On T1 MRI, cortical bone is dark (hypointense), fluid and muscle are intermediate, and fat is bright (hyperintense). On T2 FS MRI, cortical bone and fat (including bone marrow) are dark, muscle is intermediate, and fluid is bright. Other common MRI techniques where the images look like T2 FS MRI include PD FS MRI (proton density fat-suppressed MRI) and STIR MRI (short tau inversion recovery MRI). On T2 MRI (T2-weighted MRI without fat-suppression) or PD MRI (proton density MRI without fat-suppression), fat is bright instead of dark, so it may be difficult to distinguish fat from fluid. On T1 FS MRI (T1-weighted MRI with fat-suppression), fat is dark instead of bright. The diagnostic quality of MRI depends not only on the quality of the scanner and the way in which it is used, but also on the ability of the patient to lie motionless during the scanning process.

Because of the strength of the magnetic fields commonly used in clinical MRI scanners, it is unsafe for metal objects to be in proximity to the scanner. A metal object may become a dangerous projectile when being attracted to the magnet. Electronics with magnetic memory may be adversely affected as well. Objects and electronics inside of patients are of particular concern as they may move under the influence of the magnetic field or heat up during the scanning process; their presence should be screened for and safety established before entering the magnetic field [1-2]. Metal, regardless of size, will also affect the imaging process and produce local artifacts.

Ultrasound (US)

US is an imaging method that uses high frequency sound waves and echoes (no ionizing radiation). For musculoskeletal applications, a hand-held transducer produces the sound waves and detects the echoes, and the device the reconstructs timing and location of the echoes into an image that corresponds to the anatomy. Materials such as gas or calcified tissue may interfere with this process, resulting in regions of absent information. The sound waves may also be attenuated as they pass through the tissue, limiting the demonstration of deep structures. The diagnostic quality of US images depends on technical factors, sonographer expertise, and patient factors.

Nuclear Imaging

Nuclear imaging is performed when a radiopharmaceutical in administered to the patient and the distribution of the radioactivity is mapped anatomically. See Nuclear Options below.

# Contrast Options

Contrast medium, called "contrast" for short, is a substance administered to a patient in conjunction with an imaging exam that is intended to increase the information available from the exam. Exams or anatomic structures made visible or more conspicuous by the use of contrast are often said to be "enhanced." Contrast for imaging modalities that use x-rays (radiography, fluoroscopy, CT) typically contain iodine, although in the gastrointestinal tract, barium may be used, and sometimes in joints, air may be used.

When iodinated contrast is injected intravenously, it circulates through the intravascular space, passing first to the right side of the heart and then successively through the pulmonary vasculature, the left side of the heart, the arterial tree, the capillary bed, and the systemic veins. As the contrast continues to circulate, it becomes diluted by blood and will be distributed according to vascularity, with hypervascular tissues appearing whiter after contrast. In the extremities, intravenous iodinated contrast agents are commonly used to evaluate soft tissue tumors or infections. A CT angiogram may be obtained by scanning while the contrast is first passing through the vascular tree. If contrast is first injected into a joint, scanning will produce a CT arthrogram. If contrast is first injected into the subdural space of the spinal canal, scanning will produce a CT myelogram. Ultimately, the contrast excreted by the kidneys.

Contrast agents used with MRI of the musculoskeletal system contain the element gadolinium (Gd) and tissues that enhance with contrast have higher signal (appear whiter) on T1. If Gd-based contrast is injected into a joint prior to scanning, an MR arthrogram is produced. On T1 FS Gd MRI (T1-weighted fat-suppressed MRI after administration of gadolinium-based contrast), regions or tissues that enhance will be bright (have high T1 signal). MR Arthrography refers to the instillation of contrast medium into a joint cavity before scanning.

Use of iodinated or gadolinium-based contrast carries a risk of various adverse reactions, including anaphylaxis. For patients with a history of previous adverse or allergic reaction to contrast, iodinated or Gd-based, appropriate strategies to mitigate the risk should be considered [3].

US contrast agents consist of gas-filled lipid microspheres (microbubbles). Intravenously administered contrast for US has not found much utility in the musculoskeletal system.

WO Contrast

Without contrast, referring to a CT or MRI exam where the patient is scanned without contrast. When there is no designation of contrast being used, it is generally assumed that the scan was performed without contrast; therefore, use of the designation may be considered redundant.

W Contrast

With intravenous contrast, typically referring to intravenously administered contrast for CT, but it may also refer to MRI. CT and MR exams where contrast is injected into a joint or other space before scanning are also considered W Contrast.

WO/W Contrast

Without and with contrast, typically referring to MRI where the patient is scanned without contrast, is administered contrast intravenously, and is scanned again, but it may also refer to a similar exam using CT.

Arthrography

Arthrography is performed when contrast is injected into a joint cavity. The contrast may be iodinated, Gd-based, or a mixture of both, and the imaging modalities may be radiography, fluoroscopy, CT, or MRI.

Angiography

Angiography is performed when contrast is injected into a blood vessel. Imaging may be performed with radiography, fluoroscopy, CT, MRI, or Nuclear methods.

# Nuclear Options

Nuclear medicine refers to using radionuclides (radioactive isotopes) to create images. There are several radionuclides in medical use, many substances that may be labeled with these radionuclides and administered to patients by a variety of routes, and several methods to detecting the distribution of radionuclide activity and creating images. The studies are commonly referred to by some combination of the radionuclide, the labeled substance, the target organ, and the imaging method.

Tc-99m Bone Scan

Nuclear imaging of the skeleton with Tc-99m methylene diphosphonate (MDP). MDP is incorporated into hydroxyapatite crystals, reflecting both blood flow and osteoblastic activity. The radiopharmaceutical is injected intravenously, and after approximately 2 hr, most of the activity has localized in bone, in calcified tissues, or has been excreted through the kidneys. The bone scan produces planar images of low spatial resolution.

Tc-99m SPECT

Single photon emission computed tomography. An imaging method that produces low resolution cross-sectional images after the administration of various radionuclides by intravenous injection, commonly Tc-99m MDP when the target tissue is bone. SPECT may be combined with an anatomically co-registered CT scan in SPECT/CT; special equipment is needed.

18-FDG PET/CT

Positron Emission Tomography/Computed Tomography. Imaging method that combines the administration of a positron-emitting radionuclide (commonly F-18 fluorodeoxyglucose, called 18-FDG) with a CT scan. 18-FDG is a glucose analog and accumulates in tissues with high metabolic rates, such as fast-growing tumors. The combination of PET with an anatomically co-registered CT scan provides metabolic information with high anatomic resolution.

Leukocyte Scan

Nuclear imaging in which autologous leukocytes (white blood cells) are labeled with In-111 or Tc-99m in order to identify sites of infection. Imaging may be performed with a planar scanner to produce images similar to a bone scan, or imaging may be performed with a SPECT scanner to produce cross-sectional images.

Gallium scan

Nuclear imaging with Ga-67 or Ga-68. Gallium accumulates nonspecifically at sites of cancer, inflammation, or chronic or acute infection. The radiopharmaceutical is injected intravenously and scanning may be performed after 6 hr; however, follow-up scans may be required at 24 or 48 hours. Imaging may be performed with a planar scanner to produce images similar to a bone scan, or imaging may be performed with a SPECT scanner to produce cross-sectional images.

# Interventional Procedures

Interventional procedures in radiology generally refers to diagnostic or therapeutic procedures in which the skin is penetrated with an instrument such as a needle under imaging guidance. Expertise in the performance and interpretation of common musculoskeletal procedures is widely available in the U.S.

Injection refers to injection of fluid into a joint or potential space. Many joints may be successfully injected by using surface anatomy and palpable landmarks, but imaging guidance provides confirmation of the needle position. Guidance may be provided by fluoroscopy, radiography, ultrasound, or CT, often depending on local availability and expertise.

Aspiration refers to the removal fluid using a needle; imaging guidance may be used. Aspiration may be performed on any fluid collection if sufficiently large, including joint effusions or soft tissue fluid collections such as bursae or abscesses.

Percutaneous imaging-guided biopsy procedures may be used to obtain tissue samples of bone or soft tissue lesions. CT guidance is usual for bone or deep-seated soft tissue lesions. Ultrasound is usual for superficial soft tissue lesions.

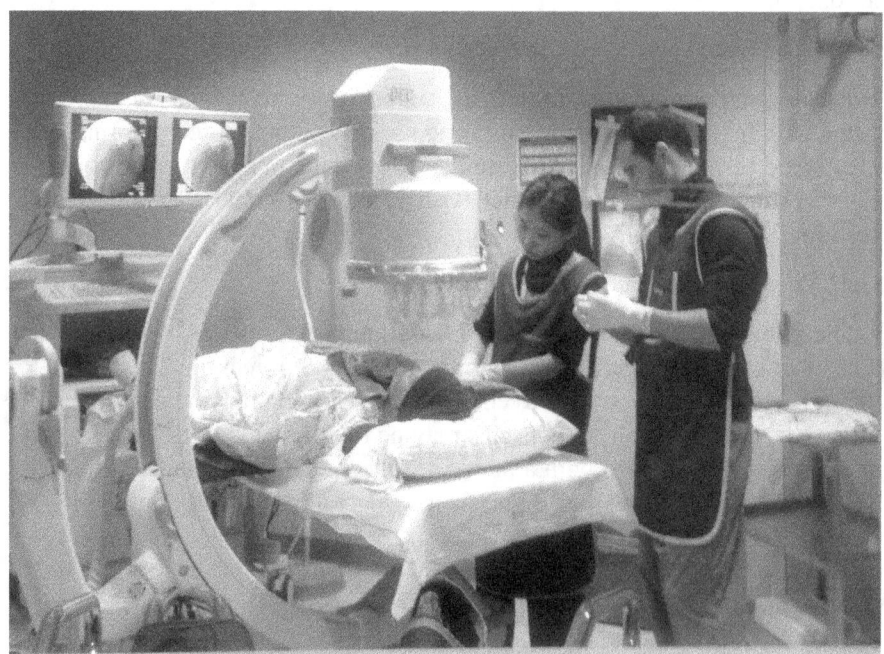

Shoulder arthrogram in progress using C-arm fluoroscopy for guidance.

# References

1.   Expert Panel on MR Safety. ACR guidance document on MR safe practices: 2013. J Magn Reson Imaging. 2013 Mar;37(3):501-30. doi: 10.1002/jmri.24011. Epub 2013 Jan 23.

2.  ACR Committee on MR Safety. ACR guidance document on MR safe practices: Updates and critical information 2019. J Magn Reson Imaging. 2020 Feb;51(2):331-338. doi: 10.1002/jmri.26880. Epub 2019 Jul 29.

3.  ACR Committee on Drugs and Contrast Media. ACR Manual on contrast media 2020. American College of Radiology, 2020. https://www.acr.org/-/media/ACR/Files/Clinical-Resources/Contrast_Media.pdf (Last accessed Apr 24, 2021).

# Chapter 2. Bayes Theorem

Michael L. Richardson, MD

## What good is Bayes theorem?

Bayes Theorem provides a simple numerical framework that allows a physician to use the best available evidence in a repeatable manner for medical decision-making. I would like to emphasize the word "repeatable". Much of the medical decision making I witness in my peers and my students is, shall we say, a "seat-of-the-pants" process. When I go with my gut on a difficult case, I may indeed make the right diagnosis. However, I am not so confident that my gut will make the same decision from the same evidence a month from now. Gut-based reasoning is also hard to teach to one's residents and fellows. Using a slightly more numeric model can make this reasoning process much more repeatable and a lot easier to teach to students.

## Bayes Theorem as a model of the diagnostic process

I think the basic formulation of Bayes Theorem is a pretty good model of the diagnostic process that goes on in a physician's brain. When we are trying to formulate a diagnosis, we take what we know about the patient and make our best estimate as to the correct diagnosis. When some new data comes in, we use that to update our original estimate and further refine our differential diagnosis. There are many formulations of Bayes theorem, and some of them are quite complex. For our purposes, we will stick to a formulation that it is utterly simple:

$$A \times B = C$$

In this formulation, $A$ is what we know when the patient hits our office door, for example, with a complaint of "knee pain". $A$ is also known as the pre-test likelihood of disease. At this point, there are a zillion possible causes for knee pain. Some are minor and some are horrible. At this point, our differential diagnosis might include all of the following:

- thrombophlebitis
- cellulitis
- necrotizing fasciitis
- osteosarcoma
- pathologic fracture from a breast cancer metastasis
- osteonecrosis due to steroid use
- osteoarthritis

- tibial plateau fracture
- stress fracture
- meniscal tear

Our next step is to gather more information. Learning that this is a 20-year-old man should move breast cancer metastases off our mental list. We have now arrived at the $C$ in our equation above, the post-test likelihood of disease. What about $B$? $B$ is an index of the credibility of our test. In this case, we consider age and gender to be very credible evidence that breast carcinoma is very unlikely. What's next in the Bayesian process? Wash, rinse, repeat. On each cycle, we get more information and use that to further refine our differential diagnosis. For example, a lack of fever or chills and a normal CBC would make inflammatory disease less likely. A radiograph of the knee could help us detect any gross skeletal pathology, such as fractures, tumors or arthritis. Finally, magnetic resonance imaging could help us demonstrate an occult stress fracture, early joint erosions, or an internal derangement such as a meniscal tear.

## Picking the right test indices to weight our diagnosis

When new data comes in the form of a diagnostic test, we have to decide how much weight we should give that test when updating our conclusions. We do this using indices of test performance such as sensitivity, specificity, accuracy, positive predictive value (PPV), negative predictive value (NPV), and likelihood ratios. A great deal of the radiology literature contains estimates of these indices for various imaging methods. Most of the time, we are trying to answer two major questions. First, given a positive test result, what is the likelihood of disease? Second, given a negative test result, what is the likelihood of no disease? At first glance, PPV and NPV seem like the perfect indices to help answer these questions. Unfortunately, both of them are extremely dependent upon disease prevalence [1]. This variability is well known to epidemiologists and statisticians, but it may not be quite so well known to many physicians. For example, the prevalence of meniscal tears at our sports medicine clinic is relatively high, (about 60%). The prevalence of meniscal tears at our cancer center is much lower (about 1%). This means that the PPV of a meniscal on knee MRI will be about 0.93 for patients from our sports medicine facility but only about 0.083 for patients at our cancer center. This large decrease in the PPV is not caused by any personal or professional failings; it is merely a result of the large decrease in disease prevalence. For this reason, I highly recommend the use of likelihood ratios (LR). These indices depend only on sensitivity and specificity, and are therefore invariant to disease prevalence. LRs for positive ($LR_{pos}$) and negative ($LR_{neg}$) test results can be calculated from sensitivity and specificity values with the use of the following simple formulas [2]:

$$LR_{pos} = \frac{sensitivity}{1 - specificity}$$

and

$$LR_{neg} = \frac{1 - sensitivity}{specificity}$$

## Bayes Theorem in practice

As mentioned earlier, I prefer to use a very simple version of Bayes Theorem. To make the math as simple as possible, one can represent the pre- and post-test likelihoods of disease in terms of odds (rather than probability). In this formulation, the weighting factor is the likelihood ratio (LR) of the test.

$$Odds_{pretest} \times LR = Odds_{posttest}$$

Let's quickly look at odds for a moment, then then we will take Bayes theorem out for a spin. Odds and probabilities are equivalent ways of expressing likelihood. Probabilities are usually expressed as a decimal fraction, and range from 0.0 (no likelihood) to 1.0 (certainty). I might express the probability of the Seattle Seahawks of winning the Super Bowl next year as 0.25, which means I expect that Seattle has a 1 in 4 chance of winning. Odds are expressed somewhat differently — as a ratio, and range from zero (no likelihood) to infinity (certainty). If I am mildly optimistic about the Seahawks' chances next year, I might estimate their odds of winning the Super Bowl as 3 to 2, which means that if the season were replayed 5 times, Seattle would win 3 times, and not win 2 times. Given either probability or odds, one can calculate the other quantity via the following simple formulas:

$$Odds = \frac{p}{1 - p}$$

and

$$p = \frac{Odds}{1 + Odds}$$

## Taking Bayes Theorem out for a spin

All we need now in order to estimate the post-test odds of disease is to know the LR and the pre-test odds of disease. The values for $LR_{pos}$ and $LR_{neg}$ are easy to estimate from the radiology literature. For medial meniscal MR, the sensitivity and specificity are each about 0.90. This means that our $LR_{pos}$ will be 9 and our $LR_{neg}$ will be 1/9. The next thing we need to know is the pre-test odds of disease. This figure usually has to come from the clinician ordering the test. I freely admit that no clinician I know has ever entered the pre-test odds of disease on the imaging requisition form. However, it's not hard to get a reasonable estimate of this from talking to them. Table 1. shows how one might translate their words into odds for a meniscal tear.

**Table 1. Translating words into odds of a meniscal tear.**

| English | odds of meniscal tear |
| --- | --- |
| I strongly doubt there is a tear | 1:10 |
| I doubt there is a tear | 1:5 |
| I am on the fence | 1:1 |
| I suspect there is a tear | 5:1 |
| I strongly suspect there is a tear | 10:1 |

Now, let's plug these numbers into Bayes Theorem to see how the numbers work out in several different clinical scenarios. If the test is negative, we use $LR_{neg}$; if the test is positive, we use $LR_{pos}$.

Scenario 1. Strong doubt with a negative MR

$$\frac{1}{10} \times \frac{1}{9} = \frac{1}{90}$$

In this scenario, the clinician's impression and the MR results are congruent. As our calculation shows, the odds of having a meniscal tear in these circumstances is only 1 to 90.

Scenario 2. On the fence with a positive MR

$$\frac{1}{1} \times 9 = 9$$

The clinical signs and symptoms are sometimes non-specific, as in this scenario. Here, the presence of a positive MR trumps the clinical information, and the odds of a meniscal tear are now about 9 to 1.

Scenario 3. Strong suspicion of tear with positive MR

$$\frac{10}{1} \times 9 = 90$$

In this scenario, the clinical exam and the MR findings both strongly suggest a meniscal tear, and our odds of a tear are now about 90 to 1. These odds should make it a lot easier to talk either a patient or their surgeon into proceeding with arthroscopy.

## Combining multiple LRs into a combined LR

Often, several tests are done on the same patient. Table 2 shows diagnostic indices for US and CT [3] versus MR with diffusion-weighted images (DWI) [4]. Bayes theorem offers us a way to combine all of this information, weighted for the efficacy of each test. This can be especially helpful when different tests give contradictory results.

**Table 2. Diagnostic efficacy of US, CT and DWI MR for diagnosis of soft tissue abscess.**

| index | US | CT | DWI MR |
|---|---|---|---|
| sensitivity | 0.967 | 0.767 | 0.923 |
| specificity | 0.857 | 0.914 | 0.727 |
| PPV | 0.853 | 0.885 | 0.923 |
| NPV | 0.968 | 0.821 | 0.727 |
| accuracy | 0.908 | 0.846 | 0.88 |
| prevalence | 0.462 | 0.462 | 0.78 |
| $LR_{pos}$ | 6.767 | 8.944 | 3.385 |
| $LR_{neg}$ | 0.039 | 0.255 | 0.106 |

As an example, let's consider several scenarios in which we are trying to decide the likelihood of patient having a soft tissue abscess. With Bayes Theorem, all we have to do to get a combined weight for our imaging tests is to multiply their LRs together. Again, if a test is negative, we use $LR_{neg}$ and we use $LR_{pos}$ if the test is positive.

Scenario 1. Abscess suspected (pre-test odds = 5:1) and all three tests are positive for abscess

$$5 \times (6.8 \times 8.9 \times 3.4) = 5 \times 206 = 1030$$

In this scenario, all the evidence is pointing in the same direction, giving us 1030 to 1 odds of there being an abscess.

Scenario 2. Clinician on the fence (pre-test odds = 1:1), US positive, but CT and DWI MR are negative

$$1 \times (6.8 \times 0.26 \times 0.11) = 0.19$$

In this scenario, we have contradictory evidence. Our best estimate is that there is actually only about a 1 in 5 odds of there being an abscess.

Scenario 3. strong suspicion of abscess (pre-test odds = 10:1), US negative but CT and DWI MR positive

$$10 \times (0.039 \times 8.9 \times 3.4) = 11.8$$

This is another scenario with contradictory evidence. However, this time, the weighted combination of evidence strongly suggests (odds = 11.8 to 1) that there is an abscess.

# References

1. Altman DG, Bland JM. Diagnostic tests 1: Sensitivity and specificity. BMJ 1994; 308:1552.
2. Glas AS, Lijmer JG, Prins MH, Bonsel GJ, Bossuyt PMM. The diagnostic odds ratio: a single indicator of test performance. J Clin Epidemiol 2003;56:1129–1135.
3. Gaspari R, Dayno M, Briones J, Blehar D. Comparison of computerized tomography and ultrasound for diagnosing soft tissue abscesses. Crit Ultrasound J 2012 Apr 17;4(1):5.
4. Unal O, Koparan HI, Avcu S, Kalender AM, Kisli E. The diagnostic value of diffusion-weighted magnetic resonance imaging in soft tissue abscesses. Eur J Radiol. 2011 Mar;77(3):490–4.

# Chapter 3. Zombie Plots

Michael L. Richardson, MD

## What is a zombie plot?

A zombie plot is a tool to tell you whether or not a diagnostic test sucks. Put slightly more formally, a zombie plot is a simple graphic method for visualizing the efficacy of a diagnostic test [1]. The slightly lurid title comes from the fact that this technique divides ROC (receiver operator characteristic) plots into "Zones *Of Mostly Bad Imaging Efficacy*" (Fig. 1).

In the previous section, Table 2 presented a big pile of numbers showing estimates of the imaging efficacy of US, CT and MR for the diagnosis of soft tissue abscess. However, it isn't immediately obvious which of these three tests does the best job from just looking at these numbers. The main point of a zombie plot is to display this same information in such a way that one's eye and brain can spot patterns that might otherwise be hard to notice from the numbers alone. There is actually a whole branch of statistics devoted to this philosophy called exploratory data analysis (EDA) [2]. A particularly vivid example of the validity of EDA is the famous Anscombe quartet [3].

## Where did these zones of efficacy come from?

From the section on Bayes Theorem, you learned that likelihood ratios are a great figure of merit for judging how much confidence we should put in an imaging test. For an ideal imaging test, we would like the likelihood of a positive test ($LR_{pos}$) to be gigantic and for the likelihood of a negative test ($LR_{neg}$) to be tiny. Since our world is not ideal, we need to decide which values of these LRs are "good enough". Kass and Raftery [4] suggest that the $LR_{pos}$ should be at least greater than 3. By the same logic, the $LR_{neg}$ should therefore be at least less than 1/3. It turns out that any straight line drawn on an ROC plot defines a line of constant LR. Therefore, if one draws lines in the appropriate spots on an ROC plot with slopes of 3 and of 1/3, these lines will demarcate the zones of acceptable and unacceptable imaging efficacy, as shown in Fig. 1 [1].

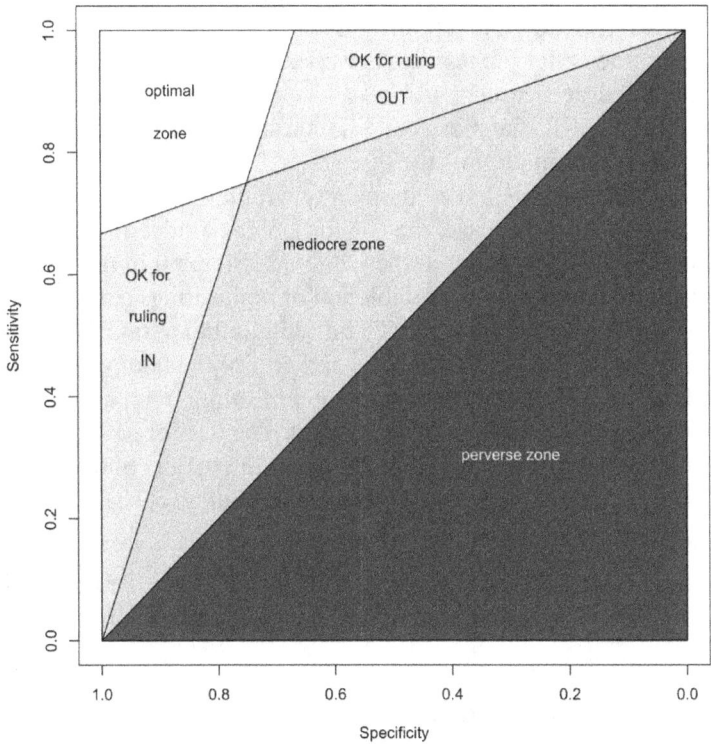

Fig. 1. ROC plot divided into zones of mostly bad imaging efficacy (75% of the area of the plot). The boomerang-shaped area formed by white and green zones defines the zones of acceptable efficacy (only 25% of the area of the plot).

## What about Confidence Intervals?

Sensitivity, specificity and other indices of imaging efficacy are not numbers handed down from the deity on a stone tablet. Rather, they are estimates made by fallible humans and can vary considerably due to chance alone. Therefore, these estimates are not simply displayed as points on the zombie plot, but as the 95% confidence regions (CR) for these estimates. The smaller the CR, the more credible we consider the estimate to be. If the CR for sensitivity and specificity lie well within the zones of efficacy on a zombie plot, life is good, and our test is a credible one. However, if a considerable portion of the CR lies outside the zones of efficacy, the test should be considered much less credible.

As an example, let's take the information from Table 2 and use it to create a zombie plot (Fig. 2). How do we interpret this figure? Here are some tips:

1. An ideal test would be located at the upper left corner of the plot, and its CR would shrink down to a point. The closer a test CR lies to the upper left corner, the better the test is. As we see here, the CR for US lies closest to the upper left corner.

2. The smaller the CR, the more certain the estimate. In this example the CR for US is the smallest of the three.

3. The CR of the test should lie completely within the acceptable zones of the zombie plot. In this case, the CR for US does indeed lie almost entirely within the optimal zone (the white quadrilateral in the upper left), indicating that it does an acceptable job of both ruling in and ruling out an abscess. Much of the CR for CT lies within the optimal zone, but essentially all of it lies within the left hand arm of the boomerang, indicating that CT does an acceptable job of ruling in an abscess, but not an acceptable job of ruling out an abscess. The CR for MR is the largest of the three. Most of it lies within the upper arm of the boomerang, indicating that it does an acceptable job of ruling out an abscess, but not of ruling in an abscess.

Based on these three criteria and on the efficacy data from Table 2, US seems to be a better test than CT or DWI MR for the diagnosis of soft tissue abscess.

## Make your own zombie plots

It's swell to see zombie plots that I have made, but it's even better to make your own plots with data that *you* care about passionately. To that end, I have created a set of online zombie plot calculators that are located at http://uwmsk.org/zombie. These calculators will allow you to take data either from a standard 2 x 2 contingency table or from a meta-analysis and produce and download your very own zombie plots.

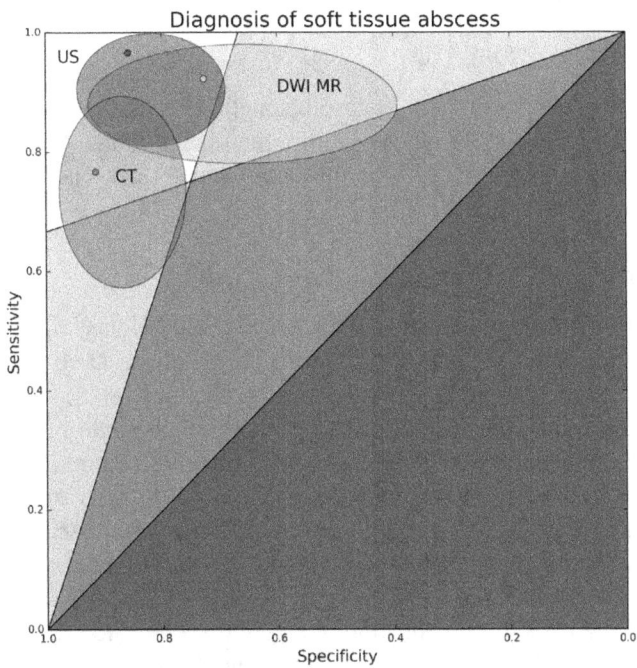

Fig. 2. A zombie plot of the information from Table 2.

# References

1. Richardson ML. The Zombie Plot: A Simple Graphic Method for Visualizing the Efficacy of a Diagnostic Test. AJR Am J Roentgenol 2016; 207:W1–W10.
2. Wikipedia contributors. Exploratory data analysis. Wikipedia, The Free Encyclopedia. Available at: https://en.wikipedia.org/wiki/Exploratory_data_analysis. (accessed Apr 24, 2021).
3. Wikipedia contributors. Anscombe's quartet. Wikipedia, The Free Encyclopedia. Available at: https://en.wikipedia.org/wiki/Anscombe%27s_quartet (accessed Apr 24, 2021).
4. Kass RE, Raftery AE. Bayes factors. J Am Stat Assoc 1995; 90:773–795.

# Chapter 4. Radiation Exposure

Michael L. Richardson, MD

Our current digital society is quite familiar with the phenomenon of ideas "going viral" and sweeping quickly across the planet via the Internet. X-rays provide a great example of this phenomenon happening a whole century before either the web or smart phones.

## A brief history of X-rays and radiation injury

On Nov 8, 1895, Wilhelm Conrad Röntgen applied a high voltage to a Crookes tube to produce X-rays. By December 28 of the same year, his paper describing this phenomenon was accepted for publication [1]. On January 6, 1896, the news went viral via the high-tech medium of its time, when a worldwide cable was sent telling the world of Röntgen's discovery. On February 4, 1896, the first clinical use of X-rays was reported from Dartmouth Medical Center, where they were used to treat an ulnar fracture [2]: "It was possible yesterday to test the method upon a broken arm. After an exposure of 20 minutes the plate on development showed the fracture in the ulna very distinctly." X-rays thus moved from discovery to clinical implementation in only two months. Early signs of possible side effects showed up almost as quickly. The March 5, 1896 issue of Nature contained the first reports of side effects of X-rays [3]: "Edison reports that his eyes were sore after working for several hours with his fluorescent tubes" (Fig. 1); and "Dr. Wm. J. Morton reports that he sees brilliant flashes of light after he has discontinued work ... he infers that the X-rays are injurious to the eye."

Unfortunately, it then took several years for the dangers of X-ray radiation to become apparent. One of the earliest casualties from X-ray radiation was Clarence Dally, an assistant of Thomas Edison. Dally built and tested (on himself) thousands of X-ray tubes for Edison during his career. By 1898, it was clear that something was wrong. In Edison's words [5-6]: "I soon found that the X-ray had affected poisonously my assistant, Mr. Dally so that his hair came out and his flesh commenced to ulcerate." Unfortunately, after multiple skin grafts and amputations for skin carcinoma, Dally died in 1904 due to mediastinal metastases of his disease.

X-rays were used extensively in military hospitals during World War I. Judging from Fig. 2, some radiographers of that time were well aware of the potential dangers from radiation exposure.

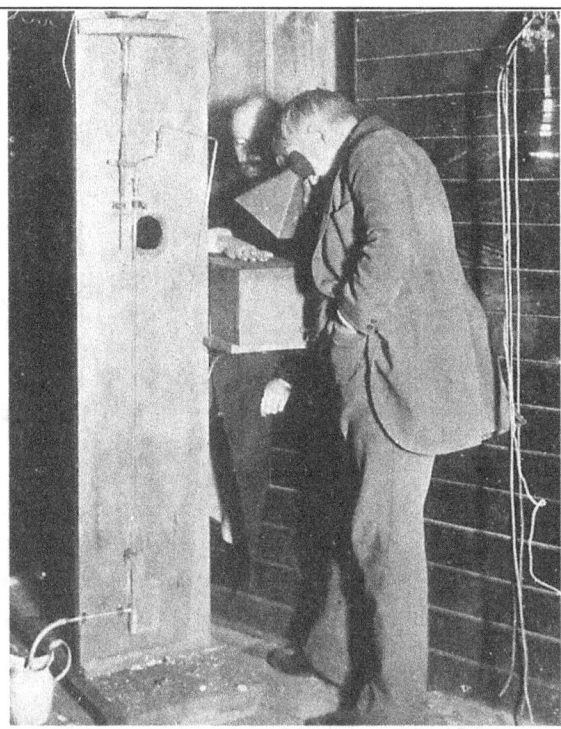

Fig. 1. Image from 1896, showing Thomas Edison examining his assistant Clarence Dally's hand with a fluoroscope of his own design. (Image licensed from Science Source — Image Number: BT6968 [4])

## Risk of cancer in radiation workers

In the 120 years since the discovery of X-rays, we have learned a lot more about the risks of radiation, and a number of epidemiologic studies have been performed on radiologists, technologists and other medical workers exposed to radiation. The balance of this evidence confirms that for members of these groups working before 1950, there was a definite link between radiation exposure and skin cancer, breast cancer and leukemia. However, there is no credible evidence of an increased risk of cancer among radiologists practicing for the last 30 or 40 years [8].

## Radiation injuries to physicians

Radiation skin burns were common among early radiologists. Fortunately, such injuries are now quite uncommon [8]. However, permanent hair loss is the distal lower extremities is still observed among interventionalists with inadequate leg shielding [9].

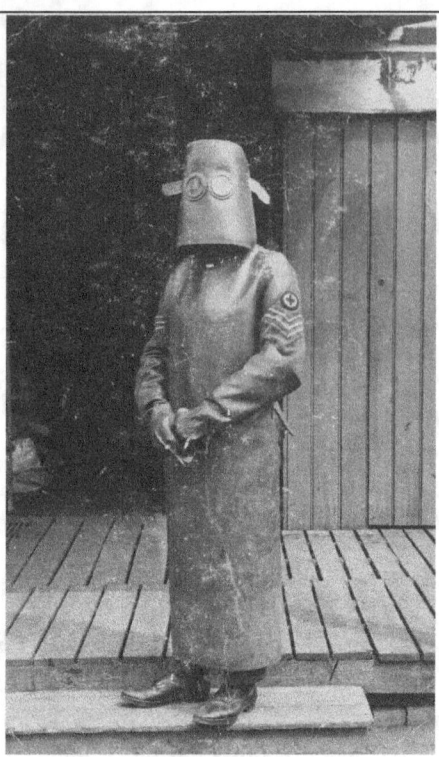

Fig. 2. World War One, France: a radiographer wearing protective clothing and headpiece. Photograph by H. J. Hickman, ca. 1918. Image from Wellcome Library, London, no. 577674i [7].

The threshold dose injury to the lens of the eye was long thought to be about 1–5 Gy [10]. However, more recent studies suggest that such a threshold, if there is one, is most likely significantly lower than previously thought [8]. With typical reported workloads, radiation doses to the lens may exceed the threshold for deterministic effects after several years of work if radiation protection tools are not used [10]. In one survey of interventional radiologists, 46% had signs of radiation-related lens changes, with posterior subcapsular cataracts in 8% [11].

Sufficiently high doses of radiation to a pregnant woman can result in major malformations and growth retardation. However, the absolute risks of fetal effects are negligible at doses less than 50 mSv [12]. Even for the childbearing interventional radiologist, fetal risk is negligible when appropriate shielding and radiation safety practices are applied [13].

The beneficial effect of protective aprons and collars is nicely shown by a study of orthopedic surgeons reported by Tsalafoutas et al [14]. A surgeon with no protective gear could carry out only about 250 procedures per year before his personal dosimeter readings exceeded the 20 mSv limit. With the appropriate protective gear, more than 2500 procedures could be carried out before exceeding the annual effective dose limit.

## Reducing radiation doses to patients and physicians

One of the prime directives for radiologists is the ALARA principle: to use radiation doses that are "as low as reasonably achievable" [15]. The Image Gently [16] and Image Wisely [17] alliances are devoted to reducing the amount of radiation received in children and in adults from medical procedures. It is worth pointing out that one of the best ways to reduce a physician's radiation dose is by reducing their patient's dose.

Other means of reducing radiation dose include time, distance and shielding. Radiation dose is directly proportional to imaging time. By keeping a light touch on the fluoroscopy control and by the use of pulsed rather than continuous fluoroscopy, radiation doses from procedures can be decreased dramatically. Radiation dosage follows the inverse square law, so standing farther from the source can have a substantial protective effect. Appropriate shielding should be applied to protect a patient's eyes, thyroid, breasts and other parts that are not the primary focus of an imaging exam.

## Radiation dosage in perspective

Radiologists should be able to give accurate and easy to understand answers when patients and other physicians ask about radiation doses from imaging procedures. The American College of Radiology Appropriateness Criteria [18] contain a wealth of evidence-based recommendations as to the appropriateness of various imaging studies for a wide variety of clinical scenarios. These documents also contain guidance as to the relative radiation dose received from each imaging modality. However, these raw numbers from the ACR are a bit hard to comprehend by themselves.

A much better tool for understanding relative radiation doses is a wonderful chart by Randall Munroe of XKCD fame [19]. This chart does a brilliant job of putting radiation doses into proper perspective (Fig. 3). The chart is broken down into four parts, by color. It uses blue squares to list the radiation dose one gets from everyday activities, green squares for diagnostic radiation, red squares for doses associated with injury, and orange squares for the dose from 10 minutes at Chernobyl. I use this chart all the time to field questions about radiation dosages. It is an especially excellent tool to use with anxious parents who consider a radiograph of their child's arm equivalent to a visit to Chernobyl. It is very reassuring to them to see that the actual dose is about the same as they would get from feeding their child 10 bananas, and about 1/40th the dose their child would get during a cross-country flight to visit their grandparents.

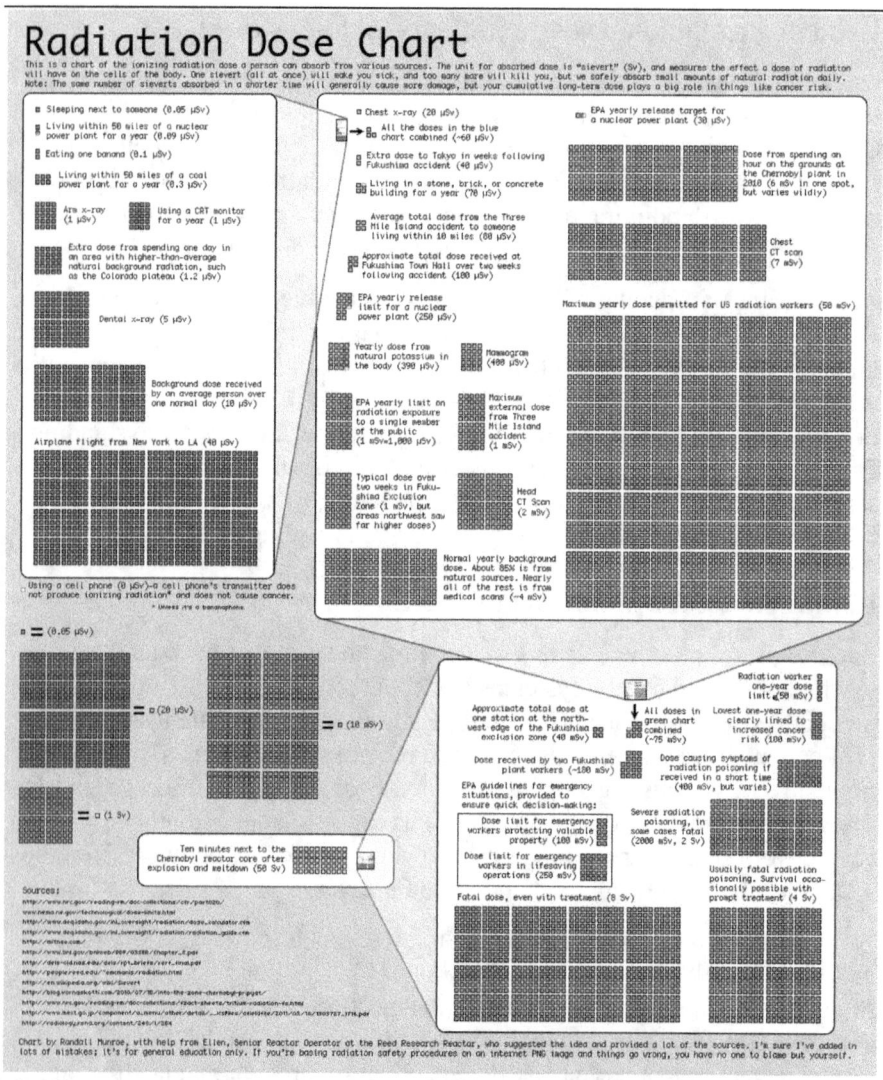

Fig. 3. A, entire XKCD Radiation Chart, placed in the public domain by its author.

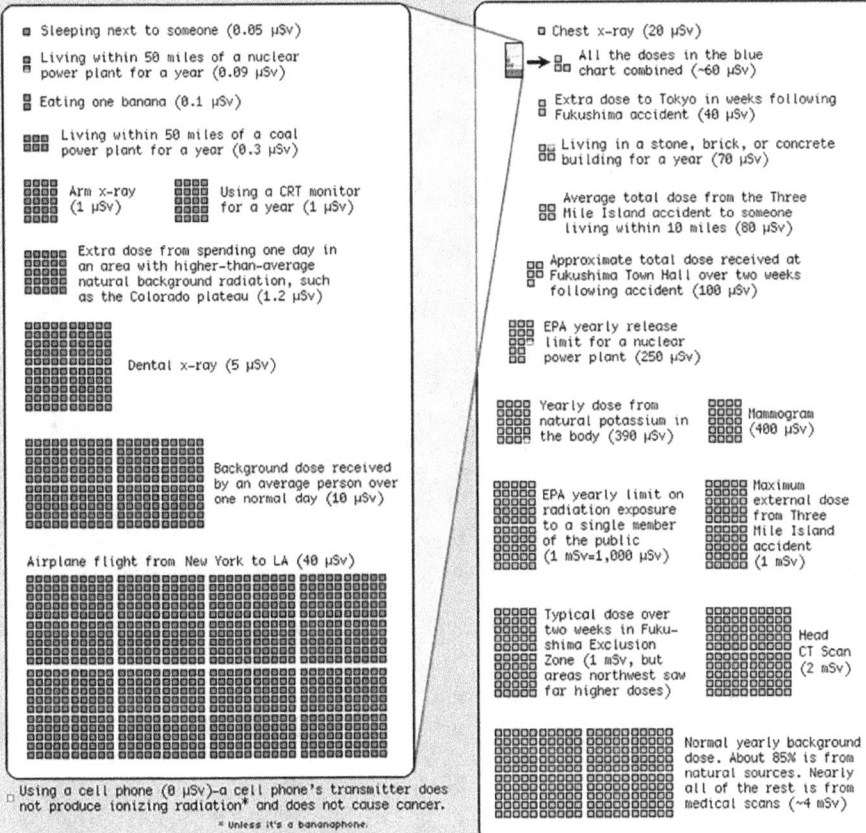

Fig. 3. B, Detail of the blue and green blocks of the Radiation Dose Chart comparing everyday exposure with medical imaging.

# References

1. Röntgen WC. On a New Kind of Rays. Science 1896;3(59):227–231.
2. Frost EB. Experiments on the X-Rays. Science 1896;3(59):235–236.
3. Notes. Nature 1896;53(1375):419–424.
4. Edison with Fluoroscope in 1896. (http://images.sciencesource.com/p/14218326/Edison-Fluoroscope–1896-BT6968.html). (accessed Jul 4, 2018).
5. Brown P. American martyrs to radiology. Clarence Madison Dally (1865–1904). 1936. Am J Roentgenol 1995;164(1):237–239.

6.  Gagliardi RA. Clarence Dally: an American pioneer. Am J Roentgenol 1991;157(5):922.
7.  Wellcome Library. World War One radiographer. Available at: http://catalogue.wellcomelibrary.org/record=b1577674~S8. (accessed Jul 4, 2018).
8.  Parikh JR, Geise RA, Bluth EI, Bender CE, Sze G, Jones AK. Potential Radiation-Related Effects on Radiologists. AJR 2017;208:595–602.
9.  Wiper A, Katira R, Roberts DH. Interventional cardiology: it's a hairy business. Heart 2005 Nov; 91(11): 1432.
10. Vano E, Gonzalez L, Fernández JM, Haskal ZJ. Eye lens exposure to radiation in interventional suites: caution is warranted. Radiology 2008;248(3):945–953.
11. Haskal ZJ, Worgul BV. Interventional radiology carries occupational risk for cataracts. RSNA News 2004;14:5–6. Available at: http://www.rsna.org/uploadedFiles/RSNA/Content/News/jun2004.pdf. (accessed Jul 4, 2018).
12. McCollough CH, Schueler BA, Atwell TD, et al. Radiation exposure and pregnancy: when should we be concerned? Radiographics 2007;27(4):909–17.
13. Vu CT, Elder DH. Pregnancy and the working interventional radiologist. Semin Intervent Radiol 2013;30(4):403–407.
14. Tsalafoutas IA, Tsapaki V, Kaliakmanis A, et al. Estimation of radiation doses to patients and surgeons from various fluoroscopically guided orthopaedic surgeries. Radiation Protection Dosimetry 2007;128(1):112–119.
15. Health Physics Society. ALARA. Available at: http://hps.org/publicinformation/radterms/radfact1.html.(accessed Jul 4, 2018).
16. Image Gently. Available at: http://www.imagegently.org/. (accessed Jul 4, 2018).
17. Image Wisely. Available at: http://www.imagewisely.org. (accessed Jul 4, 2018).
18. American College of Radiology Appropriateness Criteria. Available at: https://www.acr.org/Quality-Safety/Appropriateness-Criteria. (accessed Jun 11, 2018).
19. Munroe R. Radiation Dose Chart. 2011 Available at: https://blog.xkcd.com/2011/03/19/radiation-chart/. (accessed Jul 4, 2018).

# Part II. Acute Trauma

Acute trauma patients are typically straightforward in their presentation, although the extent of injury and sometimes even the sites of injury may not be known. In general, for patients with acute trauma to an extremity, the recommended initial imaging is radiography; the next recommendations would be CT in the acute setting and MRI in the non-acute setting. For the cervical spine, CT is the recommended initial imaging.

# Chapter 5: Acute Hand Trauma

Jack Porrino, MD, Jennifer Favinger, MD, Erin Flaherty, MD, Felix S. Chew, MD

Radiography is the initial exam for acute hand trauma and follow-up. CT may be helpful for surgical planning for intraarticular fractures, and MRI and US may have a role in evaluating soft tissue injury.

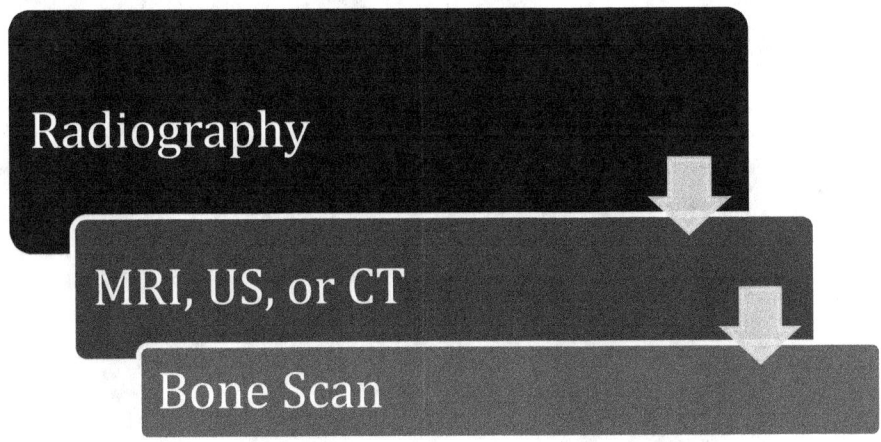

# Case 5-1.

A 20-year-old man injured his hand in a motor vehicle crash. He is being evaluated for a number of other possible injuries. What is the best initial imaging for his hand injury?

This scenario concerns a patient with blunt hand trauma and suspected fracture or dislocation.

Sensible recommendation: XR HAND 3 VIEW

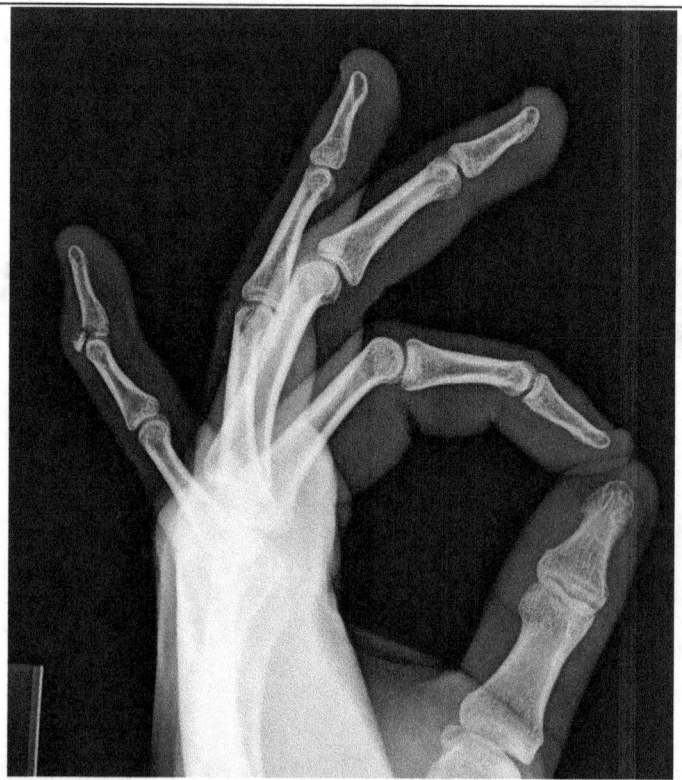

Oblique radiograph of the left hand demonstrates minimally displaced, dorsal avulsion fracture of the fifth distal phalanx.

A routine 3-view radiographic series of the hand will demonstrate most fractures and dislocations involving the hand. Where trauma has been localized to a specific finger, radiographs of just that finger will often be of higher quality than of the entire hand. Obtaining a true lateral view is important. Cross-sectional imaging with CT, MRI, or US is not recommended initially, but may be useful in limited circumstances. Nuclear imaging has no role.

# Case 5-2.

A 62-year-old man involved in a motorcycle crash with an obvious deformity of his middle finger. What is the first imaging study to evaluate the hand?

This scenario concerns a polytrauma patient with suspected finger dislocation.

Sensible recommendation: XR HAND 3 VIEW

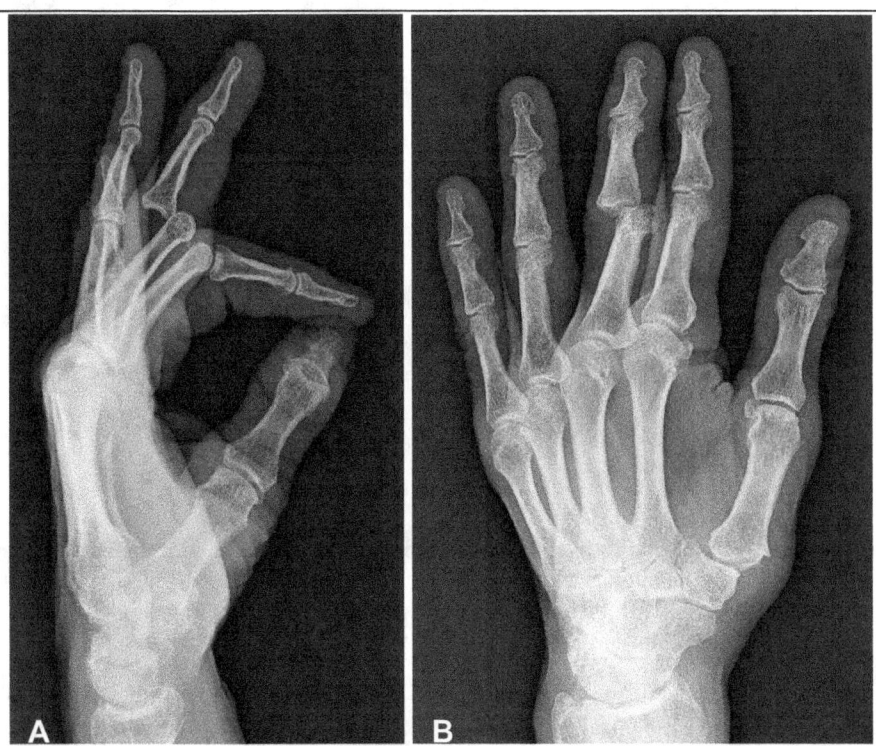

Lateral (A) and oblique (B) radiographs of the left hand demonstrate dorsal dislocation of the PIP joint of the middle finger. PA radiograph not shown.

A routine 3-view radiographic series of the hand will demonstrate most fractures and dislocations involving the hand. Where trauma has been localized to a specific finger, radiographs of just that finger will often be of higher quality than of the entire hand. Obtaining a true lateral view is important. Cross-sectional imaging with CT, MRI, or US is not recommended as an initial exam. Nuclear imaging has no role.

# Case 5-3

A 21-year-old man with hand pain and swelling that has become progressively worse since "punching a wall" with his closed fist 5 days ago. What imaging study should be performed?

Sensible recommendation: XR HAND 3 VIEW

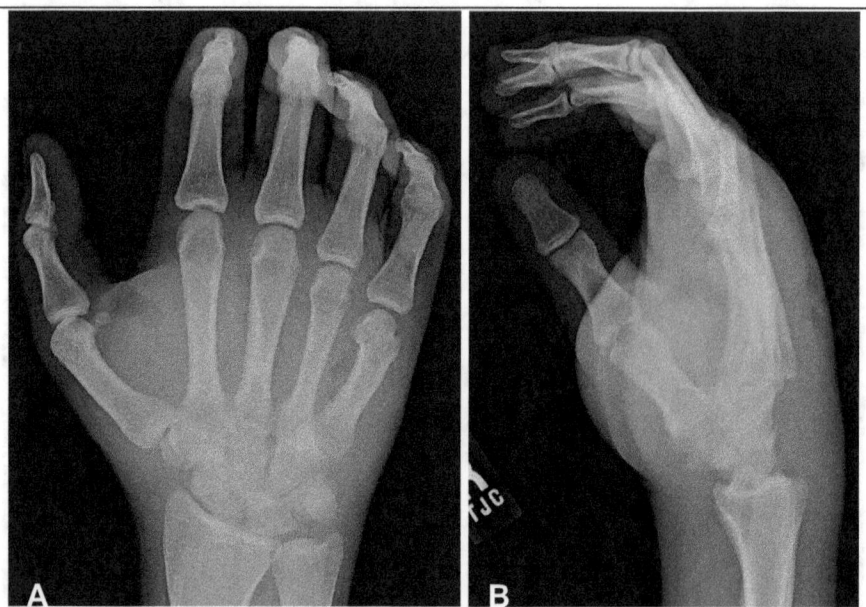

PA (A) and lateral (B) radiographs of the right hand demonstrate minimally displaced, obliquely oriented fracture of the fifth metacarpal and dorsal subluxation of the fourth and fifth MCP joints. There is massive soft tissue swelling and soft tissue defects over the dorsum of the fifth metacarpal head and first web space.

A routine 3-view radiographic series of the hand will demonstrate most fractures and dislocations involving the metacarpal bones. CT is often a useful adjunct for confirming and surgical planning for fracture-dislocation injuries involving the carpometacarpal joints or carpus. If infection is suspected, MRI wo/w contrast may be obtained.

# Case 5-4

A 29-year-old man involved in a motor vehicle collision in which he drove his vehicle into a telephone pole presents to the emergency department with facial and left hand pain. CT of the head and neck showed fracture of the nasal arch. In effort to investigate a suspected fracture of the metacarpal bones of the left hand, what is the most appropriate study?

This scenario concerns a polytrauma patient with suspected metacarpal fracture or dislocation.

Sensible recommendation: XR HAND 3 VIEW

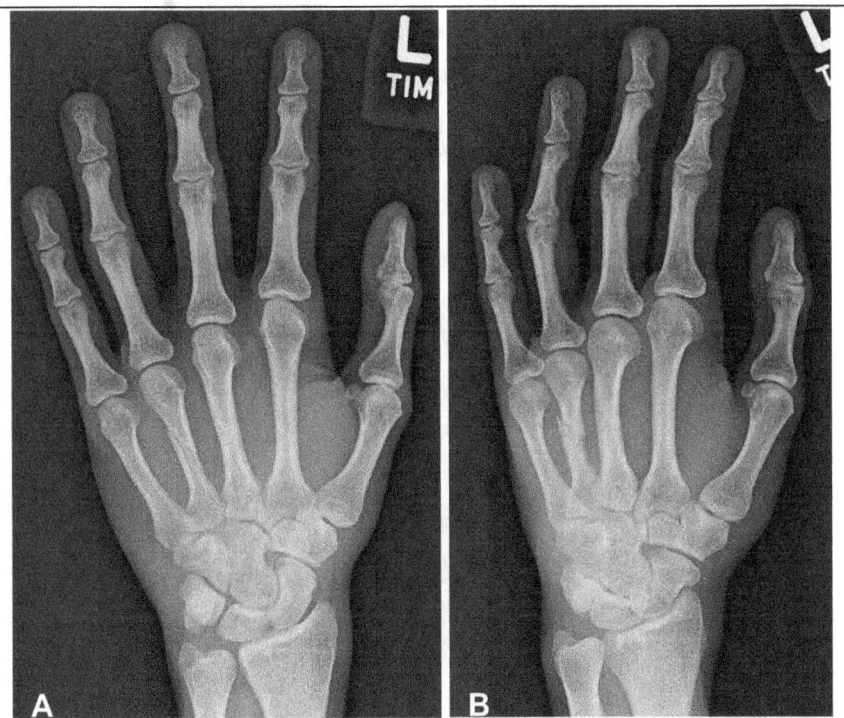

Frontal (A) and oblique (B) radiographs of the left hand demonstrate minimally displaced, obliquely oriented fractures involving the third and fourth metacarpal.

A routine 3-view radiographic series of the hand will demonstrate most fractures and dislocations involving the metacarpal bones. CT is often a useful adjunct for surgical planning in fracture-dislocation injuries involving the carpometacarpal joints.

## Case 5-5

A 56-year-old woman slipped while walking down her stairs, landing on her left outstretched hand. On examination, there is clinical concern for fracture of the phalanges of the left hand. What is the most appropriate study to obtain?

This scenario concerns a patient with blunt hand trauma and suspected phalangeal fracture or dislocation.

Sensible recommendation: XR HAND 3 VIEW

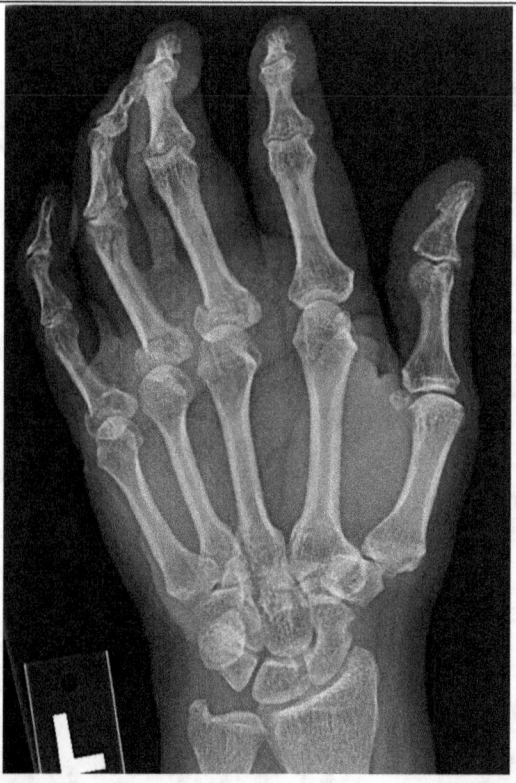

Frontal radiograph of the left hand demonstrates minimally impacted, transversely oriented fractures involving the base of the third through fifth proximal phalanges.

A routine 3-view radiographic series of the hand, or focused on the injured finger, will demonstrate most fractures and dislocations involving the phalangeal bones. An internally rotated oblique view in addition to the routine externally rotated oblique projection may increase the diagnostic confidence for phalangeal fracture.

## Case 5-6

37-year-old man slipped and fell in the shower, and now reports right distal thumb pain. A fracture of the thumb distal phalanx is suspected. What is the most appropriate image modality to obtain?

This scenario concerns a patient with blunt hand trauma and suspected thumb fracture or dislocation.

Sensible recommendation: XR HAND 3 VIEW or XR FINGER 3 VIEW

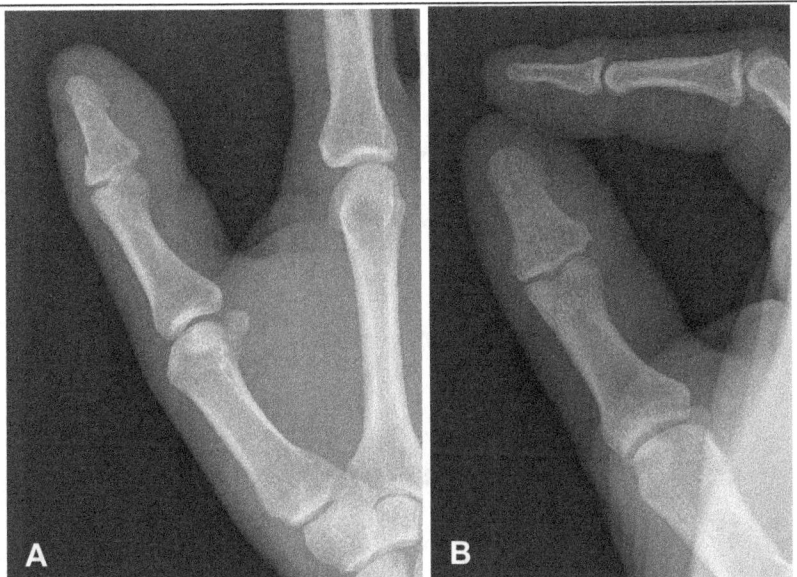

Two radiographic views of the right thumb demonstrate a minimally displaced fracture involving the base of the first distal phalanx.

Most fractures of the thumb will be detected on a 2-view radiographic series of the thumb, with slight increase in diagnostic yield with the addition of an oblique view. If the clinical exam localizes to the thumb or one finger, the finger may be adequate without the hand.

## Case 5-7

A 24-year-old man fell while skiing, at which time his left thumb was caught in the strap of the pole and he has been suffering from pain and swelling for 5 days since the injury. There is clinical concern for injury of the ulnar collateral ligament at the first metacarpophalangeal joint. What is the most appropriate study?

This scenario concerns a patient with blunt hand trauma and suspected gamekeeper's thumb injury.

Sensible recommendation: XR HAND 3 VIEW or XR FINGER 3 VIEW

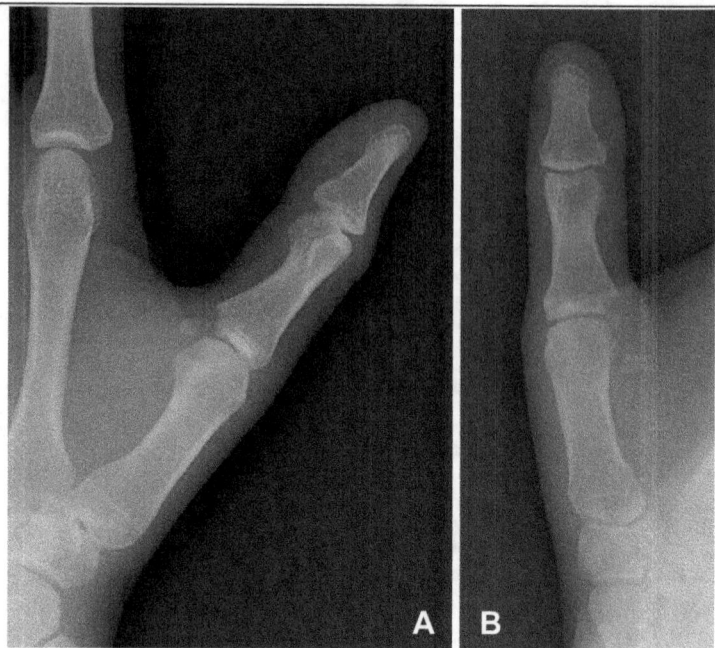

Two radiographs of the left thumb demonstrate a small, displaced fracture fragment arising from the ulnar base of the first proximal phalanx, compatible with a gamekeeper thumb injury.

The initial study to identify a gamekeeper's thumb injury (injury involving the ulnar collateral ligament of the first metacarpophalangeal joint) is a routine radiographic series of the thumb. However, unless a bony avulsion fracture arising from the distal first metacarpal and/or first proximal phalanx is present, the injury may be radiographically occult. In this scenario, a stress examination or cross-sectional imaging may be warranted. MRI is ideal for evaluating tendon injuries and helping with surgical planning. MRI is commonly used for the diagnosis of Stener lesions of the thumb and the diagnosis of pulley system injuries.

# References

1. American College of Radiology. ACR Appropriateness Criteria: Acute hand and wrist trauma. American College of Radiology, revised 2018. https://acsearch.acr.org/docs/69418/Narrative/ (accessed April 24, 2021).
2. Newberg A, Dalinka MK, Alazraki N, Berquist TH, Daffner RH, DeSmet AA, el-Khoury GY, Goergen TG, Keats TE, Manaster BJ, Pavlov H, Schweitzer ME, Haralson RH 3rd, McCabe JB. Acute hand and wrist trauma. American College of Radiology. ACR Appropriateness Criteria. Radiology. 2000 Jun;215 Suppl:375-8. PMID: 11037450.

# Chapter 6: Acute Wrist Trauma

Jack Porrino, MD, Jennifer Favinger, MD, Erin Flaherty, MD

Radiography is the initial exam for acute wrist trauma. Radiography should also be obtained after reduction of fracture. CT may be helpful for surgical planning or for diagnosis of occult or complex injuries. MRI has a role for diagnosis of occult injury.

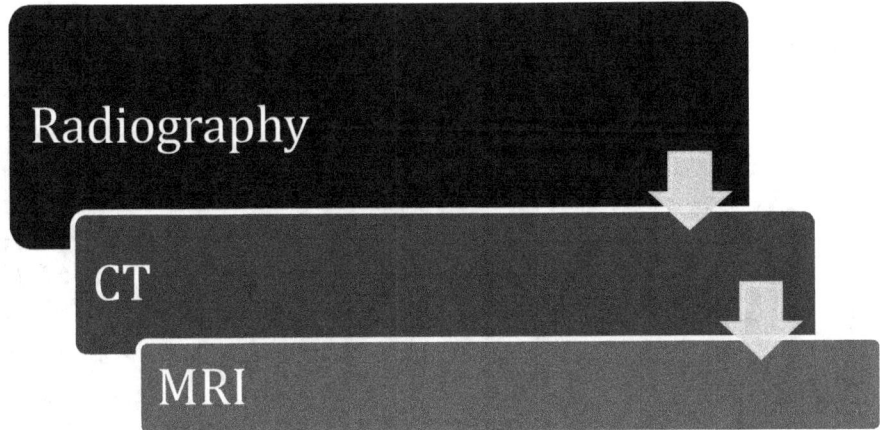

# Case 6-1

A 61-year-old woman was stuck by a slow-traveling vehicle while riding her bicycle. She landed on outstretched arms approximately 7 feet from her bike and reported pain to both wrists. She was hemodynamically normal and neurovascularly intact with no other complaints. She was wearing a helmet and denied injury to the head or loss of consciousness. What is the first examination to order with regards to her bilateral wrist pain?

This scenario concerns the first imaging exam for a patient with acute blunt wrist trauma.

Sensible recommendation: XR WRIST 3 VIEW

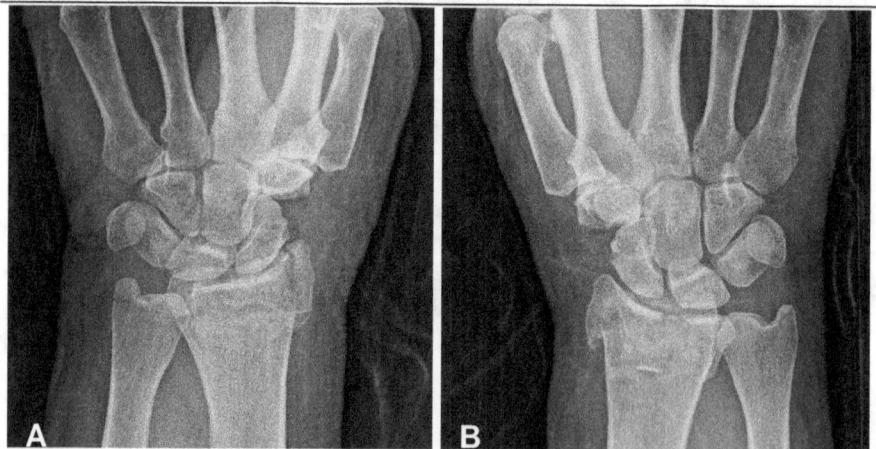

Frontal radiographs of the left (A) and right (B) wrist demonstrate comminuted fractures of the distal left and right radius.

The hand and wrist are highly vulnerable to injuries, with hand and wrist fractures and fracture-dislocations more common than those of any other part of the body. Significant long-term consequences can occur if diagnosis is delayed. Radiographs provide adequate diagnostic information and guidance for the treating physician. When initial radiographs are negative, or in the presence of certain clinical or radiographic findings, further imaging is appropriate. The standard 3-view wrist series at UW includes PA, oblique, lateral, and scaphoid views (yes, 4 actual views).

# Case 6-2

53-year-old woman who sustained injury to the right wrist after tripping over a gas pump. Radiographs acquired 4 days after injury were interpreted as normal. She is now 12 days removed from injury with persistent pain, and an acute distal radius fracture is suspected. What is the modality of choice to establish the diagnosis?

This scenario concerns the next imaging exam for a patient with suspected acute distal radius fracture. Initial radiographs are normal.

Sensible recommendation: XR WRIST, post-immobilization, or MRI WRIST WO CONTRAST, or CT WRIST WO CONTRAST

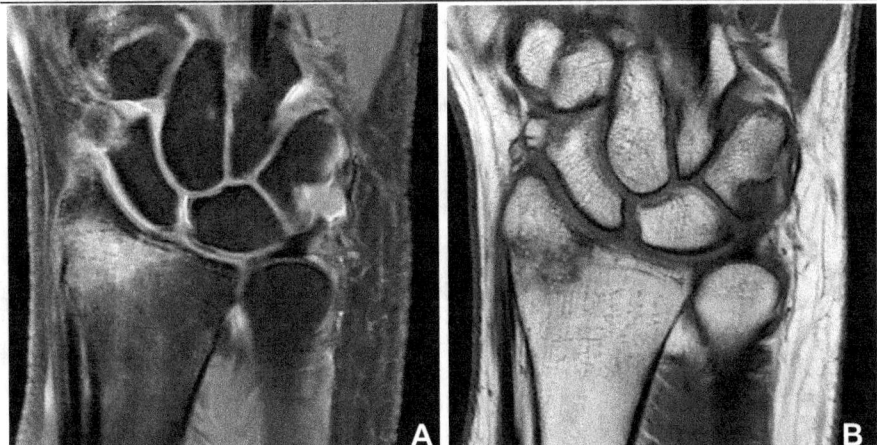

Coronal T2 FS MRI (A) and T1 MRI (B) of the right wrist demonstrate a fracture of the distal radius which was not apparent on radiographs acquired 4 days after injury.

The hand and wrist are highly vulnerable to injuries, and there are significant long-term consequences if the diagnosis is delayed or incorrect. In one particular study, fractures of the distal radius and scaphoid accounted for more delayed diagnoses than any other traumatized region in patients with initially normal emergency room radiographs. When initial radiographs are negative, or in the presence of certain clinical or radiographic findings, further imaging is appropriate. When MRI is performed in addition to radiographs, radiographically occult fractures of the distal radius as well as unsuspected fractures of the carpal bones are frequently demonstrated. MRI is a more appropriate modality to use to detect suspected radiographically occult wrist fractures before CT if there are no contraindications to MRI. Alternatively, the limb may be immobilized and follow-up radiographs may be obtained.

# Case 6-3

29-year-old man with left distal radius and ulna fractures incurred following a fall from his bicycle. He was seen in the emergency department where the fracture was diagnosed by radiographs and he was splinted. The orthopedic surgeon is interested in imaging for surgical planning. What is most appropriate?

This scenario concerns the imaging exam necessary for treatment planning of a patient with a comminuted, intra-articular distal radius fracture diagnosed on radiographs.

Sensible recommendation: CT WRIST WO CONTRAST

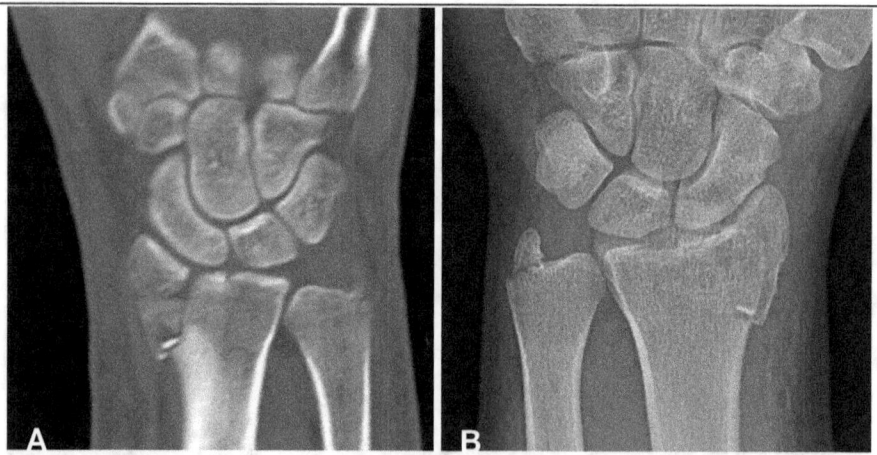

Coronal CT image of the left wrist (A) demonstrates a comminuted fracture of the distal radius with extension into the radiocarpal joint and fracture plane distraction. The complex nature of the fracture is seen to better advantage when compared with the radiograph (B).

With regards to fractures of the distal radius, CT reveals involvement of the radiocarpal and distal radioulnar articular surfaces, intra-articular displacements and depressions, and comminution more accurately than radiographs. When there is a high likelihood of intra-articular incongruence, selective or even routine use of CT to supplement the standard radiographic examination is warranted. CT is recommended over MRI for surgical planning of complex, intra-articular distal radius fractures.

# Case 6-4

A 34-year-old man was involved in a bicycle crash in which he T-boned a car while traveling approximately 20 miles per hour. He was separated from the bicycle and presents to the hospital hemodynamically stable but with left lower extremity and bilateral wrist pain. With regards to his right wrist, there is clinical suspicion of fracture of the scaphoid. What is the most appropriate first examination?

This scenario concerns the first imaging exam for a patient with a suspected acute scaphoid fracture.

Sensible recommendation: XR WRIST 3 VIEW

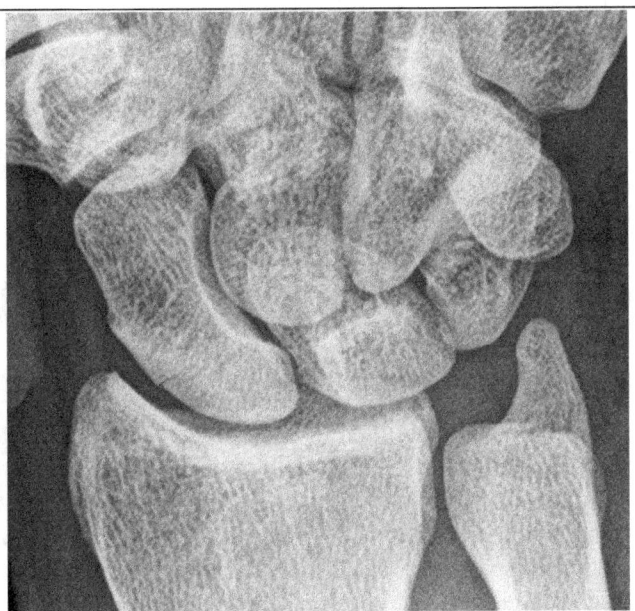

Scaphoid view of the wrist demonstrates a subtle, minimally displaced transversely oriented fracture of the scaphoid waist.

Although fractures of the scaphoid are notoriously difficult to identify on initial radiographs, the first examination to obtain when fracture of the scaphoid is suspected is a radiographic series. A projection optimized for assessment of the scaphoid, as pictured above, is routinely recommended whenever there is a clinical suspicion of a scaphoid fracture. Not only is identification of a scaphoid fracture important, but many surgeons recommend immediate operative intervention when the fracture is displaced.

## Case 6-5

35-year-old man fell off of his bicycle while avoiding a pothole, landing onto his right wrist. Upon presentation, radiographs were interpreted as normal. However, there is strong clinical concern for a radiographically occult scaphoid fracture. What is the most appropriate next procedure?

This scenario concerns the next imaging exam for a patient with a suspected acute scaphoid fracture where initial radiographs are negative.

Sensible recommendation: XR WRIST, post-immobilization, or MRI WRIST WO CONTRAST, or CT WRIST WO CONTRAST

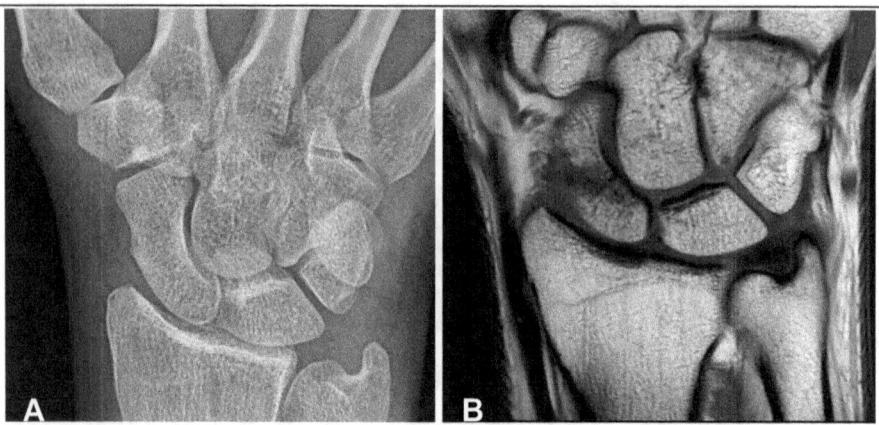

Radiograph of the wrist (scaphoid view) (A) fails to demonstrate a non-displaced fracture of the scaphoid waist that is readily apparent on the coronal T1 MRI (B).

Standard practice in patients with clinically suspected scaphoid fractures but normal initial radiographs is to apply a cast and repeat the clinical evaluation and radiographs in 10-14 days, at which time resorption about the fracture line may make the fracture visible. However, MRI can obviate the need for presumptive casting and allow for definitive care earlier for fractures, a more cost-effective alternative when considering the total cost of presumptive care and productivity lost from work. Accuracy for scaphoid fracture detection with MRI is superior when compared with CT, bone scintigraphy, and sonography. Immediate operative intervention for fractures of the scaphoid is often recommended when there is as little as 1 mm of displacement.

# Case 6-6

38-year-old woman with backward ground level fall on an outstretched hand with snuff box tenderness. Initial radiographs were normal, but because of clinical suspicion for radiographically occult scaphoid fracture, she was casted and follow-up radiographs were obtained 5 days later. The second set of radiographs is also normal, but there is continued clinical suspicion of scaphoid fracture. What is the appropriate next procedure?

This scenario concerns a suspected radiographically occult scaphoid fracture in a patient whose initial radiographs and follow-up radiographs are negative.

Sensible recommendation: MRI WRIST WO CONTRAST

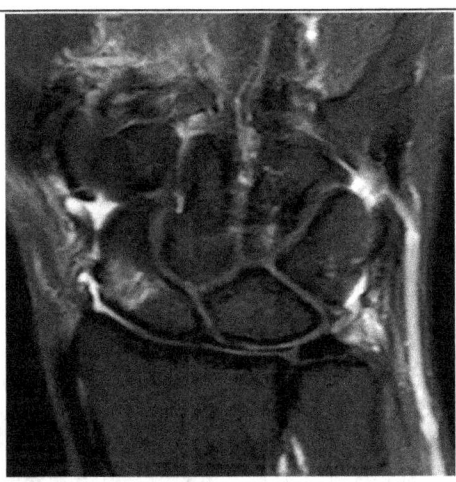

Coronal T2 FS MRI of the wrist showing non-displaced scaphoid waist fracture.

With negative follow-up radiographs in hand, if there is still suspicion for a radiographically occult fracture, the recommendation for further imaging is MRI WO CONTRAST. Although a case may be made for CT or radionuclide bone scan, or even further radiographic follow-up, a positive or negative MRI would be considered definitive. Additionally, MRI may identify soft tissue injuries that would not be seen with other imaging modalities.

# Case 6-7

35-year-old man with ulnar sided wrist pain and concern for left-sided distal radioulnar joint instability. The treating orthopedic surgeon is interested in imaging to establish the diagnosis. What is the most appropriate study to recommend?

This scenario concerns a patient with suspected distal radioulnar joint subluxation.

Sensible recommendation: CT WRIST WO CONTRAST, bilateral

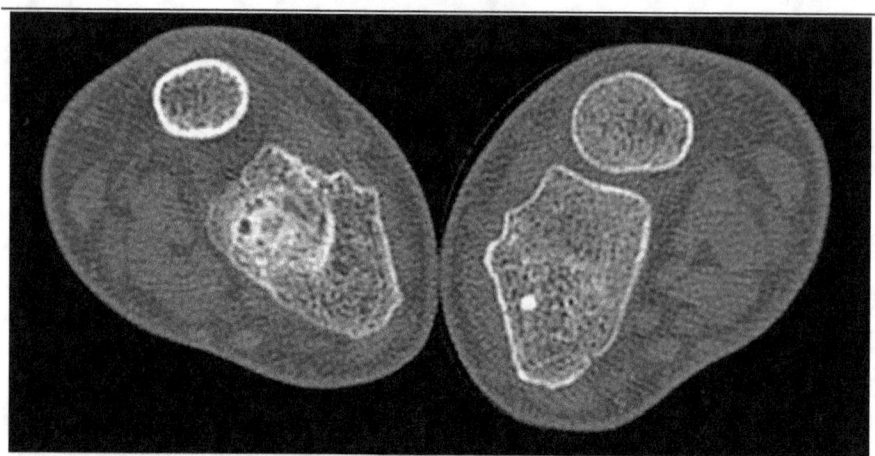

Bilateral axial CT image of the left and right wrist with pronation demonstrating left sided (wrist situated on the left side of the image) distal radioulnar joint widening.

Distal radioulnar joint subluxation is difficult to confirm radiographically, and it may be present only in certain positions. Instead, CT of both wrists scanned simultaneously in both pronated and supinated positions can be performed to establish the diagnosis. Symptoms and physical findings of this abnormality are often nonspecific, and imaging such as CT in the pronated and supinated position may be necessary in order to establish the diagnosis and allow for adequate management.

## Case 6-8

A 27-year-old man reports pain over the region of the hook of the left hamate following fall, however a traditional 3-view radiographic series of the hand was interpreted as normal. What is the appropriate study to establish the diagnosis of fracture of the hook of the hamate?

This scenario concerns a patient with suspected hook of the hamate fracture. The initial radiographs did not show such a fracture.

Sensible recommendation: CT WRIST WO CONTRAST or XR WRIST, special views

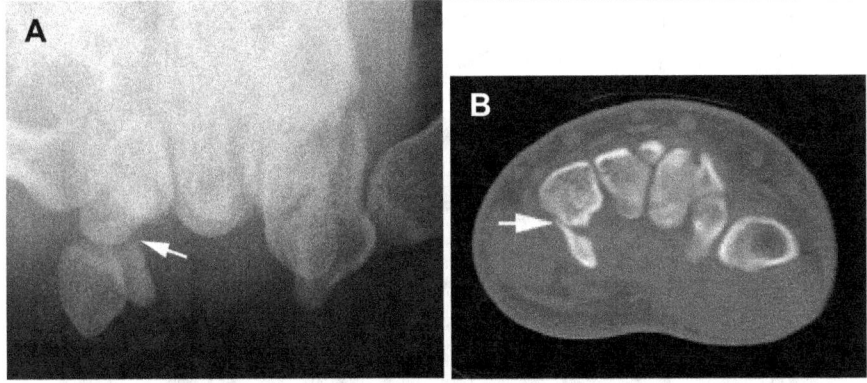

(A) Carpal tunnel radiograph of the left wrist demonstrates a transversely oriented fracture (arrow) through the hook of the hamate. (B) Axial CT also shows the hook of the hamate fracture (arrow).

While diagnosis of alternative carpal bone fractures is less problematic when compared to fractures of the scaphoid, evaluation of certain carpal bones benefits from supplemental studies in addition to the standard views. Fractures involving the hook of the hamate may be best depicted on semi-supinated AP or carpal tunnel views of the wrist. However, if these supplemental views fail to demonstrate a fracture that is strongly suspected clinically, or if obtaining these views is problematic, then CT is recommended as the alternative. MRI would also show hook of the hamate fractures.

## Case 6-9

A 38-year- old man presents with pain in his right palm. He states that approximately 4 months ago, he was using a jet ski and somehow injured himself on the dock. He thinks that he has a piece of wood in his hand. His hand radiographs were negative. What is the most appropriate next imaging study?

This scenario concerns a patient with suspected penetrating trauma with a foreign body in the soft tissues of the hand or wrist. Initial radiographs are negative. Next imaging study.

Sensible recommendation: US, region of interest

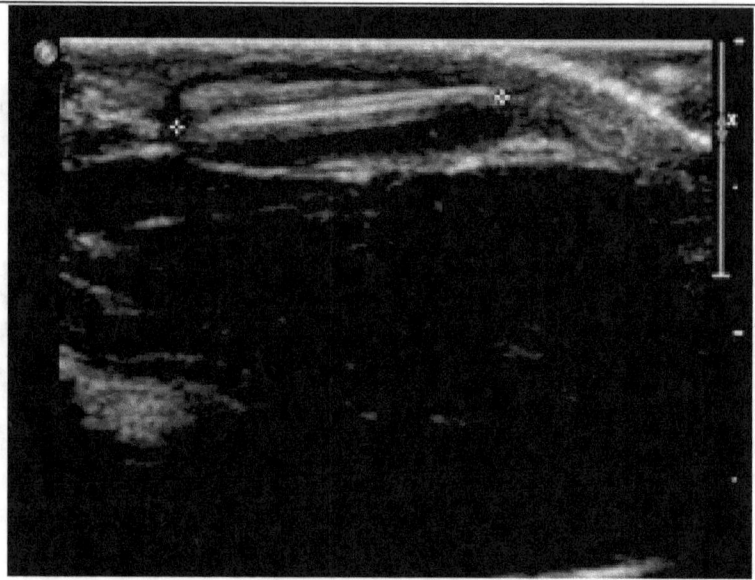

US of thenar eminence demonstrates a linear hyperechoic lesion in the superficial fat (calipers), in keeping with a foreign body.

US is superior to radiography for detection of radiolucent foreign bodies and is recommended as the first choice when the foreign body is located within the superficial soft tissues with no bone around it. US guidance may also be used for removal of the foreign body.

## References

1. American College of Radiology. ACR Appropriateness Criteria: Acute hand and wrist trauma. American College of Radiology, revised 2018. https://acsearch.acr.org/docs/69418/Narrative/ (accessed April 24, 2021).
2. Newberg A, Dalinka MK, Alazraki N, Berquist TH, Daffner RH, DeSmet AA, el-Khoury GY, Goergen TG, Keats TE, Manaster BJ, Pavlov H, Schweitzer ME, Haralson RH 3rd, McCabe JB. Acute hand and wrist trauma. American College of Radiology. ACR Appropriateness Criteria. Radiology. 2000 Jun;215 Suppl:375-8. PMID: 11037450.

# Chapter 7. Acute Elbow Trauma

Lindsay Stratchko, DO, Eric Walker, MD, Jonelle Petscavage-Thomas, MD, Felix S. Chew, MD

Radiography is the best initial exam for acute elbow trauma. Radiography should also be obtained after reduction of dislocations. CT may be helpful for surgical planning for complex fractures, and MRI has a role for diagnosis of occult fractures and soft tissue injuries.

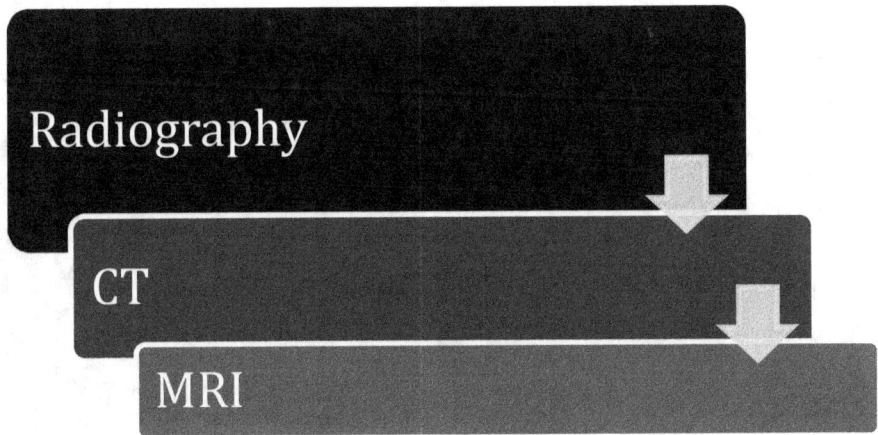

## Case 7-1

39-year-old man who injured his elbow in a bicycle crash. He complains of pain and restricted range of motion. What is the best initial imaging exam?

This scenario concerns the initial imaging study in a patient with acute trauma and elbow pain.

Sensible recommendation: XR ELBOW 3 VIEW

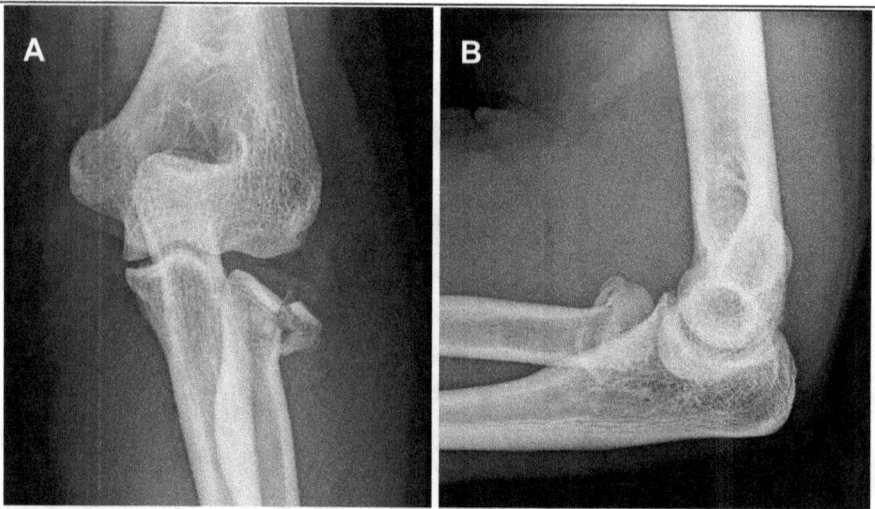

AP (A) and lateral (B) radiographs of elbow demonstrates comminuted, and depressed radial head fracture.

Post-traumatic elbow pain should initially be evaluated with radiography. The routine 3-view elbow includes AP, lateral, and oblique (radial head) views. Significant long-term consequences can occur if diagnosis is delayed. Radiographs provide adequate diagnostic information and guidance for the treating physician. When initial radiographs are negative, or in the presence of certain clinical or radiographic findings, further imaging is appropriate.

## Case 7-2

An 80-year-old woman presents for continued right elbow pain after a fall on her outstretched hand two weeks prior. The patient was evaluated in the emergency department after her initial fall and radiographs at that time showed an elbow effusion. Since her fall, the patient states her pain has persisted without improvement. What is the most appropriate next imaging test?

This scenario concerns the next imaging study in a patient with acute elbow pain and suspected radiographically occult fracture.

Sensible recommendation: MRI ELBOW WO CONTRAST

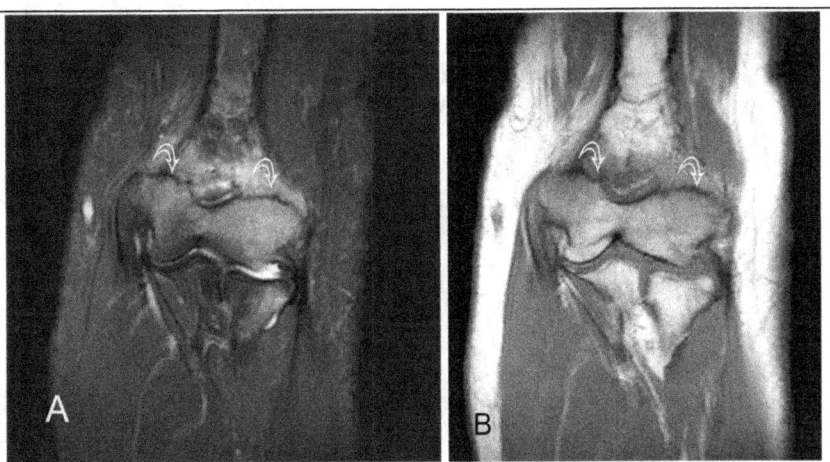

Coronal T2 FS MRI (A) and T1 MRI (B) demonstrate edema of the distal humeral metaphysis with low signal supracondylar fracture line. Additionally, there is mild edema of the radial head with associated subtle fracture line.

Post-traumatic elbow pain should initially be evaluated with radiography. In the setting of negative radiographs, elbow MRI is the most appropriate next imaging examination for suspected occult fracture. MRI is favored over CT due to its increased sensitivity for detecting stress fractures. CT can be used in the acute setting or in cases where MRI is contraindicated or not tolerated. Intra-articular contrast is of limited utility in this setting, making arthrography less appropriate. The three-phase bone scan is an alternative imaging modality in the evaluation for stress fractures, however, it is less specific and anatomic detail is limited.

# Case 7-3

38-year-old man presents with acute onset right elbow pain after feeling a popping sensation while lifting a piece of furniture. On examination, the patient has asymmetric contours of his biceps muscles and decreased supination of the right arm. The patient complains of pain primarily at the proximal radius. Radiographs were performed to evaluate suspected biceps rupture, however, only showed soft tissue swelling about the elbow. What is the most appropriate next examination to evaluate for distal biceps tendon tear?

This scenario concerns acute elbow pain with suspected tendon tear and negative radiographs.

Sensible recommendation: MRI ELBOW WO CONTRAST

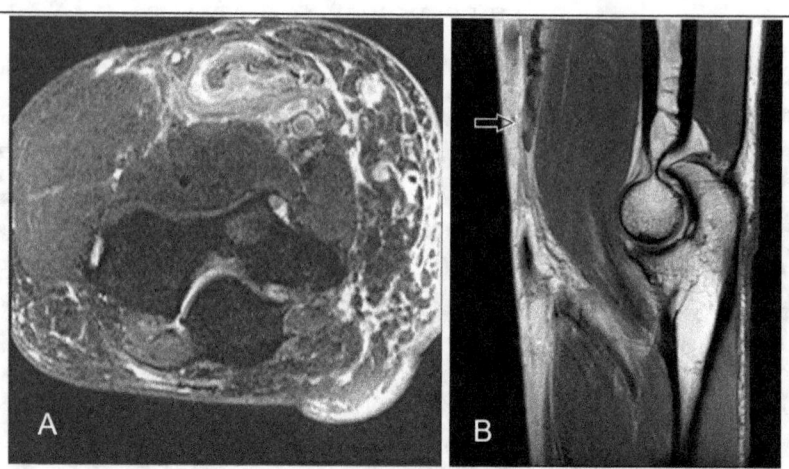

Axial T2 FS MRI (A) shows marked edema surrounding the distal biceps muscle. The sagittal PD MRI (B) identifies the torn and retracted biceps tendon, which is abnormally thickened and irregular in appearance (arrow).

Biceps tendon injuries often require further imaging beyond initial elbow radiographs. Magnetic resonance imaging plays an important role in direct visualization of the biceps tendon and evaluation of degree of tendon injury. Sagittal images allow estimation of tendon retraction and assessment of the lacertus fibrosus. Intravenous and/or intra-articular contrast does not aid in diagnosis. Ultrasound can also be used to assess for biceps tendon tear at its distal insertion, which can be used as an alternative to MRI. The degree of soft tissue detail on CT is often not sufficient for diagnosis.

# Case 7-4

17-year-old high school football athlete presents with acute onset left elbow pain after tackling a player at a recent game. The patient is tender to palpation along the lateral joint line and laxity is noted on varus stress. Left elbow radiographs show a joint effusion without evidence of fracture. What is the most appropriate next imaging test to perform?

This scenario concerns acute elbow pain with suspected ligament tear and negative radiographs.

Sensible recommendation: MRI ARTHROGRAHY ELBOW or MRI ELBOW WO CONTRAST

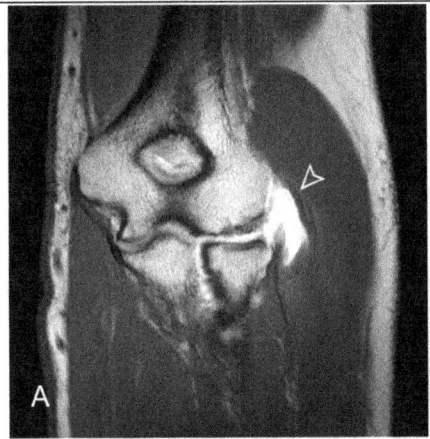
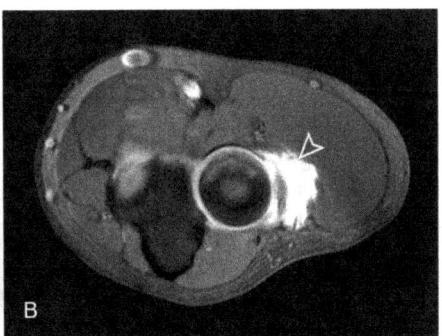

Coronal T1 (A) and axial T1 FS (B) MR arthrogram images demonstrate detachment of the radial collateral ligament from its humeral attachment with contrast extravasation outside the joint capsule.

Heterotopic ossification can occasionally be seen on radiographs in patients with history of partial or complete collateral ligament tears. When radiographs are negative, MRI is used in further evaluation of elbow instability and collateral ligament injuries. In the acute setting, elbow effusion distends the joint capsule and can aid in identifying ligamentous defects. When an effusion is absent, intra-articular contrast can be injected to expand the joint. While partial tears demonstrate high signal within the ligamentous fibers, complete tears show contrast extending beyond the confines of the joint capsule. CT arthrography may be appropriate if MRI is contraindicated.

# References

1.  American College of Radiology. ACR Appropriateness Criteria: Chronic Elbow Pain. American College of Radiology, reviewed 2015. https://acsearch.acr.org/docs/69423/Narrative/ (accessed April 24, 2021).
2.  Chew ML, Giuffre BM. Disorders of the Distal Biceps Brachii Tendon. Radiographics. 2005;25 (5): 1227-37.

# Chapter 8. Acute Shoulder Trauma

Jack Porrino, MD, Erin Flaherty, MD, Jennifer Favinger, MD, Hyojeong Lee, MD.

Radiography is the best initial exam for acute shoulder trauma. Radiography should also be obtained after reduction of dislocations. CT may be helpful for evaluation of complex, intraarticular, or scapular fractures, and MRI has a role in evaluating soft tissue injury.

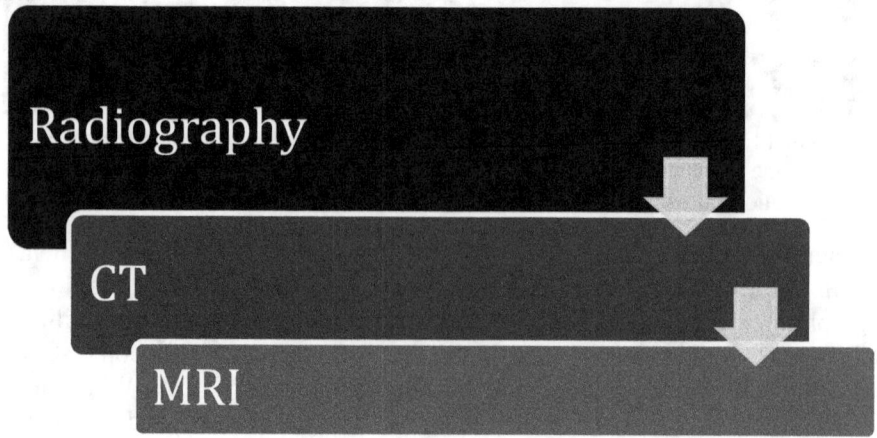

# Case 8-1

20-year-old man crashed while riding his skateboard downhill at relatively high speed. His right shoulder is painful, and he refuses to move it. There is a visible deformity. What is the best initial study of choice?

This scenario concerns the most appropriate initial imaging study for a patient with acute shoulder trauma.

Sensible recommendation: XR SHOULDER 3 VIEW

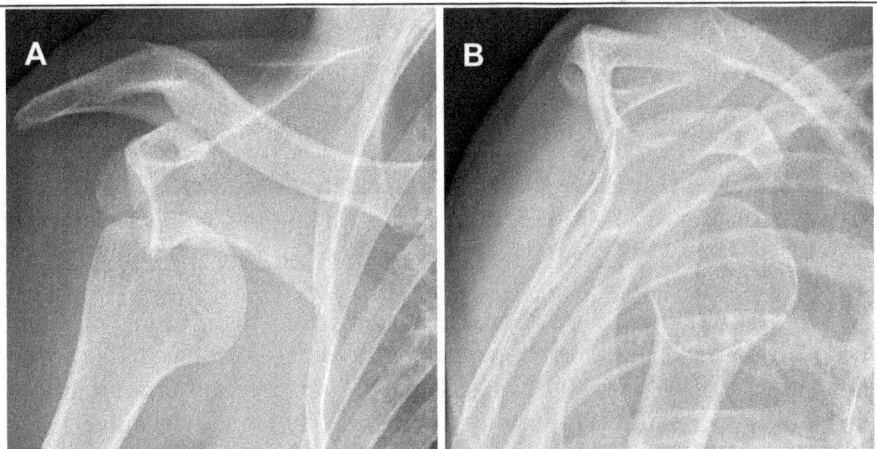

(A-B) AP and Y-view radiographs of the right shoulder demonstrate anterior dislocation of the glenohumeral joint. The humeral head has come to rest in a subcoracoid position.

For the initial screening of acute shoulder pain, radiography is most appropriate. All radiographic series of the shoulder should include a frontal view in combination with one or more orthogonal views. Although radiologists should recognize dislocations on the basis of the AP radiograph alone, the orthogonal view, usually an axillary lateral or a Y-view, increases confidence that a dislocation is present or absent. Radiography also provides a quick, inexpensive evaluation for fractures.

# Case 8-2

A 49-year-old man presents with left shoulder pain. He injured his shoulder after a fall while skiing. Initial radiographs were negative, but he continued to have pain when he placed the arm out to the side or tries to lift his arm. What is the next appropriate study?

This scenario concerns acute traumatic nonlocalized shoulder pain with negative radiographs.

Sensible recommendation: MRI SHOULDER WO CONTRAST

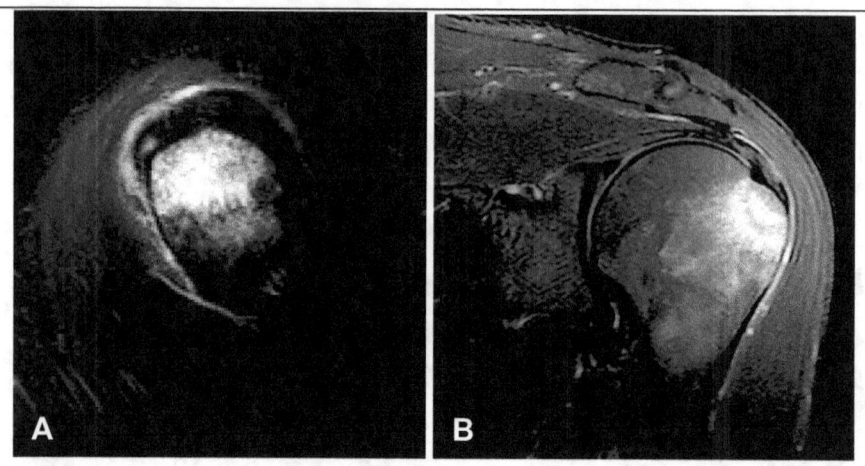

Sagittal (A) and coroal (B) T2-weighted fat saturated MRI of shoulder demonstrate non-displaced fracture of greater tuberosity and a rim rent tear of supraspinatus.

MRI WO CONTRAST is a reasonable imaging study in the setting of acute nonlocalized traumatic shoulder pain and negative radiographs. In the acute trauma setting, MRI WO CONTRAST may be preferred to MR arthrography, as acute intra-articular pathology will typically produce significant joint effusion that helps visualize intra-articular soft tissue structures. MRI is the preferred imaging modality in assessing extra-articular soft tissue traumatic pathology. MRI is also sensitive for diagnosing bone marrow contusion or an occult fracture.

# Case 8-3

A 49-year-old man presents with right shoulder pain. He flew over the handlebars of his bicycle and hit his right shoulder. Shoulder radiographs were taken and demonstrated a humeral head fracture. What is the most appropriate exam to evaluate his fracture?

This scenario concerns traumatic shoulder pain. Radiographs show humeral head or neck fracture. Next imaging study.

Sensible recommendation: CT SHOULDER WO CONTRAST

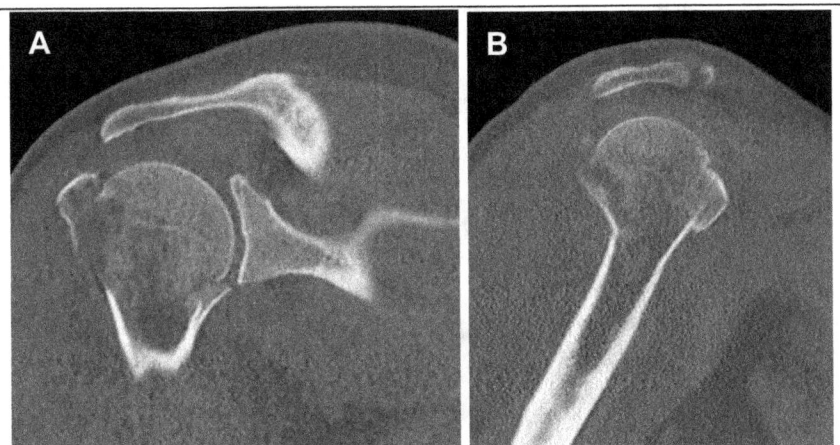

CT shoulder coronal (A) and sagittal (B) reformatted images demonstrate proximal humeral fracture.

Proximal humerus fractures of the head and neck are relatively common. These fractures have a bimodal age distribution, occurring in young patients as the result of high-energy trauma and older patients with low-energy trauma, such as falls from a standing position. The most commonly used classification for humeral head fractures is the Neer classification system. Nondisplaced fracture planes and complex bony anatomy can result in underappreciation of the extent of proximal humeral fractures on radiographs. CT is the best examination for delineating fracture patterns and has been shown to be equivocal to MRI in identifying nondisplaced fractures, making it the preferred study for characterizing proximal humeral fractures. Contrast is generally not necessary unless there is concern for arterial injury. 3-D volume-rendered CT images may be obtained to better characterize fracture patterns and humeral neck angulation, which can affect functional outcomes.

## Case 8-4

A 60-year-old man presents with acute left shoulder pain. He was riding a motocyle and hit by a semitruck. Plain radiograph of left scapula demonstrates a comminuted fracture. What is the most appropriate next imaging study?

This scenario concerns traumatic shoulder pain. Radiographs show scapula fracture. Next imaging study.

Sensible recommendation: CT SHOULDER WO CONTRAST

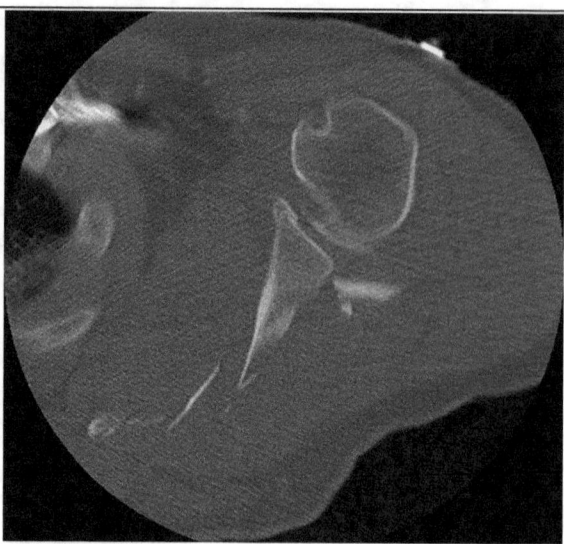

Axial CT image of left shoulder demonstrates a comminuted and displaced left scapula fracture. The glenoid articular surface is intact.

There is no consensus on indications for surgical fixation of scapula fractures. In general, isolated scapula body fractures heal well without surgical fixation, although associated rib fractures or higher injury severity score are associated with worse clinical outcomes and may benefit from more aggressive surgical fixation. Scapula fractures involving the glenoid articular surface or glenoid neck may also require surgical fixation. Because of the scapula's complex osteology and overlying ribs, scapula fractures can be easily missed or underappreciate on conventional radiographs. CT is the best imaging modality for identifying and characterizing scapula fracture patterns. Intra-articular extension, glenopolar angulation, AP angulation, and lateral border offset can all be better assessed on CT compared with conventional radiographs. Contrast is generally not necessary, unless there is concern for arterial injury. 3-D–reformatted CT images can better visualize scapula fracture displacement and angulation.

## Case 8-5

A 19-year-old man presents with acute shoulder pain. He was playing basketball a week ago and it was pulled behind him and slipped out of joint, then back into joint spontaneously about ten seconds later. His left shoulder radiographs demonstrate bony Bankart lesion. What is the most appropriate next imaging study?

This scenario concerns traumatic shoulder pain. Radiographs show Bankart or Hill-Sachs lesion. Next imaging study.

Sensible recommendation: MRI ARTHROGRAPHY SHOULDER or MRI SHOULDER WO CONTRAST

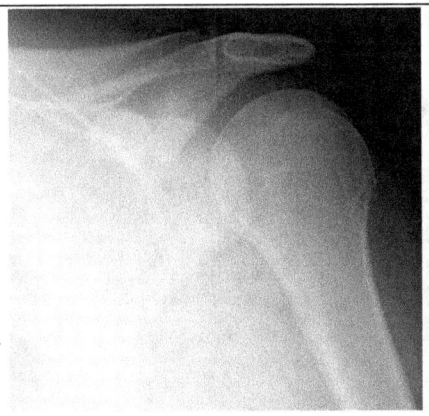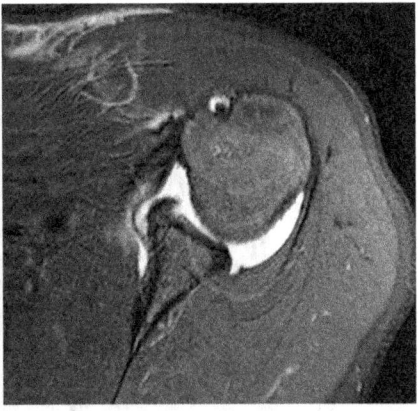

AP radiograph of left shoulder (A) demonstrates a small bony fragment at the inferior aspect of the glenoid. Axial T1-fat saturated MR arthrogram image (B) of left shoulder demonstrates a bony Bankart lesion.

Bankart and Hill-Sachs lesions are common findings associated with transient shoulder dislocation. Bankart lesions have a particularly high association with transient shoulder dislocations, and a transient shoulder dislocation should be presumed if a Bankart lesion is present. A close association exists between Bankart and Hill-Sachs lesions, and one should be sought out whenever the other is identified on radiographs. MR arthrography is the preferred study for evaluating subacute or chronic Bankart lesions because of its soft- tissue contrast. Multiple studies have shown MR arthrography to be reliable in diagnosing labroligamentous injuries and superior to MRI WO CONTRAST for this indication. MR arthrography has been shown to be equivalent to CT in the assessment of glenoid and humeral head bone loss, while being superior to CT in assessment of labroligamentous injuries.

## Case 8-6

A 30-year-old man presented with acute right shoulder pain after motor vehicle crash. He was a restrained passenger in a car which struck a concrete wall at 40 mph. There were no airbags in the car. On physical exam, active forward elevation was limited to 130 degrees. Rotator cuff strength was intact in all planes. O'Brien test was distinctly positive. He also had pain over the biceps groove anteriorly and described pain that radiated anteriorly down the shoulder. The clinician was concerned about possible labral tear.

What is the most appropriate next imaging study?

This scenario concerns traumatic shoulder pain. Radiographs normal. Physical examination findings consistent with labral tear. Next imaging study.

Sensible recommendations: MRI SHOULDER ARTHROGRAPHY or MRI SHOULDER WO CONTRAST

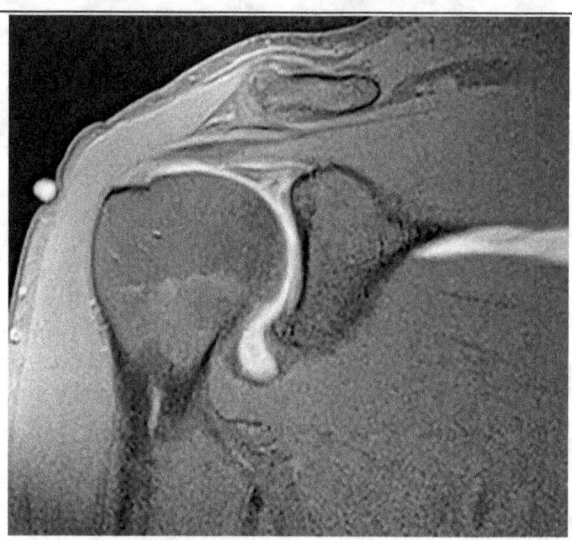

Coronal T2 FS MRI of the right shoulder demonstrates tear of bicipitolabral junction including intra-articular biceps tendon. The superior labrum shows a tear.

MR arthrography has been reported to have a high sensitivity for detection of labral injury, ranging from 86% to 100%, however, the issue of selection bias is inherent in the design of many of these retrospective studies. Compared to non-contrast MRI, MR arthrography has been shown to have increased sensitivity for detection of anterior labral and SLAP tears. MRI without contrast may be preferred to MR arthrography in the setting of acute shoulder dislocation when a post-traumatic joint effusion is typically present to provide sufficient visualization of soft tissue structures. When MRI arthrography is unavailable, CT arthrography may provide comparable sensitivity and possibly improved specificity in detection of labral lesions along with improved visualization of the bones in cases of complex trauma.

## Case 8-7

A 46-year-old man who underwent repair of his right supraspinatus and infraspinatus tendons 2 years prior to presentation. He fell from his bicycle and felt a pop in his right shoulder, followed by significant pain. Radiographs were interpreted as normal, with expected post-operative changes. What is the most appropriate procedure to establish the diagnosis of retear of the rotator cuff?

This scenario concerns a patient with a previous arthroscopic rotator cuff repair who is suspected of having a retear of the rotator cuff. Initial radiographs were negative except for previous surgery.

Sensible recommendations: MRI SHOULDER WO CONTRAST, MRI SHOULDER ARTHROGRAPHY, or US SHOULDER

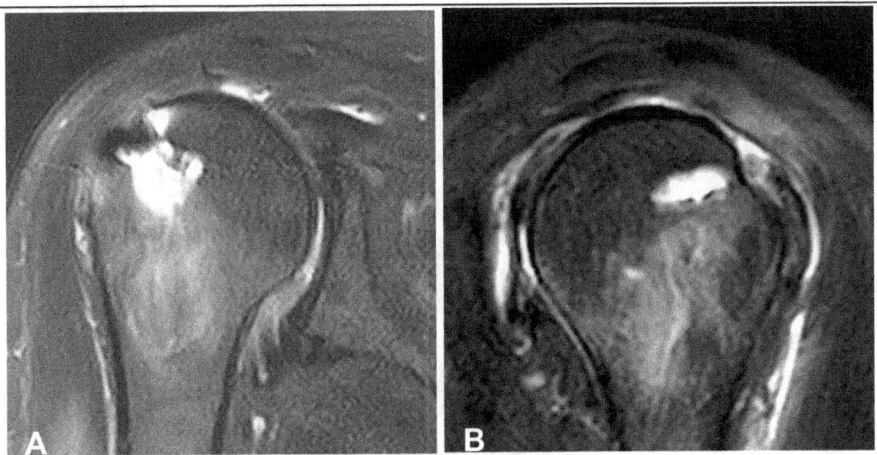

Coronal (A) and sagittal (B) T2 FS MRI of the right shoulder demonstrate susceptibility artifact within the humeral head from the prior rotator cuff repair. There is abnormal fluid signal in the expected region of the supraspinatus tendon without intact tendon fibers visualized compatible with full thickness retear.

Depending on local expertise, MRI, MRI arthrography, and US are considered equivalent for the evaluation of the rotator cuff following prior repair. All of these modalities have the ability to provide visualization of rotator cuff pathology. MRI arthrography is recommended if there is question concerning the distinction between a full-thickness and partial-thickness tear. Notably, US is limited in evaluation of the deep shoulder structures such as the labrum, as well as for assessment of bone marrow pathology. However, in the postoperative shoulder, artifacts may degrade MRI.

## Case 8-8

A 66-year-old man presents with left axillary hematoma. Radiographs of left shoulder were normal. He has history of multiple left shoulder dislocations. The clinician is concerned about vascular compromise. What is the most appropriate next imaging study?

This scenario concerns traumatic shoulder pain. Radiographs already performed. Physical examination consistent with vascular compromise. Next imaging study.

Sensible recommendation: CT ANGIOGRAPHY W CONTRAST

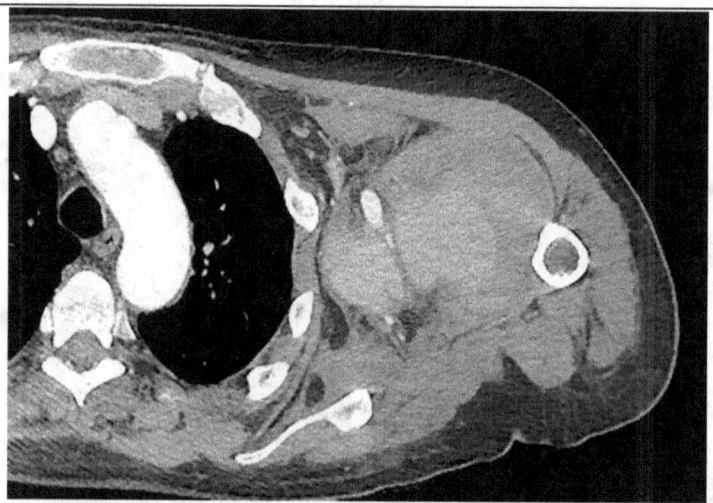

Axial image of CT arteriography demonstrates irregularity of left axillary artery with a large hematoma, in keeping with pseudoaneurysm.

The subclavian, axillary, and brachial arteries are uncommonly injured following fractures and dislocations about the shoulder; however, the consequences can be debilitating. Of these, the axillary artery is more likely to be injured in patients with proximal humeral fractures, and the risk increases in the presence of open fractures, shoulder dislocation, and fractures of the scapula and ribs. CT angiography (CTA) is a specialized protocol for contrast-enhanced CT in which image acquisition occurs during maximum arterial opacification by IV contrast. Thin-slice axial images of the region of interest is performed, which helps in detection of subtle vascular injuries. Maximum intensity projection (MIP) images in multiple planes are also commonly performed, allowing for long segments of vessels to be visualized on a single image. CTA is the preferred examination for evaluation of suspected arterial injury. It can delineate the extent of injury and has the added benefit of providing optimal assessment of osseous injuries.

# Case 8-9

A 30-year-old woman presents with left shoulder pain and weakness. She was playing flag football and dislocated her shoulder that was reduced spontaneously. Since that time, she has had difficulty lying on that shoulder and with internal rotation. Shoulder radiographs demonstrate a Hill-Sachs lesion. The clinician is concerned about neuropathy. What is the most appropriate next imaging?

This scenario concerns traumatic shoulder pain. Radiographs already performed. Neuropathic syndrome (excluding plexopathy) is suspected. Next imaging study.

Sensible recommendations: MRI SHOULDER WO CONTRAST

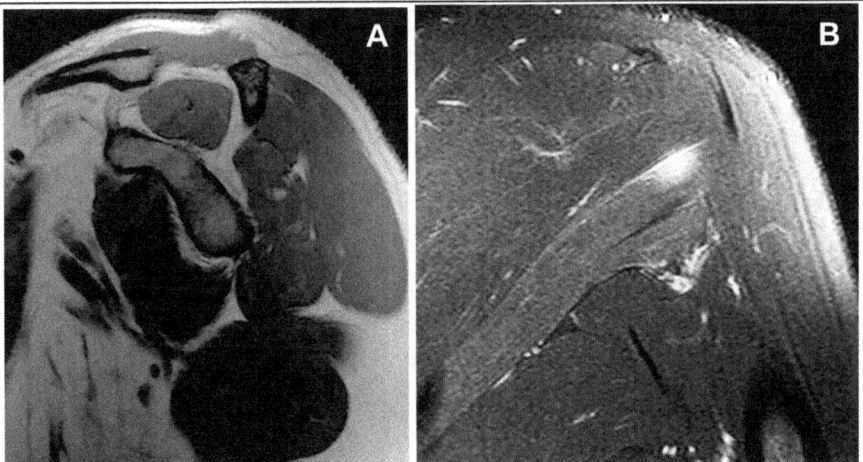

Sagittal T1-weighted (A) and coronal T2-weighted fat saturated MR images show edema along the teres minor (B) without fatty infiltration, in keeping with acute axillary neuropathy.

Neuropathic pain is defined as pain caused by a lesion or disease of the somatosensory nervous system. It is a clinical diagnosis that requires a demonstrable lesion or disease process, and can be classified as central or peripheral, depending on the level of the lesion. In the setting of trauma, neuropathic pain at the shoulder can be seen following injury to the brachial plexus or the peripheral nerves (axillary, suprascapular, radial, ulnar, and median). Electrodiagnostic studies are considered the reference standard for diagnosis; however, imaging can be helpful in delineating the extent and level of injury. Although injury to specific nerves may be suspected on radiographs and CT based on knowledge of the expected course of nerves, high-resolution MR neurography can play an important role.

# References

1.  American College of Radiology. ACR Appropriateness Criteria: Shoulder Pain-Traumatic. American College of Radiology, revised 2017. https://acsearch.acr.org/docs/69433/Narrative/ (accessed April 24, 2021).
2.  Amini B, Beckmann NM, Beaman FD, Wessell DE, Bernard SA, Cassidy RC, Czuczman GJ, Demertzis JL, Greenspan BS, Khurana B, Lee KS, Lenchik L, Motamedi K, Sharma A, Walker EA, Kransdorf MJ. ACR Appropriateness Criteria(®) Shoulder Pain-Traumatic. J Am Coll Radiol. 2018 May;15(5S):S171-S188. doi: 10.1016/j.jacr.2018.03.013. PMID: 29724420.

# Chapter 9. Acute Spine Trauma

Ryan P. Joyce, MD, Majid Chalian, MD

CT is the best initial exam for suspected acute spine trauma. Radiography is a less sensitive modality that is sometimes used as an initial exam, but should be avoided if possible, particularly in older patients and in patients with high-risk mechanisms of injury. For example, up to two-thirds of cervical spine fractures depicted by CT are radiographically occult (1). Radiographic sensitivity for thoracolumbar spine fractures ranges from 49% to 82%, compared with 94% to 100% sensitivity of CT (2, 3, 4). Even when abnormalities are identified on initial radiographs, they often warrant further characterization with a subsequent CT for definitive classification and treatment planning. The risk that a missed spine injury imposes is sufficiently high to warrant more sensitive initial imaging with CT, so as not to miss clinically significant but radiographically occult injuries.

Two clinical criteria, the NEXUS criteria and Canadian C-spine rule, are commonly used to determine the necessity of cervical spine imaging in trauma patients. Both criteria were developed and validated to be highly sensitive for the detection of cervical spine injury. That is, if the criteria are not met, then a significant cervical spine injury is highly unlikely to be present.

**NEXUS Criteria for Cervical Spine Imaging (8)**

| |
|---|
| **Focal neurologic deficit** |
| **Midline spinal tenderness** |
| **Altered level of consciousness** |
| **Intoxication** |
| **Distracting injury** |

*If any of the above criteria are present, then the C-spine cannot be cleared clinically, and imaging should be considered.*

**Canadian C-Spine Rule (CCR) for Cervical Spine Injury (7)**
The CCR essentially applies 3 separate tests to determine if the cervical spine can be cleared clinically.
First, one should determine if a high-risk factor for injury is present. If one is present, then the cervical spine cannot be cleared clinically. CCR describes the following high-risk factors:

| |
|---|
| Age > 65 years |
| Paresthesias in extremities |
| Dangerous mechanism: <ul><li>Falls from ≥ 3 feet/5 stairs</li><li>Axial load to head</li><li>Motor vehicle crash with high speed, roll-over, or ejection</li><li>Bicycle collision</li><li>Motorized recreational vehicle accident</li></ul> |

Second, one should determine if a low risk factor is present. If none are present, then the cervical spine cannot be cleared clinically. CCR describes the following low-risk factors:

| |
|---|
| Sitting position in the ED |
| Ambulatory at any time |
| Delayed onset neck pain (not immediate onset) |
| No midline tenderness |
| Simple rear-end motor vehicle collision <ul><li>Not pushed into traffic</li><li>Not hit by bus or large truck</li><li>Not rollover or high-speed collision</li></ul> |

Lastly, if the application of tests one and two suggest that the cervical spine may be cleared clinically, a final test is applied. Test if the patient can actively rotate the neck 45° to the left and right. If the patient can do so, the cervical spine can be cleared clinically, and no imaging is required. If unable to do so, the cervical spine cannot be cleared clinically, and imaging should be considered.

Thoracolumbar spine injuries are more challenging to identify clinically, and there are no well-established clinical criteria to determine when thoracolumbar imaging is appropriate in the setting of blunt traumatic injury. Since clinical examination has poor sensitivity for identifying thoracolumbar injuries, any high-risk patient (midline thoracolumbar tenderness, high-energy mechanism of injury, or >60 years of age), as well as unexaminable patients (intoxicated, GCS <15, distracting injury), should undergo imaging of the thoracolumbar spine (ACR).

Since an estimated 20% of spine injuries will have a second associated spinal injury at a noncontiguous level (i.e. concomitant cervicothoracic and thoracolumbar injuries), total spine imaging is generally advised (5, 6). Spine imaging should rarely be limited to a particular segment in the setting of acute blunt trauma.

MRI has a role in the evaluation for concomitant nerve root or spinal cord injury. It is also useful in select cases where there is concern for CT-occult ligamentous injury resulting in spinal instability, or in cases where there is concern for neural injury without CT evidence of fracture or malalignment.

CTA and/or MRA of the head and neck play a role when there are clinical or imaging findings suggestive of a cervical arterial injury. The revised Denver criteria have been validated to be 97% sensitive for detecting blunt cerebrovascular injury, with a negative predictive value of 99.6%. (10) According to the 2011 revised Denver screen criteria, signs and symptoms of blunt cerebrovascular injury include potential arterial hemorrhage from the neck/face, cervical bruit in a patient < 50 years of age, expanding cervical hematoma, focal neurologic deficit (TIA, hemiparesis, vertebrobasilar symptoms, Horner syndrome), neurologic deficit inconsistent with head CT, and infarct on CT or MRI. Denver criteria risk factors for blunt cerebrovascular injury include displaced LeFort II or III midface fracture, mandible fracture, complex skull fracture/basilar skull fracture/occipital condyle fracture, traumatic brain injury with GCS < 6, cervical spine subluxation/dislocation, cervical spine fractures at C1-3 or that involve the transverse foramen at any level, near hanging with anoxic brain injury, clothesline-type injury or seat belt abrasion with significant swelling, pain, or altered mental status, TBI with thoracic injuries, scalp degloving, thoracic vascular injuries, blunt cardiac rupture, and upper rib fractures. (9)

# Case 9-1

A 21-year-old male was brought in by ambulance after a motor vehicle collision. Per EMS, the patient was stopped at a stoplight, and was rear-ended at low velocity by another motorist. On physical exam, he has no midline spinal tenderness, is not intoxicated, and has no clear distracting injury. He is neurologically intact, alert, and oriented. He can actively rotate his neck to the left and right.

This scenario concerns the first imaging study of the cervical spine after blunt force trauma when the patient does not meet NEXUS or CCR criteria for imaging.

Sensible recommendation: NO IMAGING

The patient does not meet NEXUS or CCR criteria for imaging, which are very sensitive for cervical spine injury. When these criteria are not met, a significant cervical spine injury is extremely unlikely, and imaging evaluation is not indicated.

# Case 9-2

A 26-year-old male was brought in by EMS, unconscious. He awoke in the ED intoxicated and stated that he had been heavily drinking alcohol. He complained of 8/10 "head pain", with a laceration on his right eyebrow. Aside from the laceration, physical exam was unrevealing. What is the initial imaging examination to order regarding potential spine trauma?

This scenario concerns initial imaging for patients with suspected acute cervical spine blunt trauma as indicated by the NEXUS or CCR clinical criteria.

Sensible recommendation: CT CERVICAL SPINE WO CONTRAST

This patient meets criteria for cervical spine imaging given his altered level of consciousness, intoxication, and distracting injury. Fortunately, in his case, no injury of the cervical spine was demonstrated on CT imaging. This case illustrates that the NEXUS and CCR clinical criteria, while highly sensitive for injury, have very low specificity. Recall that radiographs have largely been supplanted by CT for the detection of acute spine injury, as CT is significantly more sensitive than radiography.

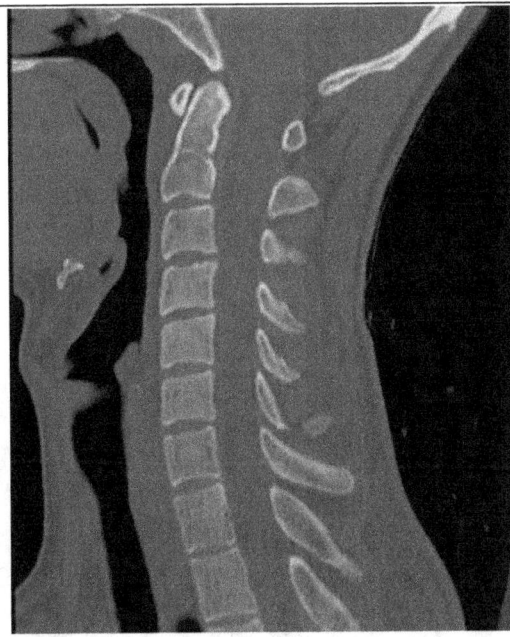

Sagittal reconstruction CT image of the cervical spine, without acute fracture or traumatic subluxation.

## Case 9-3

A 66-year-old male was brought in by EMS after a bicycle collision. He reportedly flew over his handlebars and loss consciousness on impact. He was helmeted and had a crack in his helmet. In the field, he was hypotensive with systolic blood pressures in the 70s, his GCS was 3, and he was placed in a cervical collar and intubated by EMS for inability to protect his airway. In the ER trauma bay, he was noted to have upper greater than lower extremity weakness and upper extremity sensory changes. Initial CT of the spine did not reveal an acute fracture or traumatic subluxation. What is the next imaging examination to order regarding potential cervical spinal cord or nerve root injury in the setting of trauma?

This scenario concerns the next imaging exam in a patient with suspected acute cervical spine blunt trauma with confirmed or suspected cervical spinal cord or nerve root injury, with or without traumatic injury identified on cervical CT.

Sensible recommendation: MRI CERVICAL SPINE WO CONTRAST

This patient presented with altered level of consciousness, focal neurologic deficits, and extremity paresthesia. He also had dangerous mechanisms of injury – axial load to the head and bicycle collision. Whenever there is clinical concern for neural injury, MRI should be performed to depict these potential injuries. MRI is markedly superior to CT for the detection and characterization of neural and other soft tissue injuries such as spinal cord contusion, cord transection, epidural hematoma, dural tear, and nerve root avulsion, among other lesions. The MRI in this patient demonstrated a cervical cord contusion without hemorrhage. Follow-up imaging a few months later demonstrated progressive post-traumatic cervical cord myelomalacia.

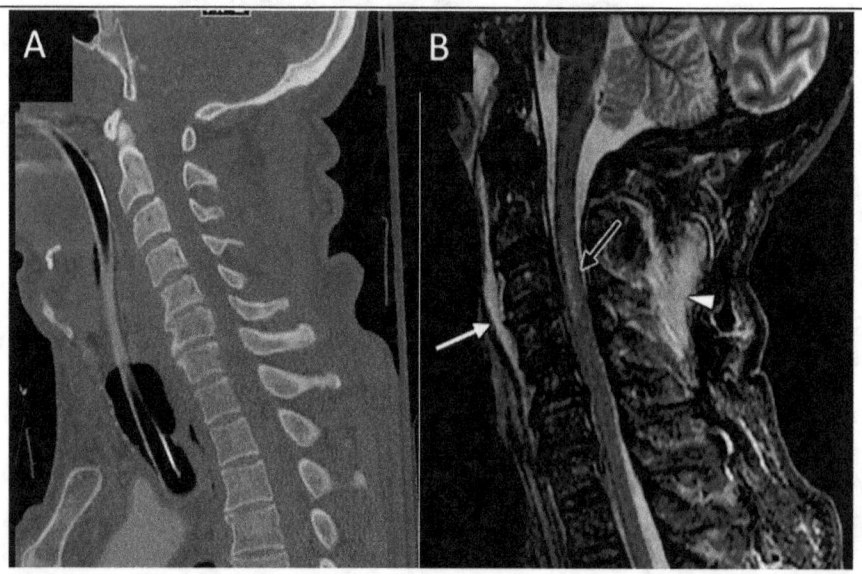

Sagittal CT reconstruction (A) of the spine is without evidence of fracture or traumatic subluxation. Sagittal STIR image (B) demonstrates at C3-C4 a focal tear of the anterior longitudinal ligament with associated prevertebral edema (white arrow), focal STIR hyperintense signal within the spinal cord in keeping with cord contusion (black arrow), and posterior paraspinal soft tissue edema (white arrowhead).

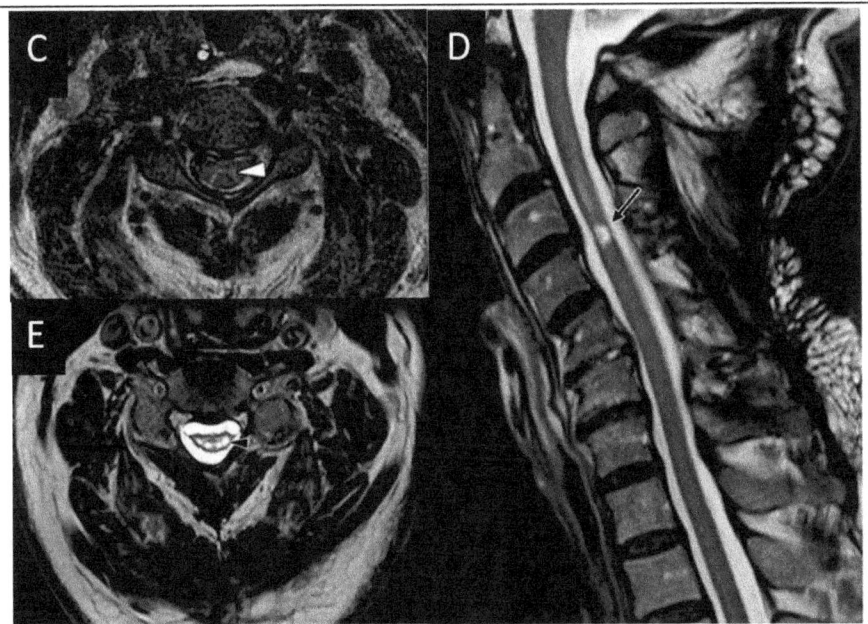

Axial T2 image (C) demonstrates at C3-C4 central spinal cord signal hyperintensity involving the gray matter in keeping with cord contusion (white arrowhead). A follow-up MRI (D) a few months later demonstrates progressive cystic change and volume loss at the injured cord, consistent with progressive post-traumatic myelomalacia (black arrow). A follow-up MRI (E) a few months later demonstrates progressive cystic change and volume loss at the injured cord (black arrowhead), consistent with progressive post-traumatic myelomalacia.

## Case 9-4

A 55-year-old male was brought in by ambulance after a fall from a ladder. He reportedly landed on his head and lost consciousness. He presented to the trauma bay on a back board with cervical collar in place. Trauma survey was notable for neck pain. As part of the radiographic trauma survey, in addition to a frontal view of the chest and pelvis, a portable cross table lateral radiograph of the cervical spine was obtained and demonstrated an acute hangman's fracture (figure A). What is the next imaging examination to order regarding the acute cervical spine fracture?

This scenario concerns the next imaging exam after radiographic detection of an acute cervical spine injury, most importantly in the context of treatment planning for a potentially mechanically unstable spine injury.

Sensible recommendation: CT CERVICAL SPINE WO CONTRAST

Many acute spine injuries, when detected radiographically, warrant further characterization with cross-sectional imaging. Exceptions include single-column compression fractures or transverse process fractures. Osseous and soft tissue injuries are best characterized by CT and MRI, respectively, and frequently occur together; it is not uncommon for a single injury to warrant evaluation with both modalities to fully characterize its extent. Complete characterization of spine injuries is of greatest interest in the treatment planning for fixation of the mechanically unstable spine, as the pattern of injury impacts the surgical approach and instrumentation technique required to achieve stability.

This patient's unstable spine injury was imaged with radiography, CT, and MRI, with the strength of each modality highlighted in the images below.

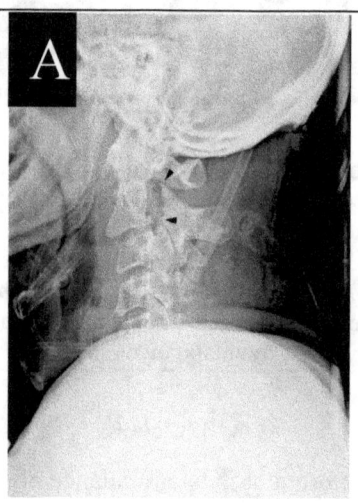

Lateral radiograph (A) demonstrates an acute C2 Hangman's fracture (black arrowheads). Although this injury is demonstrable on radiography, nondisplaced fractures are often suboptimally visualized on radiographs. Also note the patient's shoulders obscure the C5-C7 levels, resulting in an incomplete examination of the cervical spine.

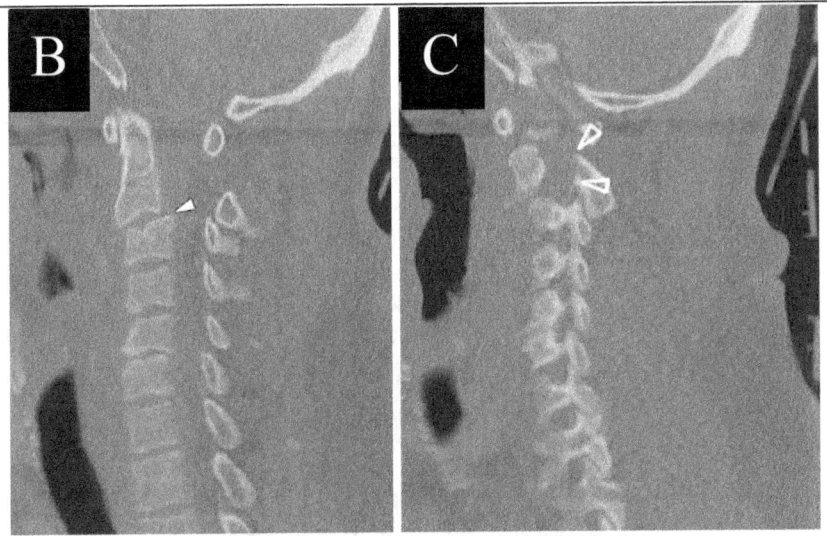

Sagittal CT (B) demonstrates an associated C2 on C3 grade 1 traumatic anterolisthesis (white arrowhead) with greater detail. Note the improved visualization of the lower cervical and T1 vertebral bodies. Sagittal CT image (C) clearly demonstrates the longitudinal fracture plane through the C2 pars interarticularis (open white arrowheads).

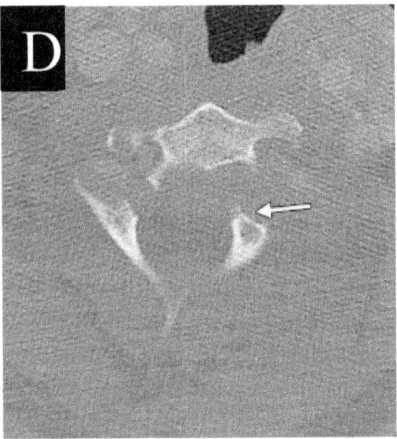

Axial CT image (D) reveals there is mild lateral displacement of the posterior elemental fracture fragment (white arrow) relative to the C2 vertebral body.

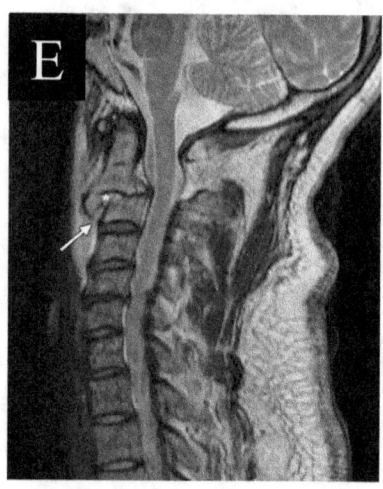

Sagittal T2-weighted MR image (E) demonstrates a focal avulsion tear of the anterior longitudinal ligament from its attachment site at the anteroinferior aspect of the C3 vertebral body (white arrow). The C2-C3 intervertebral disc has been largely extruded anteriorly (asterisk). These soft tissue abnormalities are not well visualized on the corresponding CT images, highlighting the excellent soft tissue contrast MR imaging provides.

# Case 9-5

A 25-year-old male was brought in by ambulance after a motorcycle collision. He slid and impacted a parked car at ~25 MPH. He reported some initial pain and remained on the ground until medics arrived. He was helmeted and denied loss of consciousness. He arrived at the trauma bay complaining of right-sided abdominal pain, as well as bilateral wrist, right elbow, and left foot pain. On physical exam, his vital signs were normal, and he had abrasions to bilateral knees, left foot, and right abdomen. He had no spinal tenderness or step offs, and no neurologic deficits. GCS was 15. Appropriate initial imaging, including CT pan-scan protocol for trauma and appropriate total spine CT reconstruction and interpretation, was performed. No fracture or traumatic subluxation was present within the cervical, thoracic, lumbar, or sacral spine. However, the imaged soft tissues of the neck were reported to demonstrate findings "suggestive" of injury to the right internal carotid artery. What is the next imaging examination to order regarding the potential arterial injury?

This scenario concerns the next imaging exam for a patient with suspected acute blunt cervical spine trauma with clinical or imaging findings suggestive of arterial injury, with or without positive cervical spine CT.

Sensible recommendation: CTA HEAD AND NECK W CONTRAST

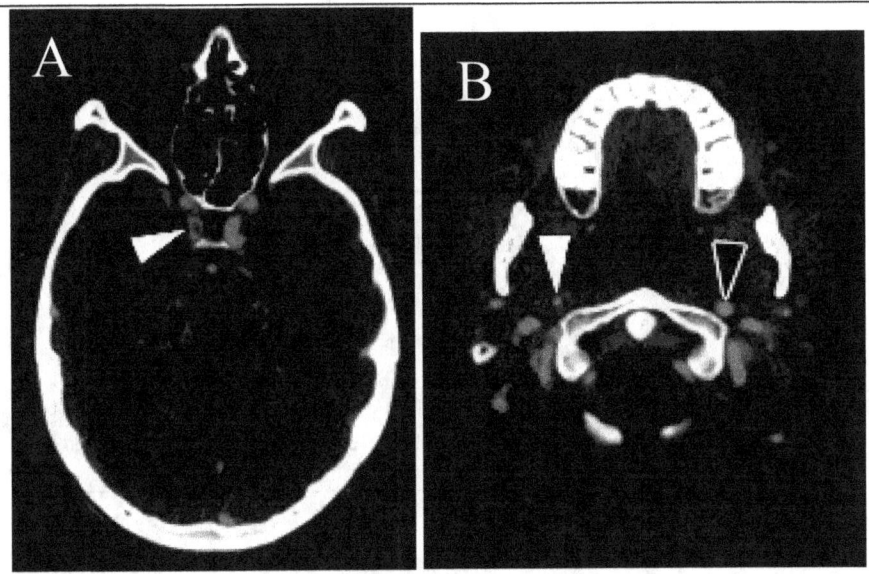

(A) A small filling defect is seen within the cavernous segment of the right internal carotid artery (arrowhead), consistent with nonocclusive thrombus. (B) More inferiorly within the neck, the right internal carotid artery (white arrowhead) demonstrates greater than 25% luminal narrowing, more conspicuous when compared to the contralateral internal carotid artery (black arrowhead).

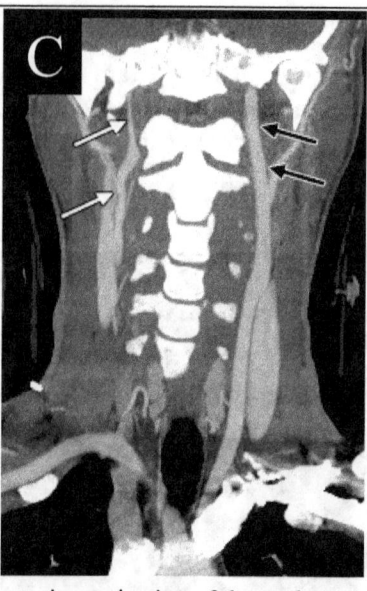

(C) Coronal maximum intensity projection of the neck vessels on head and neck CTA demonstrates long-segment greater than 25% irregular luminal narrowing and undulating contour of the right internal carotid artery (white arrows) compared to the left (black arrows), consistent with a grade 2 blunt cerebrovascular injury.

Although this patient did not complain of neck pain, he does have distracting injuries involving his abdomen, wrists, right elbow, and left foot. There are imaging findings suggestive of an arterial injury. When clinical or imaging findings suggest an arterial injury, further evaluation with dedicated CTA or MRA is warranted.

In addition to the grade 2 blunt cerebrovascular injury of the right internal carotid artery, this patient had bilateral wrist fractures, liver lacerations, splenic lacerations, and a right adrenal hemorrhage.

Biffl Scale for blunt cerebrovascular injury

| Injury grade | Description |
|---|---|
| 1 | Luminal irregularity or dissection with <25% luminal narrowing |
| 2 | Dissection of intramural hematoma with >25% luminal narrowing, intraluminal |
| 3 | Pseudoaneurysm |
| 4 | Occlusion |
| 5 | Transection with free extravasation, hemodynamically significant arteriovenous fistulae |

# Case 9-6

A young-adult male of unknown was brought in by ambulance after he was found down in his apartment complex unresponsive, followed by an episode of witnessed generalized tonic-clonic seizures. He was intubated at the scene and a cervical collar was placed. He presented normotensive but tachycardic. Additional history was not obtainable. Physical exam was notable for a right eyebrow ecchymosis, as well as left hand and knee abrasions. He had a GCS of 3T. An initial cervical spine CT was performed and demonstrated a C4 Schmorl's node, however, there was no CT evidence of a traumatic cervical spine injury. What is the next imaging examination to order regarding potential spine trauma in this obtunded patient?

This scenario concerns the next imaging study in an obtunded patient with no traumatic injury identified on cervical spine CT.

Sensible recommendation: MRI CERVICAL SPINE WO CONTRAST

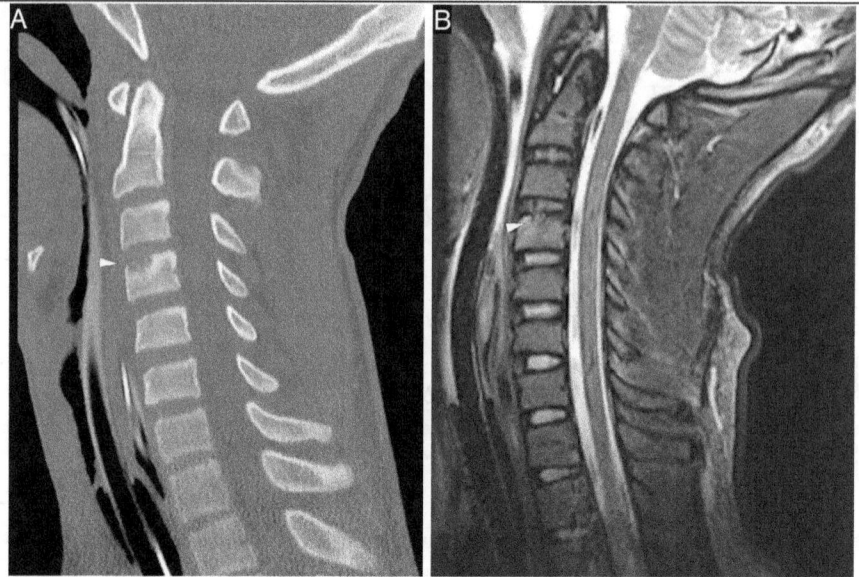

Sagittal CT image (A) demonstrates a well circumscribed lucent lesion abutting the C4 superior endplate, with mild surrounding vertebral body sclerosis (arrowhead). This appearance is typical of an inflammatory Schmorl's node, an incidental finding of little clinical significance in the context of acute trauma. The acute fracture or traumatic subluxation is identified. Sagittal MR image (B) demonstrates low-grade signal change within the C4 vertebral body near the superior endplate, compatible with the findings of a Schmorl's node on CT. Importantly, there is no evidence of cord contusion, epidural hematoma, or ligament injury – effectively excluding a traumatic injury to the cervical spine in this obtunded patient.

Since the obtunded patient cannot complete a full physical and neurological exam, it is important to exclude occult spine injuries in this patient population when presenting after acute trauma. When initial CT imaging is negative, we can be confident there is no fracture, malalignment, or focal soft tissue swelling. However, other soft tissue injuries, including cord contusion, ligamentous tears, and small epidural hematomas may be occult on CT imaging. Thus, it is appropriate to perform more sensitive soft tissue imaging in this patient population with MRI.

## Case 9-7

An 11-year-old female was brought in by ambulance after a motor vehicle collision. She was a lap-belt-only restrained passenger in the backseat of a minivan which was rear-ended by a semi-truck traveling 60 mph. At the scene, she was able to protect her airway and did not require intubation. She was placed in a cervical collar. She presented to the ED in mild distress and pain, with facial bruising and a left scalp hematoma. Her vital signs were stable. Initial CT of the head, cervical spine, chest, abdomen, and pelvis was performed, revealing a small subdural hematoma, as well as fractures of the C3 and C4 vertebral bodies. Additionally, there was subtle widening of the interspinous distance at the C3-C4 level, suggestive of a possible ligamentous injury. What is the next imaging examination to order regarding the potential cervical spine ligamentous injury?

This scenario concerns the next imaging study after when clinical or imaging findings suggest a spinal ligamentous injury.

Sensible recommendation: MRI CERVICAL SPINE WO CONTRAST

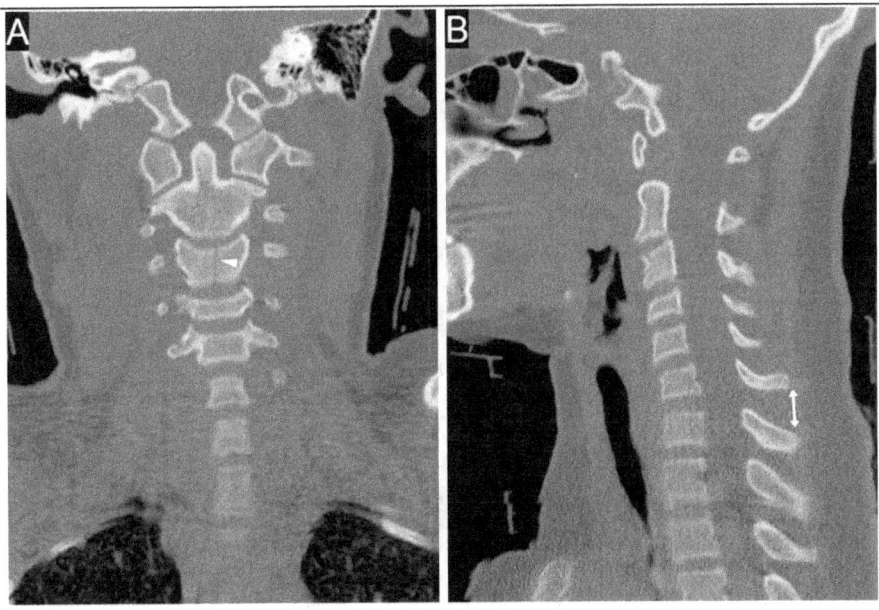

Coronal CT (A) demonstrates sagittal split fracture of the C3 vertebral body (white arrowhead), indicating high-energy trauma. Radiologists should deploy a heightened sensitivity for subtle malalignment and subluxation in this context, in order to suggest the presence of ligament injury. Sagittal CT (B) demonstrates subtle widening of the C6-C7 interspinous distance (double-headed arrow) compared to the levels above and below, along with subtle focal kyphosis at C6-C7. These findings are suggestive of ligamentous injury.

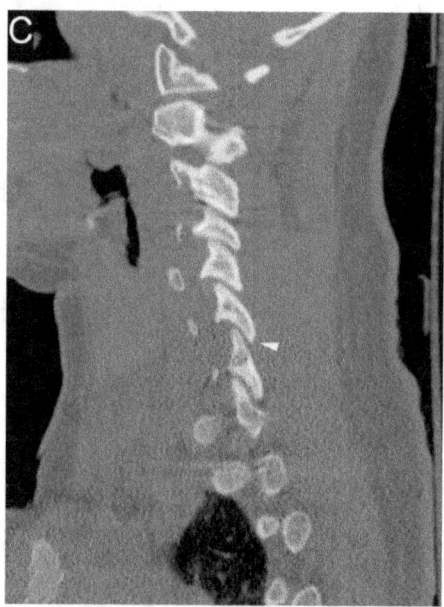

Sagittal CT (C) of the facet joints demonstrates subtle superior subluxation of the C6 facet relative to C7 (white arrowhead) compared to the levels above and below, also suggestive of ligamentous injury. This finding was present bilaterally.

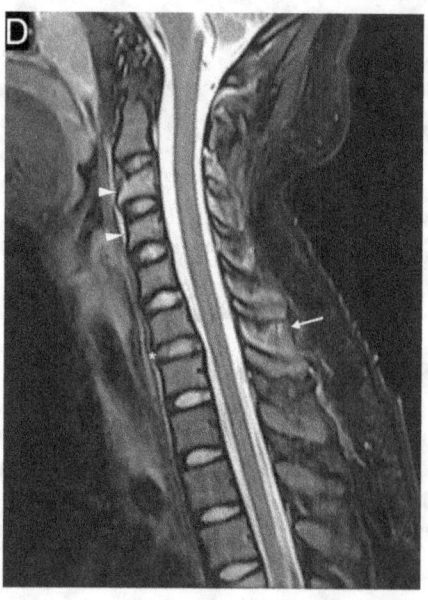

Sagittal MR image (D) demonstrates edema within the posterior paraspinal soft tissues at C6-C7, indicative of an acute injury in the region (white arrow). Slightly altered C6-C7 intervertebral disc signal also suggests a low-grade disc contusion (asterisk). Note the hyperintense marrow edema within the C3 and C4 vertebral bodies (white arrowheads), concordant with the acute fractures seen on CT.

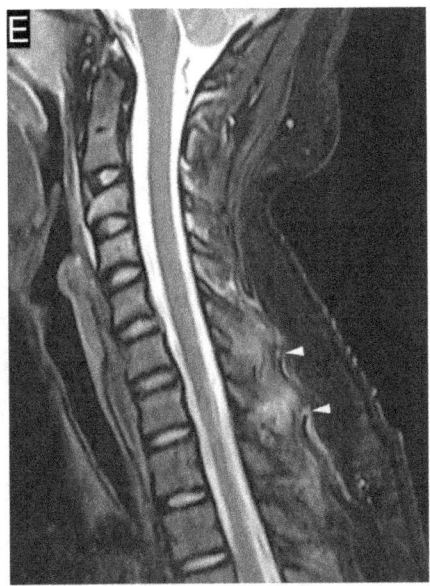

Sagittal MR image (E) slightly lateral to (D) clearly demonstrates a small focal tear involving the supraspinous ligament at the C6 and C7 levels (white arrowheads) with surrounding edema, consistent with a hyperflexion sprain.

Ligamentous and other soft tissue injuries are poorly visualized with radiography and CT. In some cases, an occult ligament injury can contribute to clinically significant spine instability, and these injuries are important to detect in the setting of acute trauma for appropriate treatment planning. When clinical or imaging findings suggest ligamentous injury may be present, it is appropriate to further evaluate with MRI. MRI accurately depicts soft tissue injuries, including ligament tears, epidural collections, and spinal cord injuries.

## Case 9-8

A 17-year-old male with no past medical history presented after a fall related to a snowboarding accident. He states he went off a jump, estimated he was about 15 feet in the air, and landed flat onto his back. He had a reported

15-second loss of consciousness on impact. Ski patrol was called and promptly packaged him with spinal precautions and transferred him to the hospital.

Initial CT of the spine for trauma was unrevealing, but upon removal of cervical collar he complained of neck pain. He was discharged with the collar in place. At his follow up appointment one week later, he had persistent complaint of neck pain with head and neck motion upon removal of the collar.

This scenario concerns the best follow-up imaging for a patient with suspected acute cervical blunt trauma, no unstable injury demonstrated on initial imaging, but kept in cervical collar for neck pain.

Sensible recommendation: MRI CERVICAL SPINE WO CONTRAST

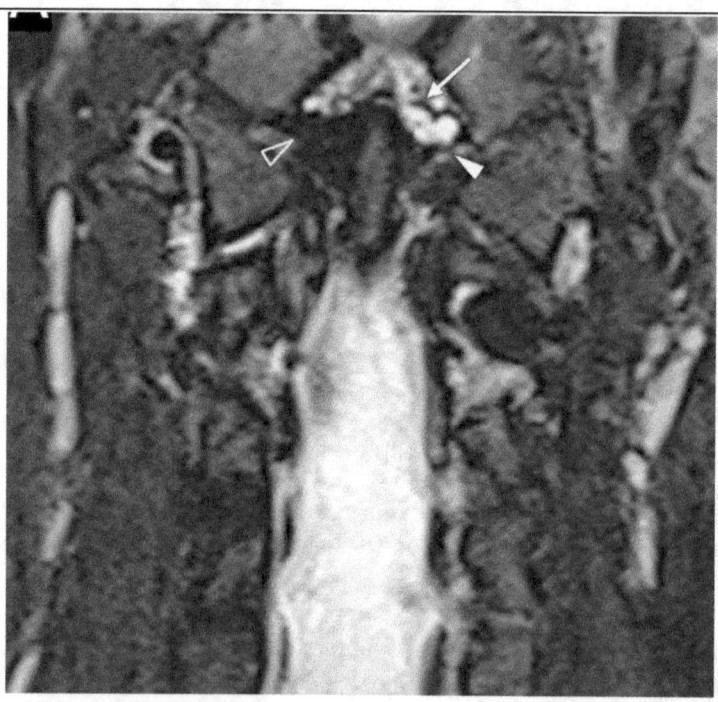

Coronal T2-weighted MR image demonstrates a high-grade partial versus complete tear of the left alar ligament (white arrowhead). Note the intact, homogenously T2 hypointense right alar ligament (open arrowhead). Redundant torn alar ligament fibers can be seen within the interval between the left occipital condyle and the dens (white arrow). Alar ligament tear is frequently associated with whiplash mechanisms of injury.

Since CT has poor sensitivity for isolated ligamentous injuries, when neck pain persists despite initial negative imaging and conservative management, follow-up imaging with MRI is warranted to detect occult ligamentous injuries.

# Case 9-9

A 35-year-old female was brought in by airlift after scene response for rollover MVC. Per EMS, the patient was found down near the vehicle, having apparently been ejected from the vehicle. She had lacerations to the head, was confused with a GCS of 14, but was hemodynamically stable and able to move all extremities. She was placed in a cervical collar with an intraosseous catheter to the right tibia and given ketamine prior to arrival. On ER trauma team evaluation, the patient was in pain, yelling, not responding appropriately to questioning, and only intermittently following commands. She was notably tender over the thoracolumbar spine. What is the first imaging examination to order regarding the potential spine trauma?

This scenario concerns the initial imaging exam for a patient with acute blunt trauma meeting criteria for thoracic and lumbar spine imaging.

Sensible recommendation: CT FULL SPINE WO CONTRAST

Since clinical examination has poor sensitivity for identifying thoracolumbar injuries, any high-risk patient (midline thoracolumbar tenderness, high-energy mechanism of injury, or >60 years of age), as well as unexaminable patients (intoxicated, GCS <15, distracting injury), should undergo imaging of the thoracolumbar spine. Radiographic sensitivity for thoracolumbar spine fractures is low, ranging from 49% to 82%, compared with 94% to 100% sensitivity of CT. For this reason, CT is preferred over radiographs for initial imaging of the thoracolumbar spine in the setting of acute trauma, and since there is a high association of multilevel spine injuries (concomitant cervicothoracic and thoracolumbar injuries), total spine imaging is generally advised. The respective portions of the cervical, thoracic, lumbar, and sacral spine are usually included within the confines of CT scans of the neck, chest, abdomen, and pelvis – all of which are included within the pan-scan protocol at most trauma centers in the US. When indicated, this imaging technique allows rapid retrospective evaluation of the entire spine at no additional radiation dose.

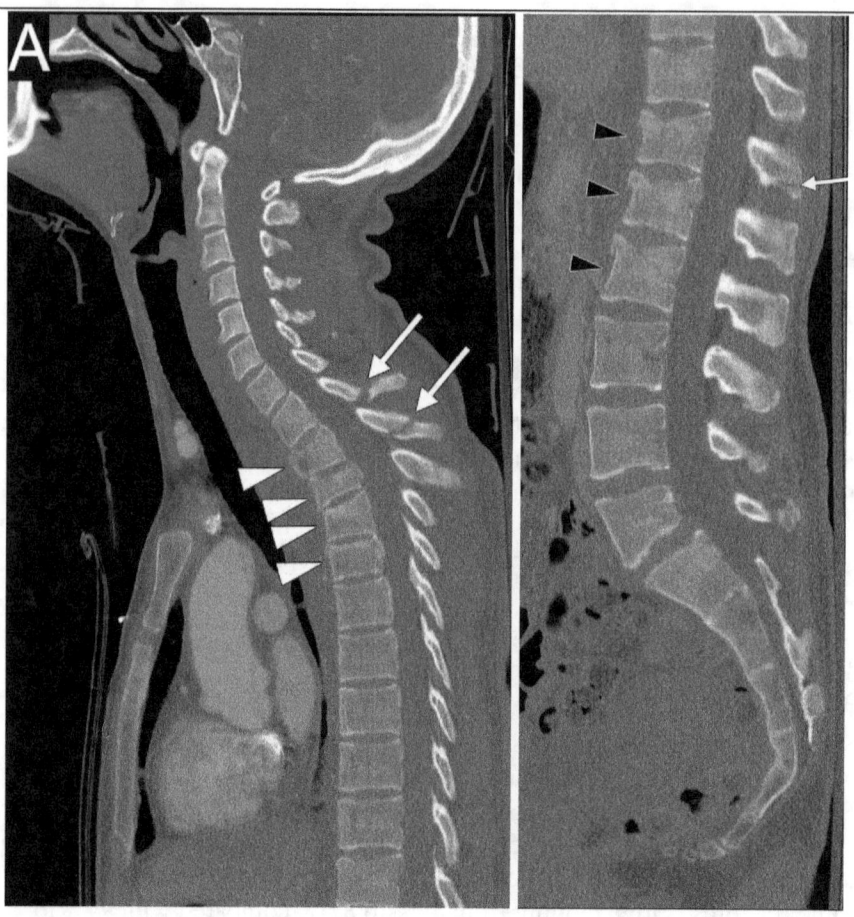

Sagittal reconstructions (A and B) of the spine demonstrate multiple acute fractures of the T1 through T5 vertebrae (white arrowheads) and T12 through L2 vertebrae (black arrowheads). Note there is posterior elemental involvement at some levels (white arrows), consistent with flexion-distraction injuries typical of motor vehicle collisions.

## Case 9-10

A 26-year-old female was brought in by ambulance after she was hit by a car while riding her motorcycle. She lost consciousness on impact. Per EMS, she was hemodynamically stable upon initial assessment but was insensate below the umbilicus and was unable to move her lower extremities. She was placed in a cervical collar and transported to the ER. Upon arrival, she was noted to have thoracolumbar spine tenderness and swelling, in addition to several cuts, scrapes, and abrasions. CT of the full spine revealed an acute 3-coluimn flexon-distraction fracture at T7-T8 with focal kyphosis, 60% anterior vertebral height loss, mild posterior cortical retropulsion, facet joint widening, interspinous distance widening, and a large paraspinal hematoma.

What is the next imaging examination to order regarding assessment of the patient's neurologic abnormalities?

This scenario concerns the next imaging study to perform when neurologic abnormalities are present in the setting of an acute thoracic or lumbar spine injury detected on radiographs or CT.

Sensible recommendation: MRI OF THE THORACIC/LUMBAR SPINE WO CONTRAST

Whenever patients exhibit neurologic deficits in the setting of acute spine trauma, and especially when an injury has been detected by CT or radiography, further evaluation with MRI is warranted. MRI can fully characterize the extent of soft tissue injury, including spinal cord contusion, cord transection, epidural hematoma, and ligamentous injury. This information has clinical value in treatment planning and prognostication.

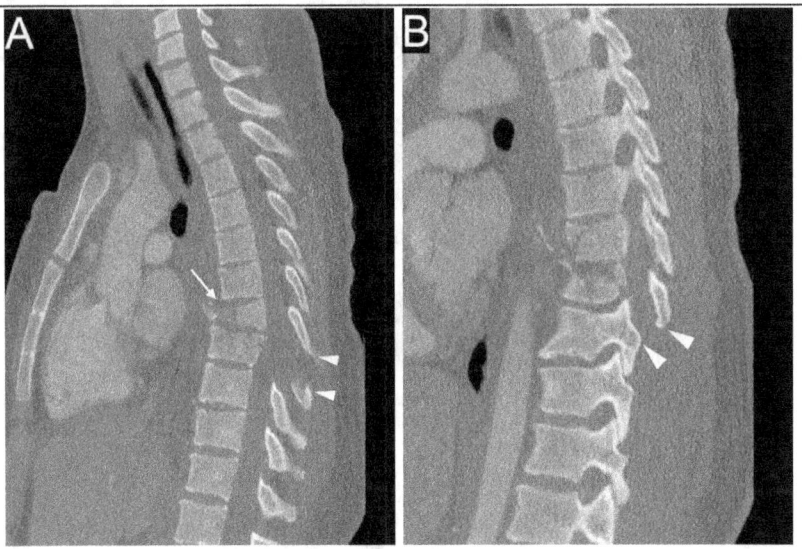

Sagittal CT (A) demonstrates the T7 fracture with ~60% height loss anteriorly (white arrow). Note that these is significant widening of the interval between the T7 and T8 spinous processes, indicating associated distraction injury at this level (arrowheads). Sagittal CT (B) demonstrates significant widening between the T7-T8 facet joints (arrowheads). This finding was present bilaterally.

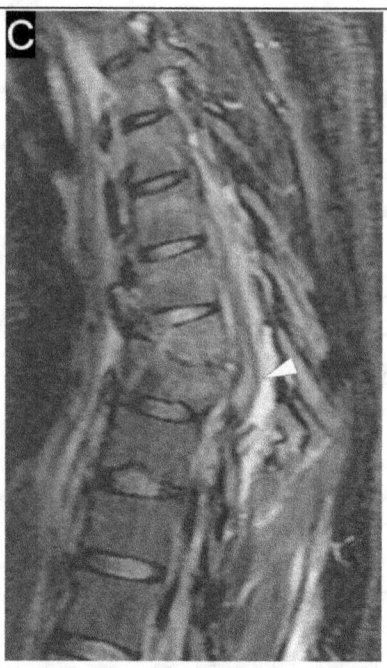

Sagittal STIR MR image (C) demonstrates focal T2 hyperintense cord signal and swelling (arrowhead), consistent with focal cord contusion at the T7-T8 level.

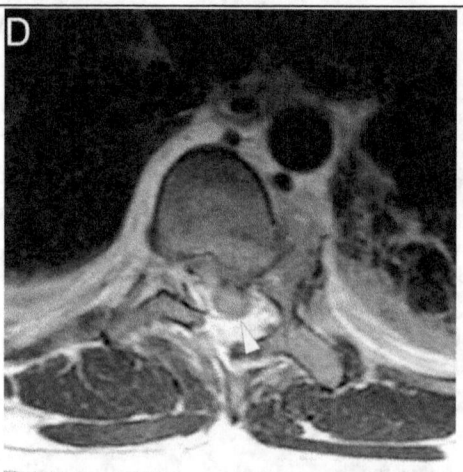

Axial T2-weight image (D) again demonstrates the T2 hyperintense cord signal, consistent with cord contusion (arrowhead). Note the absence of low-signal intensity foci within the cord, indicating there is no associated cord hemorrhage.

# References

1. Bailitz J, Starr F, Beecroft M, et al. CT should replace three-view radiographs as the initial screening test in patients at high, moderate, and low risk for blunt cervical spine injury: a prospective comparison. J Trauma 2009;66:1605-9.
2. Karul M, Bannas P, Schoennagel BP, et al. Fractures of the thoracic spine in patients with minor trauma: comparison of diagnostic accuracy and dose of biplane radiography and MDCT. Eur J Radiol 2013;82:1273-7.
3. Rhea JT, Sheridan RL, Mullins ME, Novelline RA. Can chest and abdominal trauma CT eliminate the need for plain films of the spine?—Experience with 329 multiple trauma patients. Emerg Radiol 2001;8:99-104.
4. Sheridan R, Peralta R, Rhea J, Ptak T, Novelline R. Reformatted visceral protocol helical computed tomographic scanning allows conventional radiographs of the thoracic and lumbar spine to be eliminated in the evaluation of blunt trauma patients. J Trauma 2003;55:665-9.
5. Miller CP, Brubacher JW, Biswas D, Lawrence BD, Whang PG, Grauer JN. The incidence of noncontiguous spinal fractures and other traumatic injuries associated with cervical spine fractures: a 10-year experience at an academic medical center. Spine (Phila Pa 1976) 2011;36:1532-40.
6. Nelson DW, Martin MJ, Martin ND, Beekley A. Evaluation of the risk of noncontiguous fractures of the spine in blunt trauma. J Trauma Acute Care Surg 2013;75:135-9.
7. Stiell IG, Wells GA, Vandemheen KL, et al. The Canadian C-spine rule for radiography in alert and stable trauma patients. JAMA 2001;286:1841-8.
8. Hoffman JR, Mower WR, Wolfson AB, Todd KH, Zucker MI. Validity of a set of clinical criteria to rule out injury to the cervical spine in patients with blunt trauma. National Emergency X-Radiography Utilization Study Group. N Engl J Med 2000;343:94-9.
9. Burlew CC, Biffl WL, Moore EE, Barnett CC, Johnson JL, Bensard DD. Blunt cerebrovascular injuries: redefining screening criteria in the era of noninvasive diagnosis. J Trauma Acute Care Surg 2012;72:330-5; discussion 36-7, quiz 539.
10. Geddes AE, Burlew CC, Wagenaar AE, et al. Expanded screening criteria for blunt cerebrovascular injury: a bigger impact than anticipated. Am J Surg 2016;212:1167-74.

# Chapter 10. Acute Pelvis and Hip Trauma

Felix S. Chew, MD

Radiography is the initial exam for acute pelvis and hip trauma and should also be obtained after reduction of dislocations and placement of hardware. CT is indicated for evaluation of pelvic ring and acetabular fractures, and MRI has a role for diagnosis of occult hip fractures and injuries.

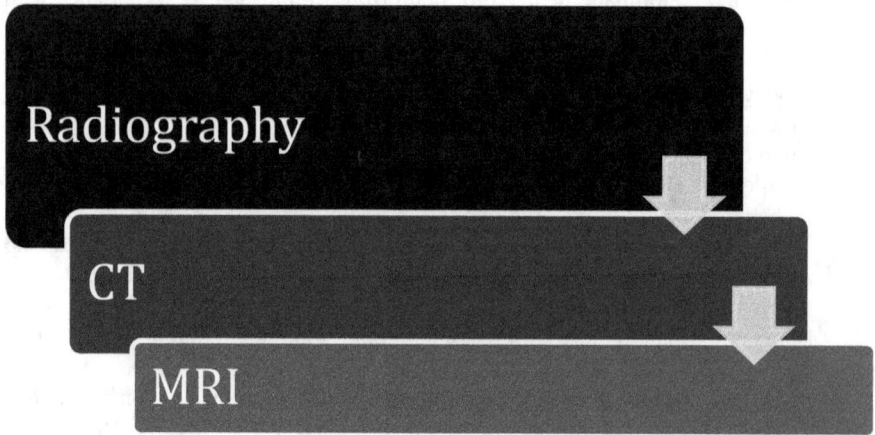

# Case 10-1.

A 54-year-old woman was injured in a motor vehicle crash. She was the re-strained driver of a car that was struck from the side while attempting to traverse an intersection. She is brought to the emergency room on a back-board, conscious and responsive. Which imaging test should be the first study ordered to evaluate for pelvis trauma?

This scenario concerns the first imaging study of the pelvis in blunt force polytrauma.

Sensible recommendation: XR PELVIS

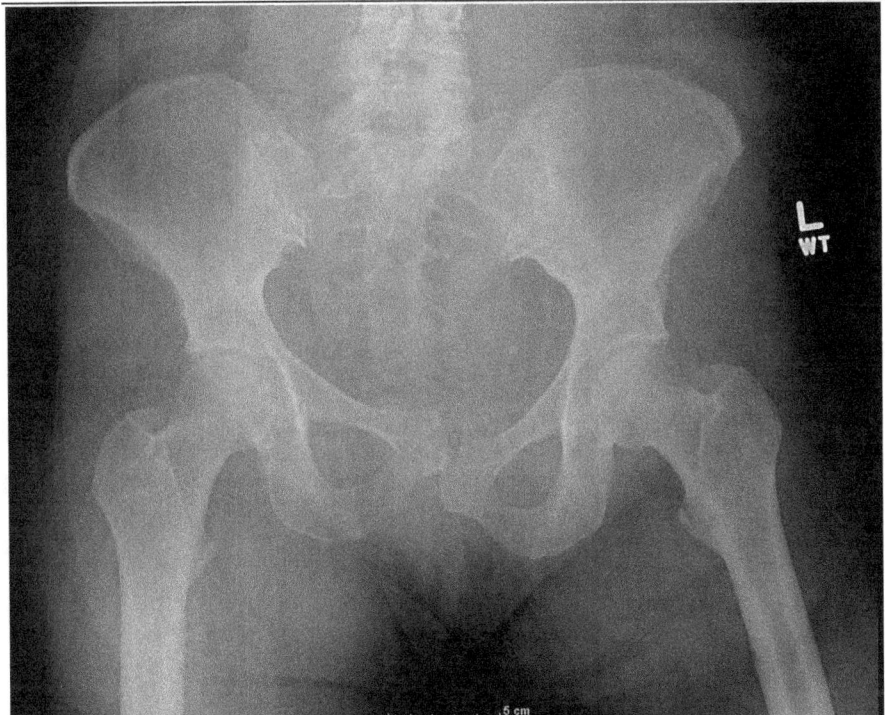

AP radiograph of the pelvis shows an impacted right sacral wing fracture and dis-ruption of the symphysis pubis.

In patients with blunt trauma following high energy trauma, the immediate concern is to determine whether life-threatening injuries are present that re-quire immediate attention. A radiographic trauma series is often the fastest study to obtain and consists of an AP chest and AP pelvis. In some circum-stances, the patient may be taken directly to the operating room or directly to the CT scanner.

# Case 10-2

A 54-year-old woman injured in a motor vehicle crash. She was the re-strained driver of a car that was struck from the side crossing an intersection. She is brought to the emergency room on a backboard, conscious and responsive. A pelvis radiograph shows a sacral fracture and disruption of the symphysis pubis. Which imaging test should be the next study ordered to evaluate the pelvic injuries?

This scenario concerns the next imaging study for further evaluation of pelvic ring injuries in the setting of blunt polytrauma.

Sensible recommendation: CT PELVIS WO CONTRAST

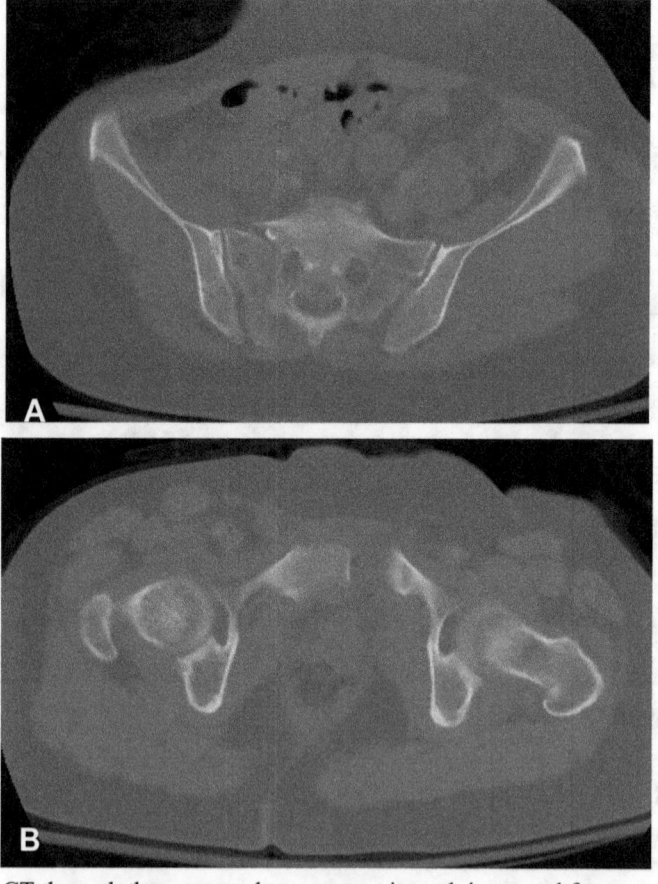

(A) Axial CT through the sacrum show a comminuted, impacted fracture of the right sacral wing extending into the S1 neural foramen. (B) Axial CT through the hips shows dislocation of the symphysis pubis, with the right public overriding the left. There is hematoma in the right gluteal region.

CT is the standard modality for evaluating blunt trauma to the abdomen and pelvis. Coronal and sagittal reformations should be done. Depending on circumstances, a pan-scan may be done, consisting of CT of the head, cervical spine, chest, abdomen, and pelvis. For the pelvis, it should be standard to obtain bone and soft tissue reconstructions, as well as coronal and sagittal reformations. Our focus here is on the musculoskeletal injuries, but obviously any visceral injuries must be identified and attended to as well.

## Case 10-3

A 54-year-old woman injured in a motor vehicle crash. She was the restrained driver of a car that was struck from the side crossing an intersection. She is brought to the emergency room on a backboard, conscious and responsive. A pelvis radiograph shows a sacral fracture and disruption of the symphysis pubis, confirmed by CT. The surgeon requests further imaging of the pelvic injuries for surgical planning. Which imaging test should be the next study ordered for surgical planning?

This scenario concerns the next imaging study for further evaluation of pelvic ring injuries in a patient for whom surgery is planned.

Sensible recommendation: CT PELVIS WO CONTRAST with 3D

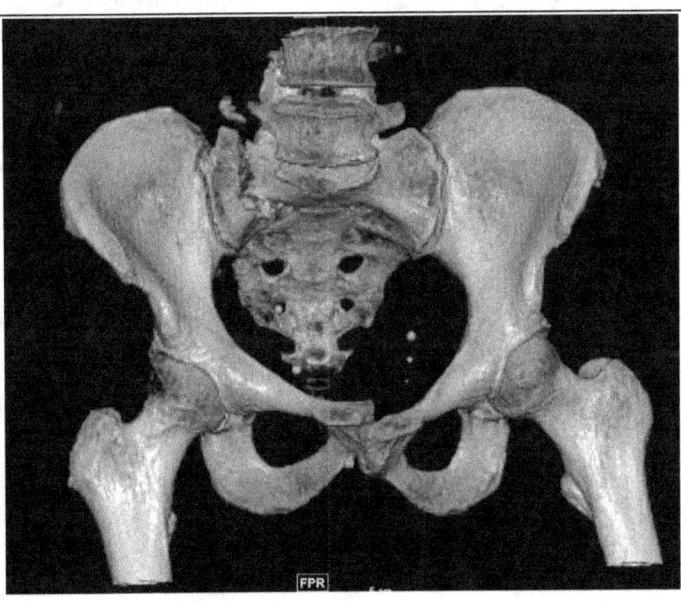

CT surface-rendered 3D reconstruction shows a right sacral wing fracture and disruption of the symphysis pubis. By rotating the image along different axes helps the surgeon understand the anatomy in three dimensions. The pelvis injuries were subsequently treated with internal fixation.

The CT images desired for surgical planning may vary from one setting to another. At the University of Washington, we typically obtain two sets of surface-rendered 3D reconstructions of the pelvis with hips, one rotating horizontally and one rotating vertically, as well as a set of volume-rendered images that simulate AP, oblique, inlet, and outlet radiographs. If there is an acetabular fracture, the ipsilateral femur may be removed from the hip for better visualization of the acetabulum.

# Case 10-4

A 46-year-old man injured in a ground-level fall onto his left hip 12 days ago. He was initially seen in the emergency room with complaints of left hip pain, but radiographs did not show any fractures. Since then he has had worsening left hip pain and is now unable to bear weight. Medical history is remarkable for chronic renal failure and a previous liver transplant. Repeat radiographs do not show any fractures, but the clinician is concerned that a radiographically occult fracture may be present. Which imaging test should now be ordered?

This scenario concerns middle-aged and elderly patients with acute hip pain where fracture is suspected, and initial radiographs are negative or indeterminant.

Sensible recommendation: MRI HIP WO CONTRAST

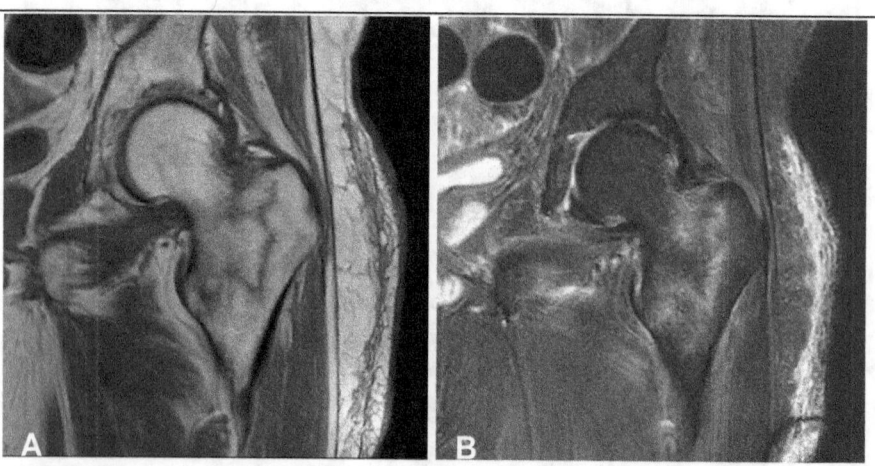

Coronal T1 MRI (A) and T2 FS MRI (B) of the left hip show an irregularly shaped nondisplaced intertrochanteric fracture of the left proximal femur, evident on the T1 image as a low-signal fracture line and on the T2 FS image as a high-signal fracture line. There is a bruise in the lateral subcutaneous tissues and, not shown on these images, a nondisplaced left pubic fracture. The fracture was subsequently treated with internal fixation.

Detection of radiographically occult hip fractures in middle-aged and elderly patients is important because treatment is usually surgical. The age range is relevant because bone and muscle loss are associated with low-energy hip fractures. Medical conditions that contribute to bone and muscle loss, including chronic renal failure and systemic corticosteroids, are similarly associated. MRI is sensitive and specific for the detection of nondisplaced hip fractures and, if negative, may identify other causes of acute posttraumatic hip pain. CT may be less accurate in this circumstance because it depends on morphologic rather than physiologic features but should be considered if MRI is unavailable or contraindicated. MRI or CT with contrast are usually no better than non-contrast studies. Radionuclide bone scan may be appropriate in circumstances where MRI and CT cannot be obtained or are non-diagnostic due to patient or technical factors.

# Case 10-5

73-year-old woman with ground level fall several weeks ago with on-going right groin and buttock pain. Radiographs were normal except for showing diffuse demineralization. Additionally, a bone scan was obtained soon after, and also interpreted as normal. She is having trouble walking given continued pain and she lives alone. What is the next appropriate study to obtain in order to exclude the clinical suspicion of pelvis insufficiency fracture?

This scenario addresses further imaging of suspected insufficiency fracture in osteoporotic patient or patient on long-term corticosteroid therapy. Radiographs and bone scan obtained within the preceding 48 hours are normal.

Sensible recommendation: MRI PELVIS WO CONTRAST

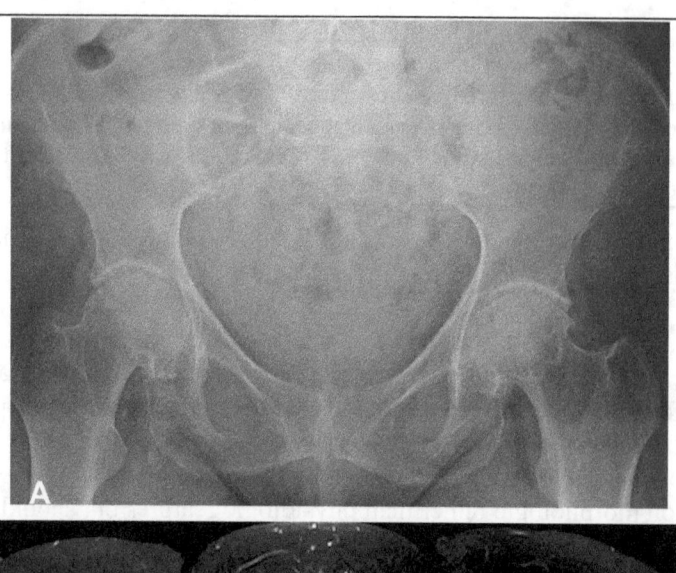

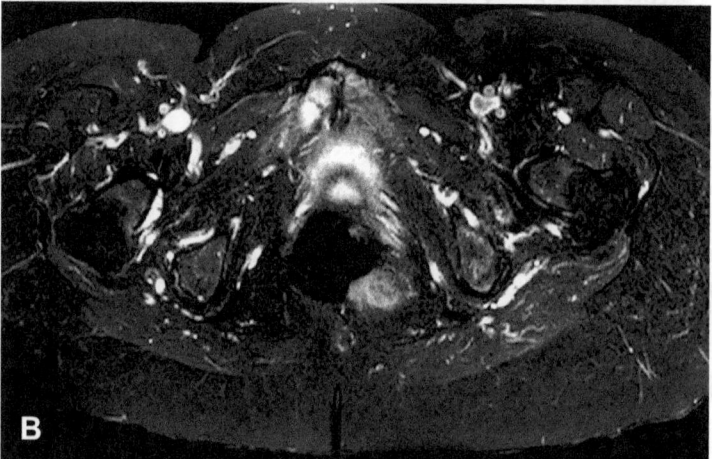

Frontal radiograph of the pelvis (A) demonstrates decreased mineralization, but no fracture. Follow-up axial T2 FS MRI (B) demonstrates an insufficiency fracture at the right parasymphyseal pubic body.

When an insufficiency fracture is suspected in an osteoporotic patient or patient on long-term corticosteroid therapy who has undergone negative radiographs and bone scan within the past 48 hours, MRI of the area of interest is recommended. If the diagnosis is non-urgent, repeat radiographs could be obtained. Bone scan may be falsely negative in this particular cohort (elderly or osteoporotic, as well as those using corticosteroids) of patients, with decreased sensitivity documented.

# References

1.  American College of Radiology. ACR Appropriateness Criteria: Acute hip pain--suspected fracture. American College of Radiology, revised 2018. https://acsearch.acr.org/docs/3082587/Narrative/ (accessed April 24, 2021).

# Chapter 11. Acute Knee Trauma

Hyojeong Lee, MD

Radiography is the initial exam for acute knee trauma. CT may be helpful for surgical planning for intraarticular fractures. MRI has a role in evaluating soft tissue injury, but usually not in the acute setting.

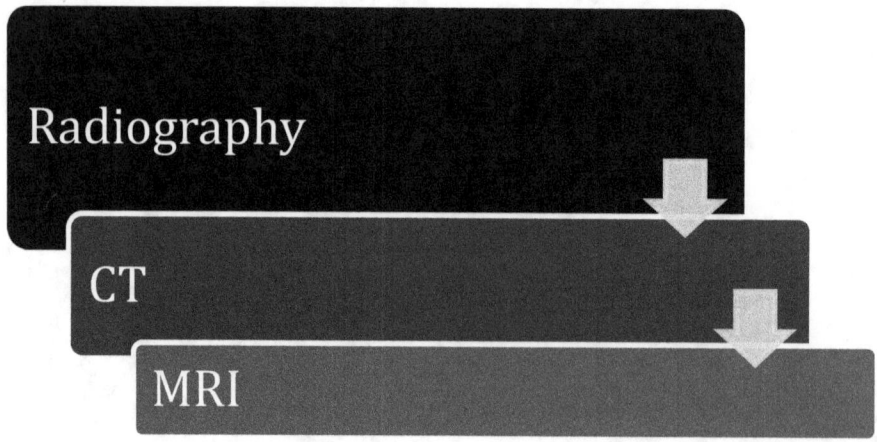

# Case 11-1

A 22-year-old woman presents with knee pain after twisting her knee during soccer. On physical exam, she doesn't have focal tenderness, or joint effusion. Which imaging tests should be ordered?

This scenario concerns the first imaging study for patients (adult or child 5 years of age or older) after fall or acute twisting trauma to the knee. No focal tenderness, no effusion, able to walk.

Sensible recommendation: NO IMAGING

With no clinical symptoms in the injured knee, including lack of focal tenderness and joint effusion, and with ability to walk, knee radiographs may be indicated if a patient >55 years old per Ottawa rules or >50 years old or <12 years old per Pittsburgh rule criteria. Radiographs are commonly performed in the setting of acute knee injuries but have a low yield for showing fractures.

# Case 11-2

A 16-year-old male gymnast comes with right knee pain. He performed a front flip during a floor routine exercise, landing directly on his feet, but his body continued moving forward, although his right foot was planted. He twisted his knee and felt an acute pop and pain in the medial aspect of his knee. He noted increased swelling and was unable to bear weight. The examination of the right knee demonstrates diffuse swelling with knee joint effusion. The patient has tenderness in the medial joint space. Which imaging tests should be ordered?

This scenario concerns the first imaging study for patients (adult or child 5 years of age or older) after fall or acute twisting trauma to the knee. One or more of the following: focal tenderness, effusion, inability to bear weight.

Sensible recommendation: XR KNEE 4 VIEW

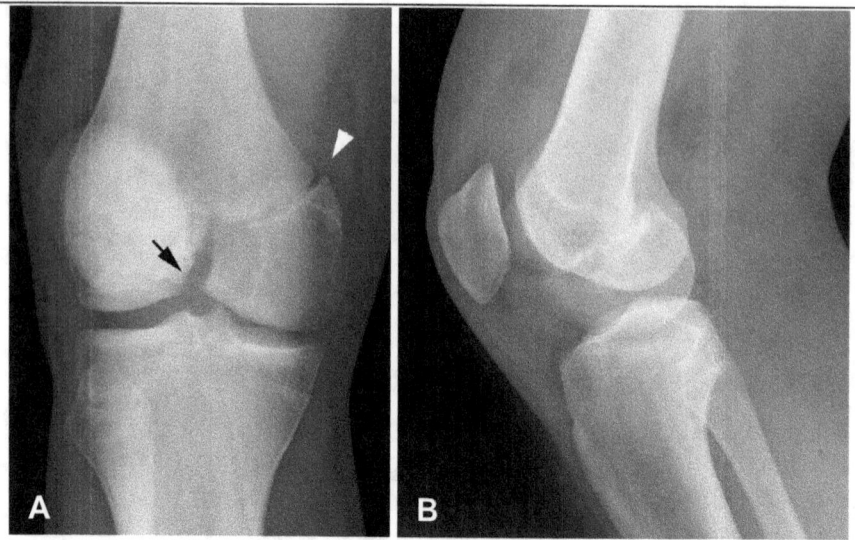

Oblique anterior posterior radiograph of the knee (A) shows intra-articular fracture of the medial femoral condyle extending into the intercondylar fossa (arrow). There is a transverse fracture separating the medial femoral condyle from the femoral metaphysis as well as a small bone fragment from the medial metaphysis (arrowhead). Lateral radiograph of the knee (B) shows large amount of suprapatellar effusion.

Clinical decision rules for the acutely injured knee suggest that radiographic examination of the knee following acute injury can be eliminated in many instances by applying specific clinical guidelines. Two of the most common clinical decision rules are the Ottawa Knee Rule and the Pittsburgh Decision Rule. The Ottawa Knee Rule states that patients more than 18 years old with acute knee pain should have knee radiographs if they meet any of the following criteria:

(A) 55 years of age or older,
(B) palpable tenderness over the head of the fibula,
(C) isolated patellar tenderness,
(D) inability to flex the knee to 90 degrees,
(E) inability to bear weight immediately following the injury, or
(F) inability to walk in the emergency room (after taking 4 steps).

# Case 11-3

A 46-year-old man presents with left knee pain after soccer injury. He was planting his left leg and the knee gave way. He heard a pop and noted fairly significant swelling quickly. Inspection of his left knee demonstrates significant swelling, and tenderness over the lateral joint line. He reaches full extension with some mild discomfort. Flexion at about 60 degrees is painful and limited by the swelling in that position. Radiographs of the knee were negative. Which imaging tests should be ordered next?

This scenario concerns the first imaging study for patients (adult or skeletally mature child) after fall or acute twisting trauma to the knee. No fracture seen on radiographs. Suspect occult fracture or internal derangement. Next study.

Sensible recommendation: MRI KNEE WO CONTRAST

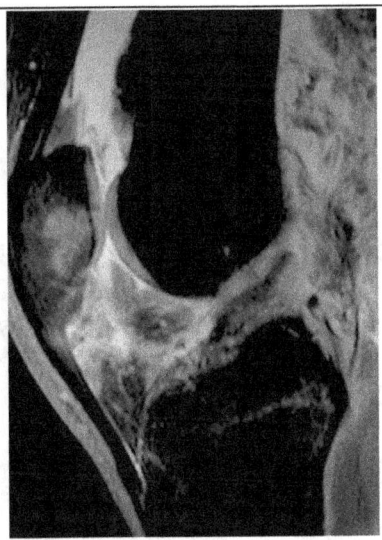

Sagittal PD FS MRI of knee shows a full-thickness tear of ACL at its proximal attachment. There is a large effusion. Also, there is bony contusion at the patella.

MRI is considered the optimal imaging modality for identifying meniscal, ligament, chondral, and nondisplaced bone injuries around the knee. Characteristic imaging patterns on MRI, including specific patterns of bone marrow edema and osteochondral injuries, help make MRI highly accurate for even subtle ligament and meniscal injuries. The anterior cruciate ligament (ACL) is a straight, predominantly low- signal ligament that fans distally as it attaches to the anterior tibial plateau. ACL tears are mechanically caused from a valgus force with a rotatory motion resulting in anteromedial rotary instability. Most commonly, ACL tears occur at its proximal femoral attachment. Characteristic bone bruise pattern includes marrow edema at the posterolateral tibial plateau and the midportion of the lateral femoral condyle. An important associated condition is the Segond fracture. This fracture is an avulsion fracture of the lateral tibial plateau at the insertion of the meniscotibial portion of the lateral capsular ligament.

## Case 11-4

A 13-year-old girl presents with right knee pain. While she was playing a soccer three days ago, she heard a pop during a kick, and felt unstable. Knee radiographs were negative. What is the most appropriate next imaging study?

This scenario concerns the next imaging study for patients (skeletally imma- ture child ) after fall or acute twisting trauma to the knee. No fracture seen on radiographs. Suspect occult fracture or internal derangement.

Sensible recommendation: MRI KNEE WO CONTRAST

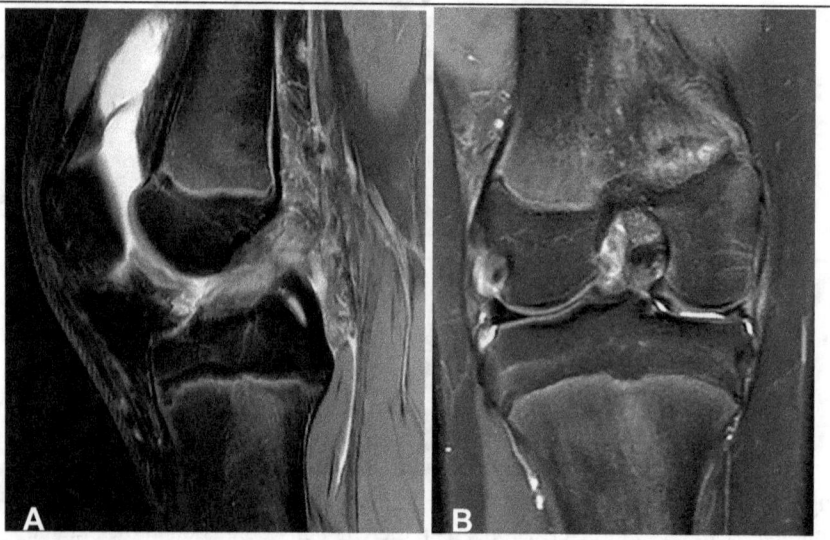

MRI of right knee sagittal (A) and coronal (B) PD fat-saturated images demonstrate full-thickness tear of anterior cruciate ligament (A), and a bucket-handle tear of me- dial meniscus (B).

MRI should be the next imaging modality to evaluate for the presence of ra- diographically occult fractures and/or internal derangements of the acutely injured knee. With its superb contrast resolution and multiplanar imaging capability, MRI is proven to be a highly accurate imaging modality in the evaluation of bone marrow contusions and occult fractures as well as menis- cal and ligamentous injuries.

## Case 11-5

A 34-year-old man presents with right knee pain secondary to motorcycle collision. Patient states he was going approximately 30 mph, losing control and attempting to swing his right leg out to control himself. Patient is some-what unsure as to the exact mechanism of injury, but after extreme rotation of his lower leg, he ended up beneath his bike and subsequently self-extri-cated. Radiographs of the knee show a tibial plateau fracture. Which imaging tests should be ordered next?

This scenario concerns the first imaging study for patients after fall or acute twisting trauma to the knee, with a tibial plateau fracture on radiographs and additional bone or soft tissue injury suspected. Next study after radiographs.

Sensible recommendation: CT KNEE WO CONTRAST

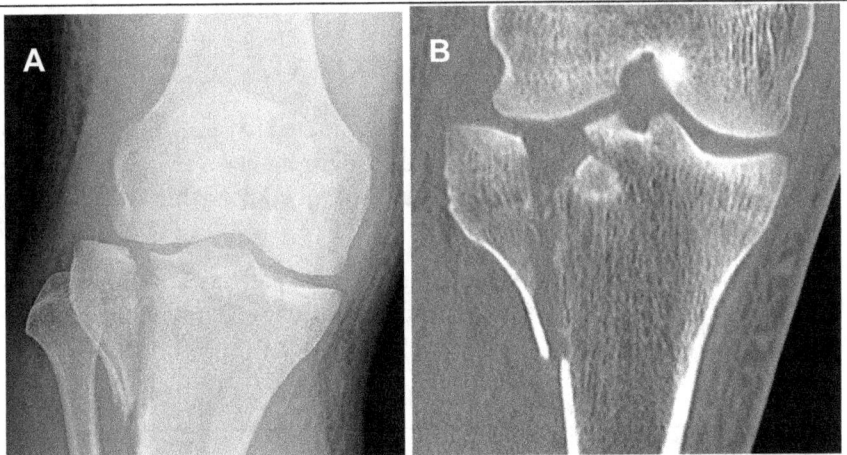

AP radiograph of the knee (A) shows vertically oriented fracture of lateral tibial plateau with minimal depression. Coronal CT reformatted image (B) shows a large lateral split fracture fragment that is laterally displaced approximately 6-7 mm. Approximately 7 mm depression of the comminuted central fracture is present (Schatzker type II).

CT with 3D reconstruction has been compared to knee radiographs and shown to be more sensitive for fracture, 100% versus 83% for radiographs, and to reflect the severity of tibial plateau fractures more accurately. In se-verely injured patients, diagnostically sufficient radiographs are sometimes difficult to obtain, and therefore a negative radiograph is not reliable in rul-ing out a fracture. In these patients, CT and MRI are helpful for complete injury assessment and for presurgical planning. The advantage of CT is that it shows cortical bone detail well, is easier to obtain if a CT scanner is near the emergency department, has a shorter total scan time, and has a lower cost. The advantage of MRI is that it can demonstrate soft tissue and bone marrow injuries while adequately demonstrating many cortical bone frac-tures.

Tibial plateau fractures are the result of compressive loading of the tibia. Approximately 76% of cases involve the lateral tibial plateau alone, 11% involve the medial condyle alone, 10% involve both condyles, and 3% of cases involve the posterior margin. The Schatzker classification system divides tibial plateau fractures into six types: lateral tibial plateau fracture without depression (I), lateral tibial plateau fracture with depression (II), compression fracture of the lateral (IIIA) or central (IIIB) tibial plateau, medial tibial plateau fracture (IV), bicondylar tibial plateau fracture (V), and tibial plateau fracture with diaphyseal discontinuity (VI). The first three types (I, II, and III) are typically the result of low-energy injury. The second three types (IV, V, and VI) are typically the result of high-energy injury.

## Case 11-6

An 18-year-old man presents with right knee pain. He twisted his knee outward while going up stairs a couple of days ago. He has a sharp pain in front area below the kneecap. He can walk but it is not comfortable. What is the most appropriate initial imaging study?

This scenario concerns the first imaging study for patients after injury of unknown mechanism. Clinical features include focal patellar tenderness, knee effusion, but able to walk.

Sensible recommendation: XR KNEE 4 VIEW

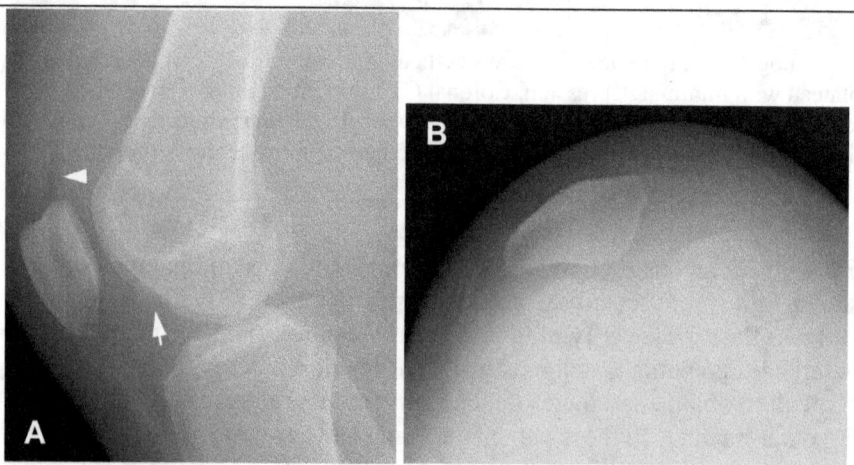

Transient lateral patellar dislocation. Lateral knee radiograph (A) shows large lipohemarthrosis with fat-fluid level (arrowhead), and small osteochondral fracture at lateral femoral condyle (arrow). Sunrise view of the knee (B) shows lateral subluxation of the patella.

Patellar pain after trauma may be from several causes, including patellar fracture and transient patellar dislocation. For patellar fractures, radiographs should include a patellar view such as a sunrise view in addition to anterior posterior and lateral radiographs.

Transient patellar dislocation is unsuspected clinically in 45 to 73 percent of patients with evidence of dislocation subsequently seen on MRI. MRI is a valuable tool in the decision-making process, altering the treatment plan and allowing earlier surgical intervention by obtaining a more accurate diagnosis. Radiographs may demonstrate a fracture of the medial patella or lateral trochlear and can also show anatomic features that predispose to dislocation such as a decreased sulcus angle, patella alta, patellar tilt, or patellar subluxation. MRI is more sensitive than radiographs for imaging findings of lateral patellar dislocation, including injury to the medial patellofemoral ligament, bone contusions, and osteochondral injuries.

## Case 11-7

A 22-year-old man presents with knee dislocation. He sustained injury to the knee in an off-roading Jeep accident. He recalls his knee striking the dashboard. Knee radiographs taken in the ER demonstrated posterior knee dislocation. His dislocation was reduced and he was placed in an immobilizer. Unfortunately, the next day when putting weight on the leg, he re-dislocated his knee. He was again taken ER, and the knee was reduced again. After reduction, patient starts to complain cold foot, and on physical exam his pedal pulse is weak. Which imaging tests should now be ordered?

This scenario concerns the first imaging study for patients (adult or child 5 years of age or older) with acute high-energy trauma to the knee, often from motor vehicle crash, with suspected knee dislocation. Next study after radiographs.

Sensible recommendation: ANGIOGRAPHY, lower extremity

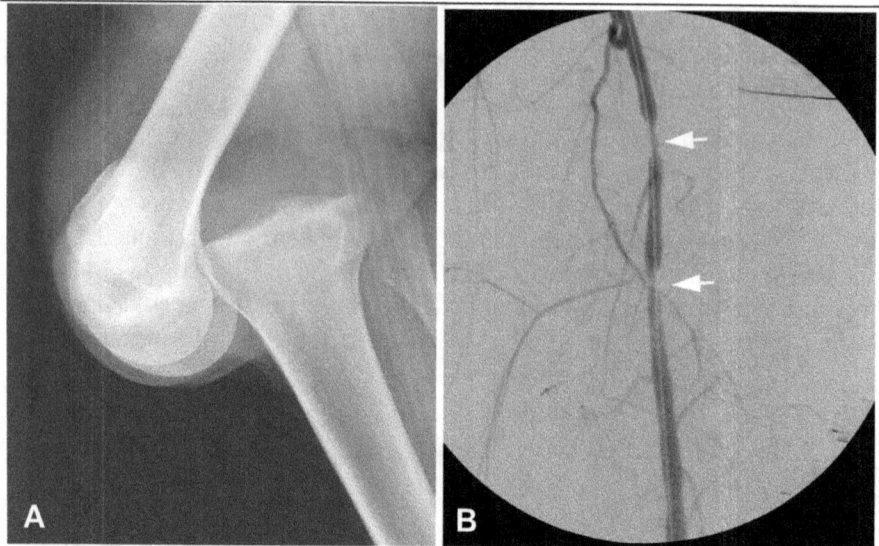

Lateral radiograph of the knee (A) shows posterior knee dislocation. Spot image of lower extremity arteriography (B) shows multifocal severe narrowing of popliteal artery (arrows). Patient was treated with balloon dilatation and stent (not shown).

Dislocation of the knee is uncommon, representing about 0.1% of orthopedic injuries. The injury typically results from a motor-vehicle accident, but can also occur from contact sports, a vehicle striking a pedestrian, falls, or even a spontaneous dislocation in morbidly obese individuals. This injury, which may reduce spontaneously, constitutes a true orthopedic emergency because of possible nerve or arterial damage.

Vascular injury may be found in about 30% of patients following posterior knee dislocation. Physical signs of clinically significant vascular injury are the absence of pulses, ischemia, active bleeding, and bruit/thrill. Although angiography is considered the gold standard for assessing for vascular injury, there is some debate whether it should be obtained in all knee dislocation patients or be used selectively. CT angiography is increasingly being used because it is less invasive, has a similar high accuracy, and involves a lower radiation dose. MR angiography has also been shown to be an accurate technique for assessing for vascular injury after knee dislocation.

# References

1.  American College of Radiology. ACR Appropriateness Criteria: Acute trauma to knee. American College of Radiology, revised 2019. https://acsearch.acr.org/docs/69419/Narrative/ (accessed April 24, 2021).

2. Beutel BG, Trehan SK, Shalvoy RM, Mello MJ. The Ottawa knee rule: examining use in an academic emergency department. West J Emerg Med. 2012;13(4):366-372.
3. Cheung TC, Tank Y, Breederveld RS, Tuinebreijer WE, de Lange-de Klerk ES, Derksen RJ. Diagnostic accuracy and reproducibility of the Ottawa Knee Rule vs the Pittsburgh Decision Rule. Am J Emerg Med. 2013;31(4):641-645.
4. Sanders TG, Miller MD. A systematic approach to magnetic resonance imaging interpretation of sports medicine injuries of the knee. Am J Sports Med. 2005;33(1):131-148.
5. Mustonen AO, Koskinen SK, Kiuru MJ. Acute knee trauma: analysis of multidetector computed tomography findings and comparison with conventional radiography. Acta Radiol. 2005;46(8):866-874.
6. Markhardt BK, Gross JM, Monu JU. Schatzker classification of tibial plateau fractures: use of CT and MR imaging improves assessment. Radiographics. 2009 Mar-Apr;29(2):585-97.
7. Kirsch MD, Fitzgerald SW, Friedman H, Rogers LF. Transient lateral patellar dislocation: diagnosis with MR imaging. AJR Am J Roentgenol. 1993;161(1):109-113.
8. Howells NR, Brunton LR, Robinson J, Porteus AJ, Eldridge JD, Murray JR. Acute knee dislocation: an evidence based approach to the management of the multiligament injured knee. Injury. 2011;42(11):1198-1204.

# Chapter 12. Acute Ankle Trauma

Kimia Kani, MD

Radiography is the initial exam for acute ankle trauma. Radiography should also be obtained after reduction of fractures and dislocations. CT may be helpful for evaluation of complex fractures, and MRI may have a role in evaluating soft tissue injuries.

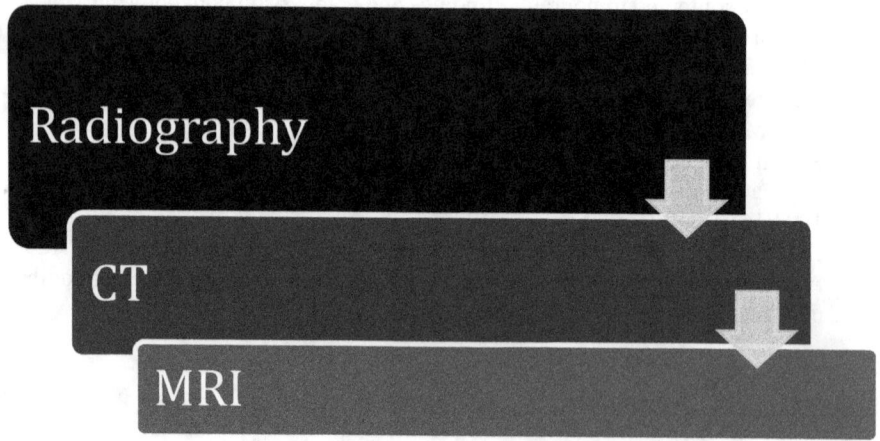

## Case 12-1

An 18-year-old woman sustained a twisting injury of her left ankle after falling from a skateboard. At the emergency department she is unable to bear weight on the injured and painful ankle. On physical examination there is tenderness along the posterior edge of the left lateral malleolus. Which imaging test should be ordered initially?

This scenario concerns the first imaging study for acute ankle trauma in an adult or child older than 5 years. These patients meet the Ottawa Ankle Rules.

Sensible recommendation: XR ANKLE 3 VIEW

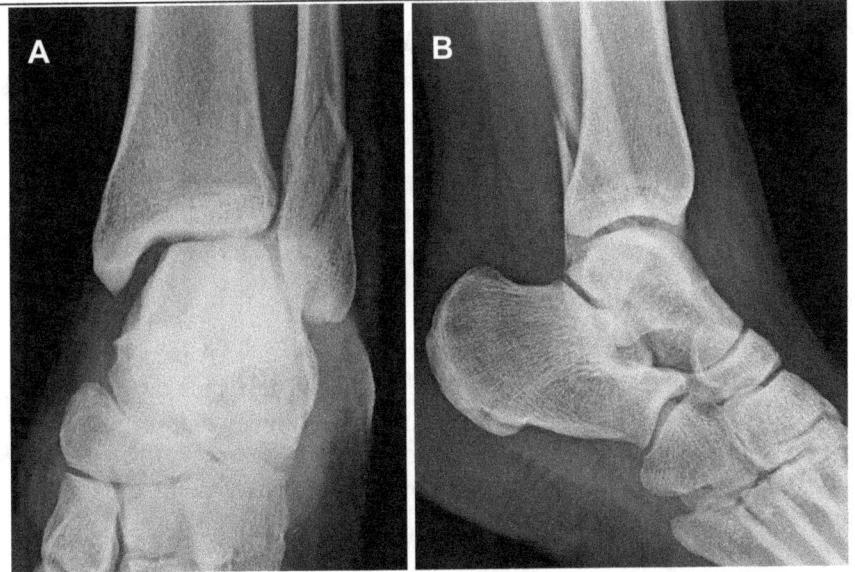

Mortise (A) and lateral (B) radiographs of the left ankle demonstrate a mildly displaced spiral distal fibular fracture at the tibial plafond level. Widening of the medial mortise on the mortise view is suggestive of deltoid ligament injury.

In patients sustaining acute ankle trauma, the immediate concern is determining whether a fracture is present. Radiographs are usually the most appropriate initial imaging study to obtain when there is a clinical suspicion for ankle fracture. The Ottawa Ankle Rules are a set of clinical guidelines commonly used for determining the necessity of radiographic evaluation in ankle and foot injuries (for the foot portion of the criteria please refer to Chapter 13). These guidelines recommend ankle x-ray series only in patients complaining of pain in the malleolar zones and any of the following find-ings: a) bone tenderness along the distal 6 cm of the posterior edge or tip of the lateral malleolus, b) bone tenderness along the distal 6 cm of the poste-rior edge or tip of the medial malleolus, or c) inability to take 4 complete steps both immediately and in the emergency department. Standard ankle ra-diographs should include anteroposterior (AP), lateral, and mortise views (the base of the fifth metatarsal distal to the tuberosity should be seen at least on one projection). Although originally described for use in adults in the emergency department setting, the Ottawa Ankle Rules have been subse-quently validated for use in children (over 5-years-old) and in outpatient settings.

# Case 12-2

A 24-year-old man presents to urgent care with left ankle pain after a twist-ing injury last night. On physical examination there is no evidence of tenderness over the posterior edges or inferior tips of the malleoli and he is able to walk four steps. Which imaging studies should be ordered initially?

This scenario concerns the first imaging study for an adult or child over 5-years-old with an acute injury to the ankle that does not meet the Ottawa Ankle Rules. The patient is neurologically intact (including no peripheral neuropathy).

Sensible recommendation: NO IMAGING

There are several clinical situations in which the Ottawa Ankle Rules should not be used or should be used with great caution. These include: pregnancy, penetrating trauma, any skin wound, gross swelling which prevents assess-ment of malleolar tenderness, polytrauma, altered sensorium, uncooperative patients, neurologic abnormality affecting the foot, underlying bone disease, transferred with radiographs already taken, greater than 10 days after trauma or a returned visit for continued traumatic foot pain. In patients who sustain acute ankle injury, do not meet the Ottawa Ankle Rules and do not have the above-mentioned exclusions, further imaging may not be necessary. In such setting, it is recommended to give patients written instructions and encour-age follow-up in 5 to 7 days, if there is no improvement in pain and ability to ambulate.

# Case 12-3

A 56-year-old diabetic man fell and lost consciousness when his defibrilla-tor discharged. He awoke with his right ankle swollen and twisted underneath him. He presented to the emergency department on the subsequent day for evaluation of his swollen ankle. He had no complaint of ankle pain. Which imaging tests should be ordered initially?

This scenario concerns the initial imaging study for an adult or child over 5-years-old with an acute injury to the ankle that does not meet the Ottawa Ankle Rules. However, the patient is not neurologically intact and/or has a peripheral neuropathy that involves the ankle and foot.

Sensible recommendation: XR ANKLE 3 VIEW

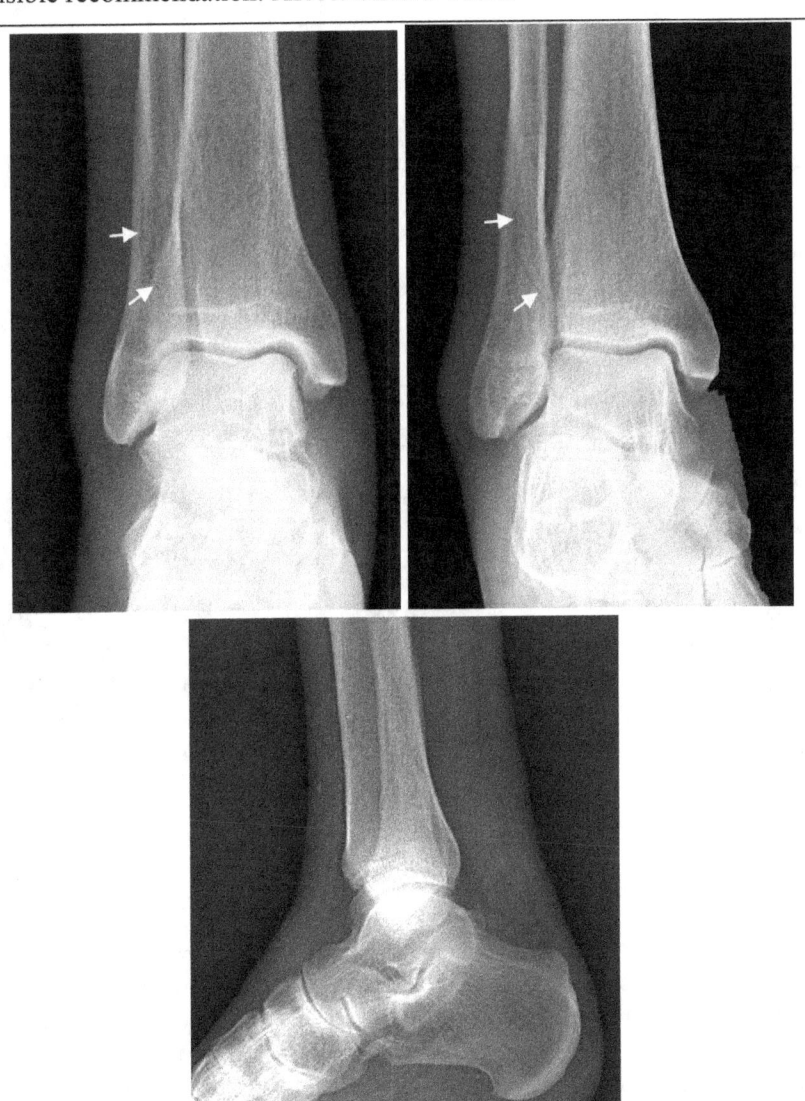

AP (A) and mortise (B) radiographs of the right ankle show a nondisplaced distal fibular fracture (arrows). On the lateral right ankle radiograph (C) observe the heavy arterial calcifications in keeping with patient's known diabetes mellitus.

As mentioned in the above section, the Ottawa Ankle Rules should not be used if the patient who has sustained an acute ankle injury has peripheral neuropathy of the ankle and foot. Standard ankle radiographs (including AP, lateral, and mortise views) are obtained as the initial imaging study in such patients.

## Case 12-4

A 20-year-old woman presents with right ankle pain after slipping on ice 1 week ago. Her pain is getting worse and she has locking events. Radiographs were not obtained at time of injury. Which imaging tests should be ordered first?

This scenario concerns the initial imaging study for an adult or child over 5-years-old with persistent pain after an acute injury to the ankle. Radiographs were not obtained at the time of injury.

Sensible recommendation: XR ANKLE 3 VIEW

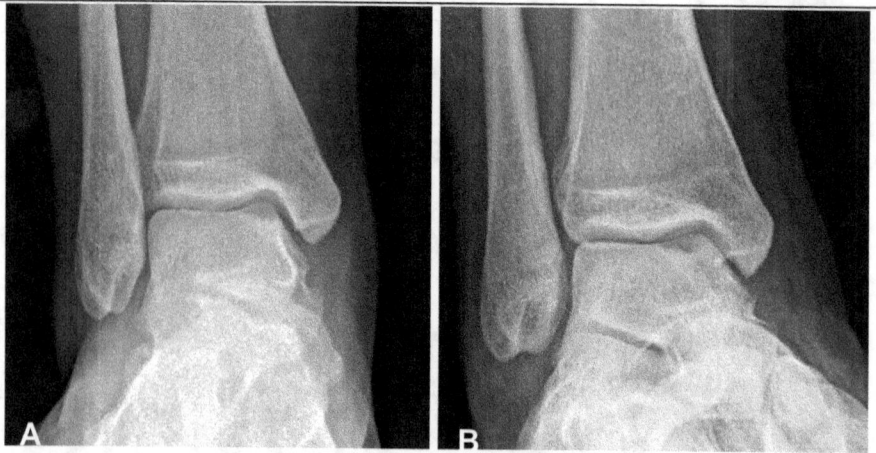

AP (A) and mortise (B) radiographs of the right ankle show an osteochondral lesion in the medial talar dome.

In patients with persistent pain after acute ankle trauma, in which radiographs were not obtained at time of injury, 3-view ankle x-ray series is the most appropriate initial imaging study. The primary concern in such patients is differentiating ankle fracture from ankle sprain. Ankle fractures usually require immobilization or referral to/management by an orthopedic specialist. While ligamentous ankle sprains (except for full thickness ligament tears that may require surgery) are usually treated with immobilization, RICE (rest, ice, compression, and elevation) and/or physical therapy.

## Case 12-5

A 41-year-old woman complains of persistent pain after sustaining an inversion injury to her right ankle while playing soccer 2 weeks ago. Initial radiographs were unremarkable. Which imaging tests should be ordered now?

This scenario concerns the next imaging study for an adult or child over 5-years-old with an acute injury to the ankle and more than 1 week of persistent pain. The initial radiographs were negative.

Sensible recommendation: MRI ANKLE WO CONTRAST

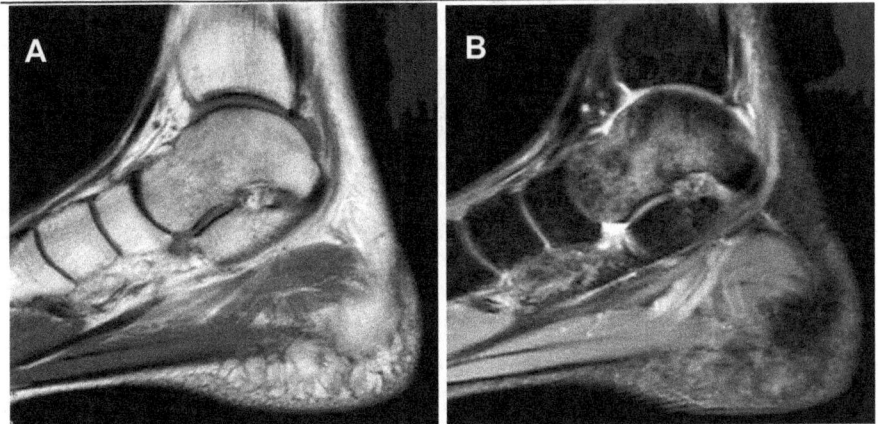

Sagittal T1 MRI (A) and T2 FS MRI (B) of the right ankle show extensive talar contusion.

Persistent pain following trauma may be associated with a radiographically occult fracture, osteochondral lesion, bone marrow contusion, or soft tissue injury. Repeat radiographs, ultrasound, CT or MRI may be appropriate for evaluation of persistent pain after acute ankle injury. MRI is especially useful as a global screening tool as it permits evaluation of soft tissues, cartilage and bone marrow.

## Case 12-6

31-year-old man was brought to the emergency department after he was hit by a vehicle while crossing the street. Patient complains of pain in his right ankle. Ankle x-ray series showed a mildly displaced fracture of the medial cortex of the talar body. Which imaging study should be ordered next?

This scenario concerns the further imaging evaluation for an adult or child over 5-years-old with an acute injury to the ankle. The initial radiographs demonstrated a talus fracture.

Sensible recommendation: CT ANKLE WO CONTRAST

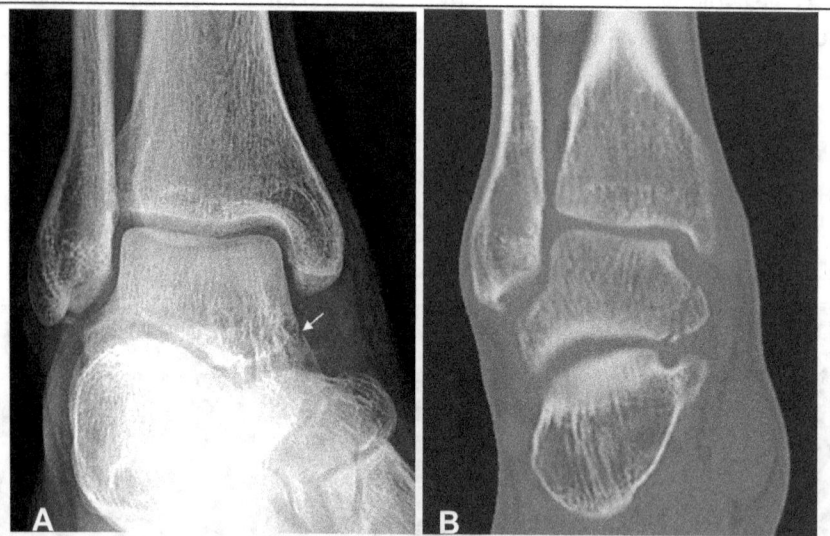

Mortise radiograph of the right ankle (A) shows a mildly displaced fracture of the medial cortex of the talar body. Coronal reconstructed CT image of the right ankle (B) shows a mildly comminuted, intra-articular fracture of the medial talar body with 1 mm displacement.

Talar fractures usually result from high energy trauma. Although an uncommon injury, talar fractures may lead to complications and long-term morbidity, especially if not diagnosed and managed appropriately. Initial evaluation is usually with standard ankle and foot radiographs. CT ankle is the most appropriate next study and is recommended for evaluation of the extent, displacement, comminution, and intra-articular extension of the fracture, determination of associated injuries and surgical planning.
Supplemental ankle x-ray views (such as Broden's view for evaluation of lateral talar process fractures, Canale view for evaluation of talar neck fractures or the Harris projection for visualization of the posterior and middle subalar joints) may be appropriate, especially when CT is not available.
MRI ankle may be an appropriate next study and would allow simultaneous evaluation of soft tissue injuries.

## Case 12-7

21-year-old female collegiate volleyball player sustained an injury to her right ankle 1 week ago. She had sharp pain, abrupt swelling and was unable to bear weight immediately. Ankle radiographs are consistent with a lateral talar dome osteochondral lesion. Which imaging test should be ordered next?

This scenario concerns the further imaging study for an adult or child over 5 years old with an acute injury to the ankle. Initial radiographs suggest an osteochondral injury of the talar dome.

Sensible recommendation: MRI ANKLE WO CONTRAST

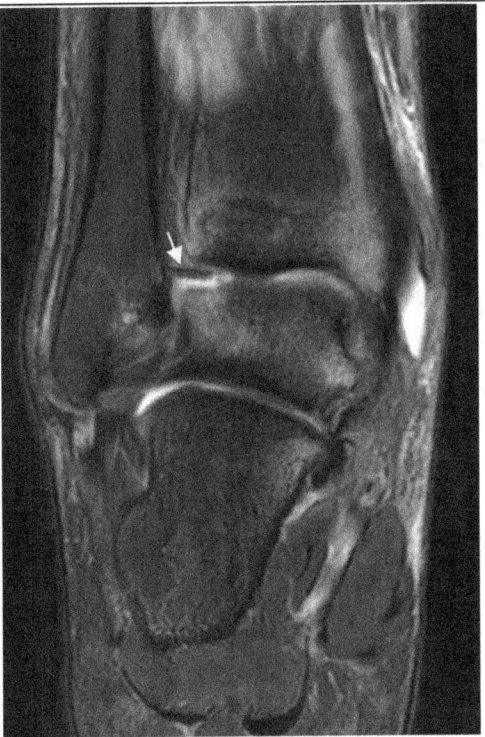

Coronal T2 FS MRI of the right ankle shows a detached and displaced osteochondral fragment arising from the posterior aspect of the lateral talar dome. Bone contusions are noted in the distal tibia, talus and to a lesser extent in the calcaneus.

Osteochondral lesions (OCLs) involve the articular surface and/or subchondral bone. Up to 50% -70% of ankle sprains and fractures may result is some form of cartilage injury. Since cartilage is avascular and has a poor healing potential, untreated OCLs can increase in size and severity, eventually resulting in ankle osteoarthritis. Ankle radiographs are the first line of imaging in suspected osteochondral injury (radiographs may fail to detect up to 50% of OCLs). When radiographs suggest an OCL or when there are persistent symptoms (such as pain, locking, clicking, stiffness and ankle swelling) after ankle injury, MRI is the study of choice. MRI can accurately evaluate and determine the stability of an OCL. However, due to bone marrow edema, the true extent of an OCL may be overestimated on MRI, which may affect treatment. CT ankle may be an appropriate study and may be useful for preoperative planning. CT can accurately evaluate the location, size and detachment of the bony component of an OCL but lacks the ability to visualize cartilage directly. CT does not overestimate the bony involvement and may be useful for comparing pre- and post-operative bony lesion size.

# Case 12-8

A 19-year-old man a left ankle injury when he fell from a height of 10 feet. He was immediately unable to bear weight and his ankle became swollen rapidly. In the emergency department, ankle radiographs showed no fractures but widening of the medial clear space of the mortise, indicating disruption of the syndesmosis and tear of the deltoid ligament. Which imaging test should be ordered next?

This scenario concerns the next imaging study for an adult or child over 5 years old with an acute injury to the ankle. The initial radiographs do not show an ankle fracture but suggested a syndesmotic injury.

Sensible recommendation: XR TIBIA-FIBULA 2 VIEW

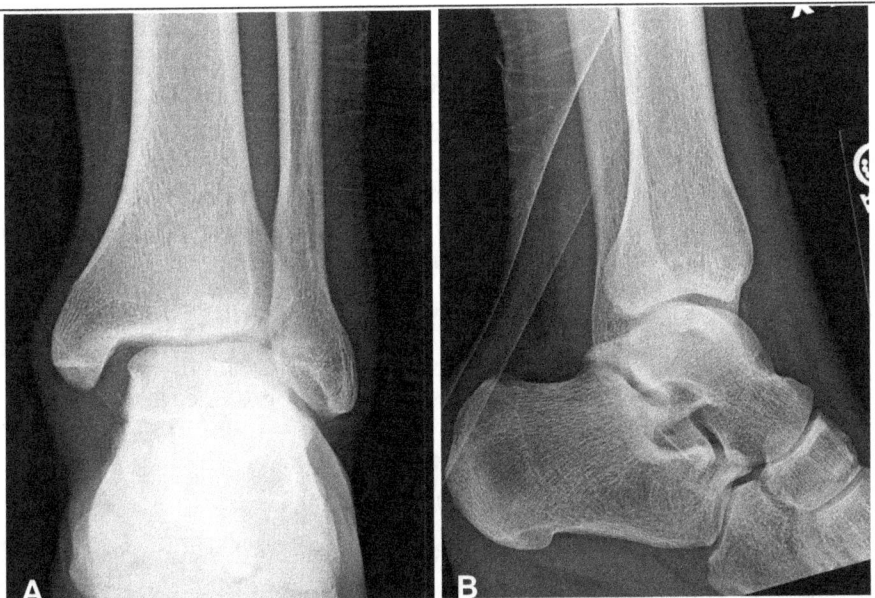

Mortise (A) and lateral (B) radiographs of the left ankle show widening of the medial clear space and lateral talar shift, without fractures.

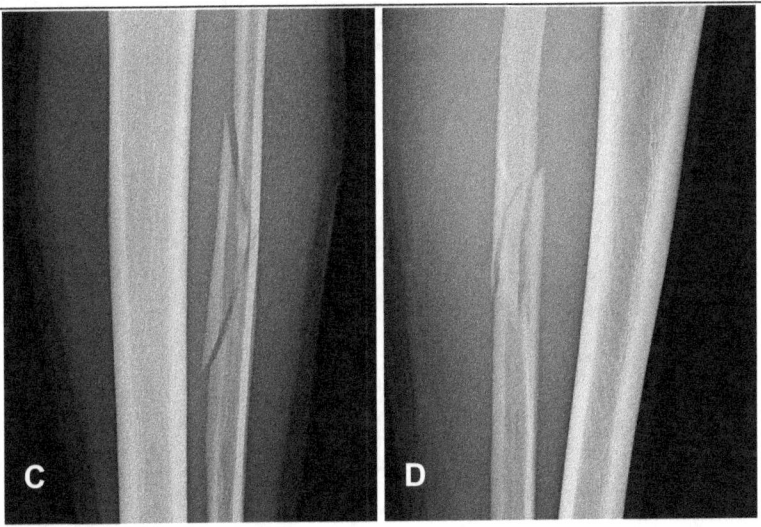

AP (C) and lateral (D) radiographs of the left leg demonstrated a comminuted midshaft spiral fracture of the fibula.

Injury of the ankle syndesmosis can occur as an isolated injury or in association with a proximal fibular fracture and/or an ankle sprain/fracture. Injury of the tibiofibular syndesmosis may result in altered ankle joint mechanics with resultant disability and prolonged recovery. Therefore, accurate identification and early treatment of injuries of the distal tibiofibular syndesmosis is of critical importance. Diagnosis of syndesmotic injury is based on careful history, clinical examination, and imaging evaluation. Syndesmotic injury may be associated with a spiral fracture of the upper third of the fibula (Maisonneuve fracture). This type of fracture result from external rotation force to the ankle, that is transmitted through the interosseous membrane and exits through a proximal fibular fracture. Such patients may not have localized rest pain at site of fibular fracture, and the severity of injury may be overlooked if the proximal fibula is not carefully palpated. When ankle radiographs and/or physical examination suggest syndesmotic injury, the most appropriate subsequent imaging study is anteroposterior and lateral radiographs of the tibia/fibula.

# References

1. American College of Radiology. ACR Appropriateness Criteria: Acute Trauma to the Ankle. American College of Radiology, revised 2020. https://acsearch.acr.org/docs/69436/Narrative/ (accessed April 24, 2021)
2. Mosher TJ, Kransdorf MJ, Adler R, Appel M, Beaman FD, Bernard SA, Bruno MA, Dempsey ME, Fries IB, Khoury V, Khurana B, Roberts CC, Tuite MJ, Ward RJ, Zoga AC, Weissman BN. ACR Appropriateness Criteria acute trauma to the ankle. J Am Coll Radiol. 2015 Mar;12(3):221-7. doi: 10.1016/j.jacr.2014.11.015. PMID: 25743919.

# Chapter 13. Acute Foot Trauma

Kimia Kani, MD

Radiography is the initial exam for acute foot trauma. Radiography should also be obtained after reduction of fractures and dislocations. CT may be helpful for complex or intraarticular fractures, and MRI may have a role in evaluating soft tissue and occult injuries.

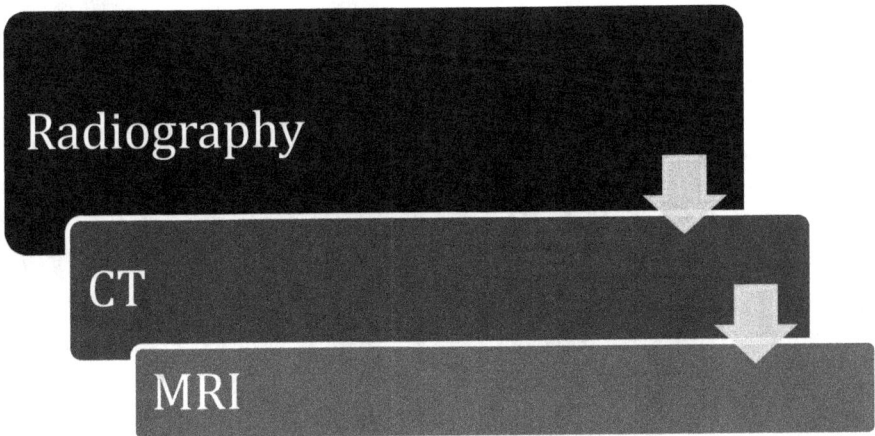

# Case 13-1

A 35-year-old woman presents with right foot pain after inversion injury last night. She is able to walk. On physical examination there is point tenderness over her fifth metatarsal base. Which imaging studies should be performed?

This scenario concerns the first imaging study for an adult or child over 5-years-old with acute injury to the foot; positive Ottawa Rules; suspicious for fracture.

Sensible recommendation: XR FOOT 3 VIEW

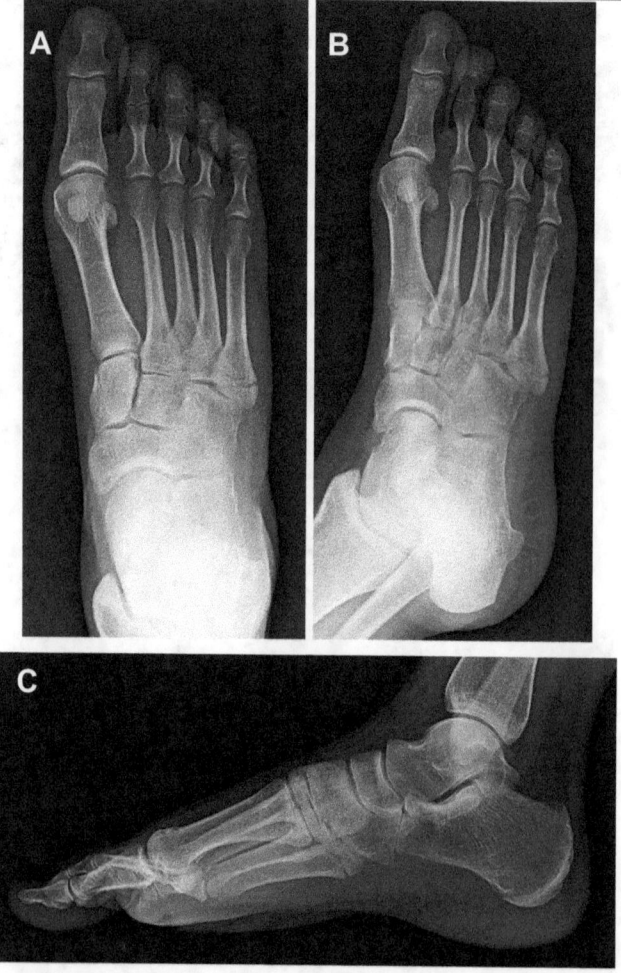

AP(A), oblique (B) and lateral (C) radiographs of the right foot demonstrate a non-displaced fracture of the fifth metatarsal base.

In patients sustaining acute foot trauma, the immediate concern is determining whether a fracture is present. Radiographs are usually the most appropriate initial imaging study to obtain when there is a clinical suspicion for foot fracture. The Ottawa Ankle Rules are a set of clinical guidelines commonly used for determining the necessity of radiographic evaluation in ankle and foot injuries. These guidelines recommend foot x-ray series only in patients complaining of pain in the midfoot zone and any one of the following: a) bone tenderness at the navicular, b) bone tenderness at the fifth metatarsal base, or c) inability to take 4 complete steps both immediately and in the emergency department. Standard radiographs should include anteroposterior (AP), lateral, and oblique views. Although originally described for use in adults in the emergency department setting, the Ottawa Rules have been subsequently validated for use in children (> 5 years old) and in outpatient settings. It must be emphasized that the Ottawa Rules do not address hindfoot, Lisfranc joint, metatarsal and toe injuries and must be used with caution or not at all in several clinical situations.

## Case 13-2

A 34-year-old man presents to urgent care with left midfoot pain after a twisting injury last night. On physical examination there is no evidence of navicular or fifth metatarsal base tenderness and he is able to walk four steps. Which imaging studies should be ordered initially?

This scenario concerns the initial imaging study for an adult or child over 5-years-old with an acute injury to the foot; does not meet Ottawa Rules; no focal tenderness in the foot or palpable abnormality of the foot on physical examination; able to walk; neurologically intact (including no peripheral neuropathy).

Sensible recommendation: NO IMAGING

There are several clinical situations in which the Ottawa Rules should not be used or should be used with great caution. These include pregnancy, penetrating trauma, any skin wound, polytrauma, altered sensorium, uncooperative patients, neurologic abnormality affecting the foot, underlying bone disease, transferred with radiographs already taken, greater than 10 days after trauma or a returned visit for continued traumatic foot pain. In patients who sustain acute midfoot zone injury, do not meet the Ottawa Rules and do not have the above-mentioned excluding conditions, further imaging may not be necessary. In such a setting, it is recommended to give patients written instructions and encourage follow-up in 5 to 7 days, if there is no improvement in pain and ability to ambulate.

## Case 13-3

A 61-year-old woman with history of diabetes mellitus presents to urgent care with a red and swollen left foot. Last night she states that she slipped and heard a crunching sound from her left foot with mild pain. The crunching sound remained as she continued to walk on her foot. She denies fevers or chills. On physical examination her left foot is red and swollen and she does not have sensation to light touch. She is unable to move her toes and she is barely able to dorsiflex or plantarflex her foot about her ankle. Which imaging test should be ordered initially?

This scenario concerns the initial imaging study for an adult or child over 5-years-old with acute injury to the foot; does not meet Ottawa Rules; however, patient is not neurologically intact and/or has a peripheral neuropathy that involves the feet.

Sensible recommendation: XR FOOT 3 VIEW

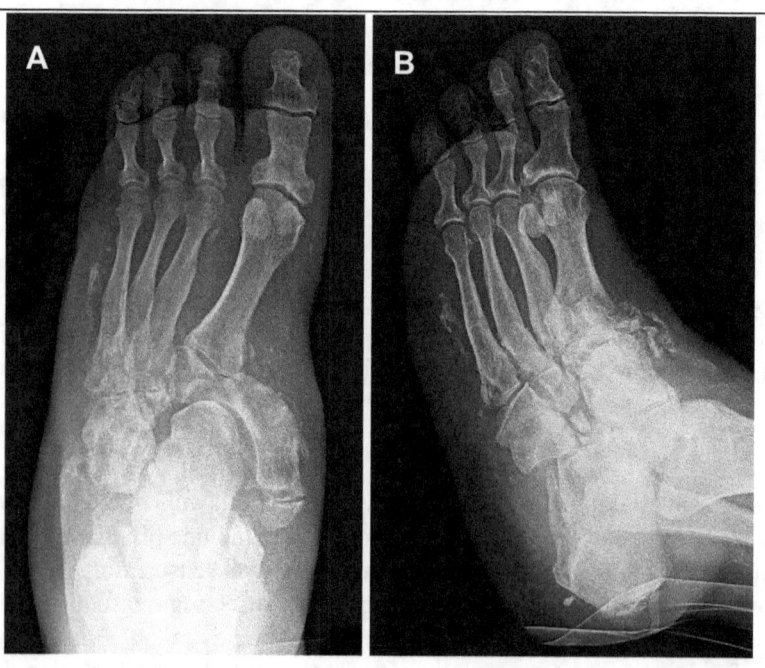

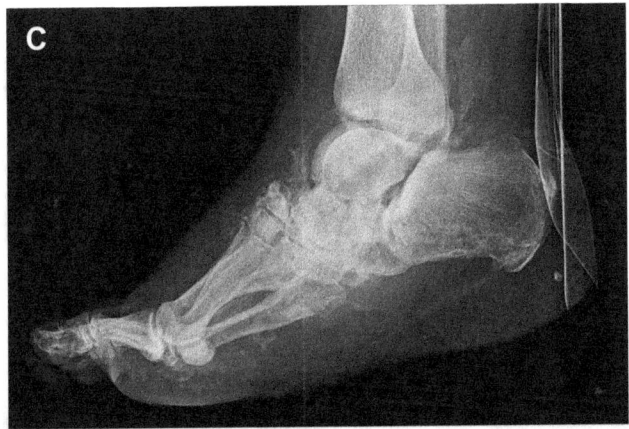

AP (A), oblique (B) and lateral (C) radiographs of the left foot. There are pronounced changes of neuropathic osteoarthropathy (including debris, disorganization, fractures, subluxation/dislocation and osseous sclerosis) especially at the level of hindfoot, midfoot and tarsometatarsal joints. There has been prior fifth ray amputation.

The Ottawa Rules should not be used if the patient who has sustained an acute foot injury is not neurologically intact and/or has a peripheral neuropathy involving the feet. Three-view study of the affected foot are obtained as the initial imaging study in such patients.

## Case 13-4

A 34-year-old man who was in a high-speed motor vehicle crash is being evaluated in the emergency department for multiple injuries. He has sustained a traumatic subdural hematoma, nasal fractures, splenic laceration, mesenteric injury, and a left open olecranon fracture. His left foot was injured but he is not complaining of foot pain. Which imaging studies should be performed initially for evaluation of the foot?

This scenario concerns an adult or child over 5-years-old with polytrauma. Acute injury to the foot; does not meet the Ottawa Rules; first study for evaluation of the foot.

Sensible recommendation: XR FOOT 3 VIEW

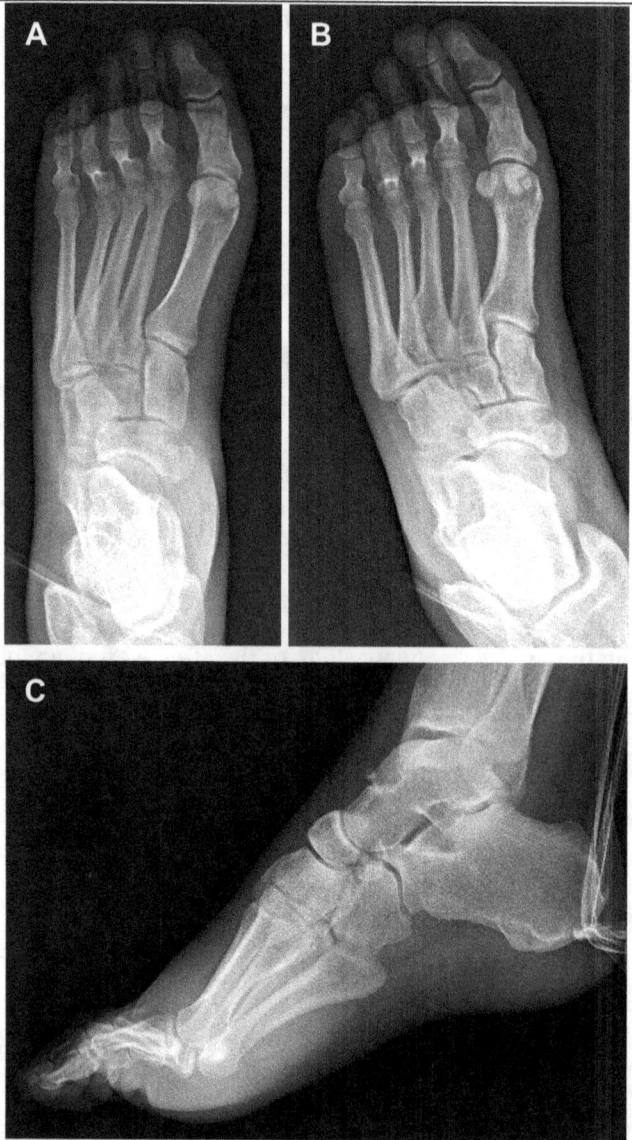

AP (A), oblique (B) and lateral (C) radiographs of the left foot show a mildly impacted navicular fracture with extension to the first naviculocuneiform joint. There are also nondisplaced to minimally displaced fractures of the second metatarsal base, medial hallux sesamoid and first proximal phalanx.

Missed foot fractures are a known problem in the care of polytrauma patients. Identifying these fractures early does not usually affect survival but may influence the long-term result and the subsequent quality of the patient's life. The Ottawa Rules should not be used or should be used with great caution in patients with polytrauma. General practice is to radiograph the injured foot in polytrauma patients with acute foot injury. However, data can support using CT of the foot (including the ankle) as the initial imaging modality in polytrauma patients. In one study of polytrauma patients, 25% of fractures detected on MDCT were not seen on radiographs. One of the causes that may contribute to missed diagnosis is that appropriate radiographic positioning may be difficult in polytrauma patients.

# Case 13-5

A 17-year-old male is brought to the emergency department after his right foot was accidentally crushed under the tire of his friend's truck. He has pain and deformity of his right foot that is concerning for Lisfranc injury. Which imaging tests should be performed initially?

This scenario concerns the initial imaging study for an adult or child over 5-years-old with an acute injury to the foot; does not meet the Ottawa Rules; physical examination is concerning for Lisfranc injury.

Sensible recommendation: XR FOOT 3 VIEW

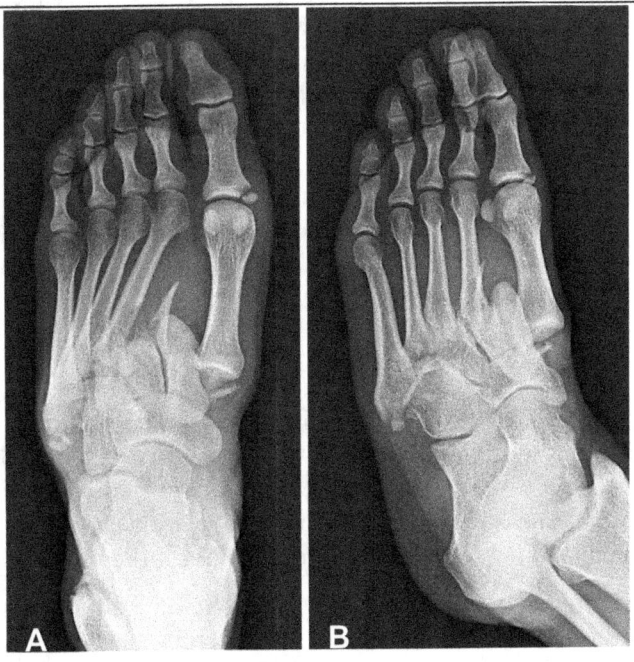

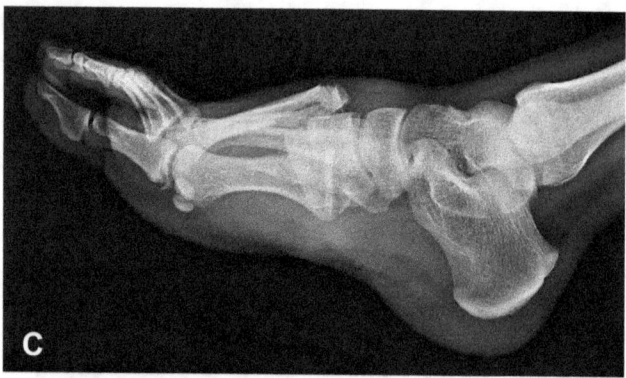

AP (A), oblique (B) and lateral (C) non-weight-bearing radiographs of the left foot demonstrate a divergent Lisfranc fracture-dislocation involving the first through fifth tarsometatarsal joints. There is also a mildly displaced fracture of the medial aspect of the first proximal phalangeal base

When there is clinical concern for acute Lisfranc injury, the most appropriate initial imaging study is the typical 3-view (AP, oblique and lateral) non-weight-bearing x-ray foot series. The most common radiographic findings of Lisfranc injury include malalignment at the second tarsometatarsal articulation, more than 2 mm diastasis between the first and second tarsometatarsal articulations, and a small bony fragment between the first and second metatarsal bases. However, Lisfranc injuries often have a subtle radiographic presentation that may be missed on initial AP and oblique foot radiographs. Weight-bearing radiographs may be obtained as the initial radiographic exam when there is a clinical suspicion for Lisfranc injury subsequent to negative or equivocal non-weight bearing 3-view foot radiographs. Weight-bearing radiographs may include AP, lateral, and oblique views of the foot (inclusion of both feet on AP radiographs can be helpful for detection of subtle malalignment on the injured side).

# Case 13-6

A 44-year-old male who was involved in a motor vehicle accident last night is being evaluated for right foot injury. On physical examination there is concern for Lisfranc injury. His non-weight bearing right foot radiographs are unremarkable, and he is unable to tolerate weight-bearing foot radiographs. Which imaging tests should be ordered for further evaluation?

This scenario concerns the next imaging study for an adult or child over 5-years-old with acute injury to the foot and physical examination is concerning for a Lisfranc injury. Initial radiographs were normal and the patient is not able to tolerate weight-bearing.

Sensible recommendation: CT FOOT WO CONTRAST or MRI FOOT WO CONTRAST

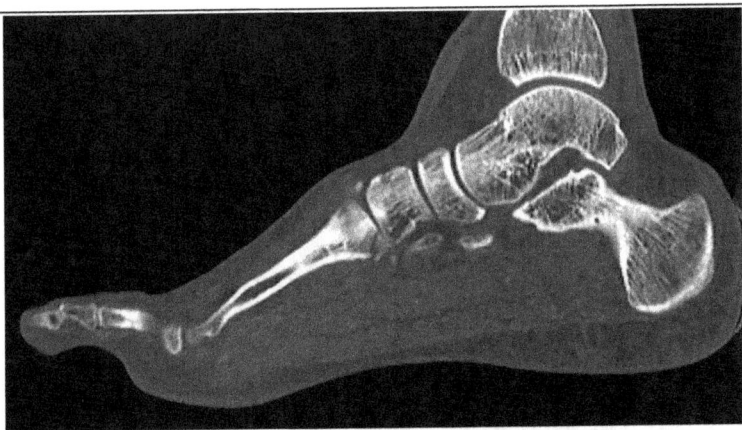

Sagittal reconstructed CT image shows a mildly displaced fracture of the second metatarsal base.

Early diagnosis and prompt appropriate management of Lisfranc injuries are important prognostic factors for prevention of potential long-term disability. When there is a clinical concern for Lisfranc injury and patient is not able to tolerate weight-bearing radiographs, further evaluation with either MRI or CT is recommended. In addition to detecting radiographically occult Lisfranc injuries, multiplanar CT can help detect some other types of radiographically occult foot fractures, verify radiographic findings, and be used for preoperative planning (especially with the addition of reformatted 3D images). MRI is slightly preferred over CT scan for evaluation of Lisfranc injuries, due to its superior ability in the evaluation of soft tissues (including direct evaluation of ligament injury), osseous contusions and at times nondisplaced fractures. However, MRI may not be available in the emergency setting.

# Case 13-7

A 46-year-old woman presents after being scratched rather deeply by her dog along the dorsal aspect of her right great toe three weeks ago. At that time, she went to urgent care and was given four stitches. The laceration has not yet fully healed but the erythema and pain have decreased. She has also noticed inability to extend her right great toe and has developed a foot drop. Right foot radiographs are unremarkable except for soft tissue swelling along the dorsal aspect of the great toe. Which imaging test should be ordered next?

This scenario concerns the next imaging study for an adult or child over 5-years-old with an acute injury to the foot; physical examination is concerning for an acute tendinous rupture or dislocation in the foot; radiographs are negative.

Sensible recommendation: MRI FOOT WO CONTRAST

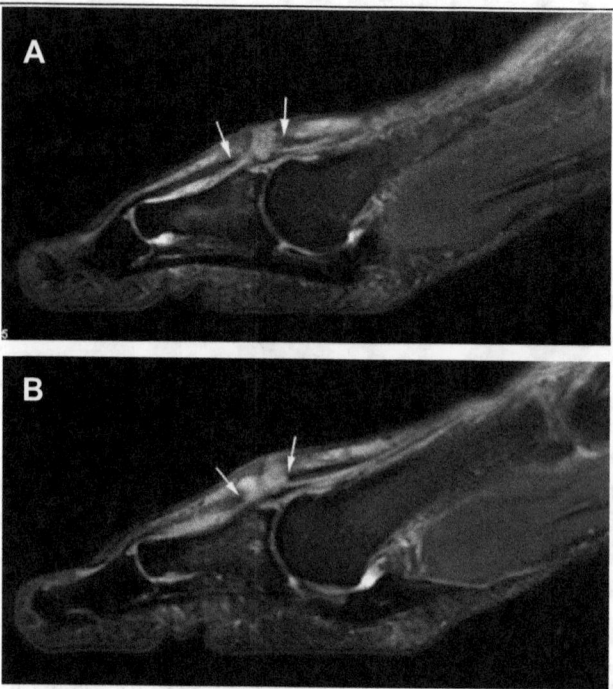

Consecutive sagittal STIR MRI of the right foot show a full thickness laceration of the extensor hallucis longus tendon at the first metatarsophalangeal joint level. The proximal and distal torn tendon stumps are marked by arrows.

Tendon abnormalities include tendinopathy, tenosynovitis, tendon tear (partial or complete) and tendon subluxation or dislocation. MRI and US can both effectively demonstrate tendon abnormalities, although US results are more dependent on operator expertise. An exception is the significant advantage of US over MRI in the dynamic evaluation of tendon subluxation or dislocation. MRI is especially useful as a global screening tool, particularly if one is not certain of the specific tendon injury or when there is suspicion of associated osseous injury. CT is typically used for evaluation and preoperative planning of fractures. Nevertheless, some soft tissue injuries can be diagnosed on CT images.

## Case 13-8

A 20-year-old wide receiver on a college football team injured his right great toe during a game. He did not notice immediate pain or a popping sensation, but after several more plays, he experienced aching on the plantar aspect of his great toe. Plantar plate injury is suspected clinically. Which imaging test should be performed initially?

This scenario concerns the initial imaging study for an adult or child over 5-years-old with a first metatarsophalangeal joint injury. Plantar plate injury is suspected.

Sensible recommendation: XR FOOT 3 VIEW

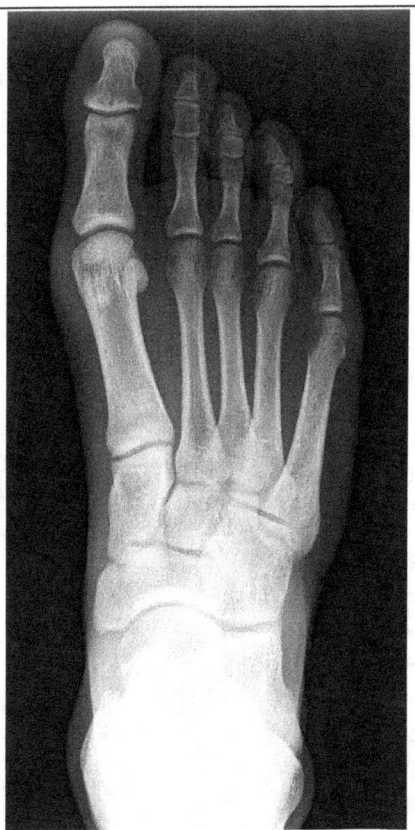

Weight-bearing AP foot radiograph shows proximal migration of the lateral hallux sesamoid and the proximal component of the bipartite medial hallux sesamoid. Findings are suggestive of hallux metatarsophalangeal plantar plate disruption.

Standard weight-bearing AP, lateral, and sesamoid axial radiographs should be obtained initially for evaluation of suspected turf toe. Patients with plantar plate disruption may demonstrate proximal migration of one or both of the hallux sesamoids. Comparison radiographs of the contralateral foot may be of value for confirming the proper positioning of the hallux sesamoids. When there is complete disruption of the plantar plate, the hallux sesamoids will not track distally with extension of the first toe and will remain beneath the first metatarsal head on a lateral stress view or fluoroscopy. The plantar plate can be further evaluated with US or preferably with MRI. MRI permits direct evaluation of the capsuloligamentous soft tissues as well as assessment of chondral and osteochondral lesions.

## Case 13-9

A 10-year-old girl presents to urgent care after stepping on something in her dining room. She has a cut on the plantar aspect of her forefoot, with pain and a foreign body feeling. On physical examination there is a puncture wound on the plantar surface of the base of her second toe. Which imaging test should be ordered initially?

This scenario concerns the initial imaging study for an adult or child over 5-years-old. Acute injury to the foot; physical examination is concerning for penetrating trauma with a foreign body in the soft tissues.

Sensible recommendation: XR FOOT 3 VIEW

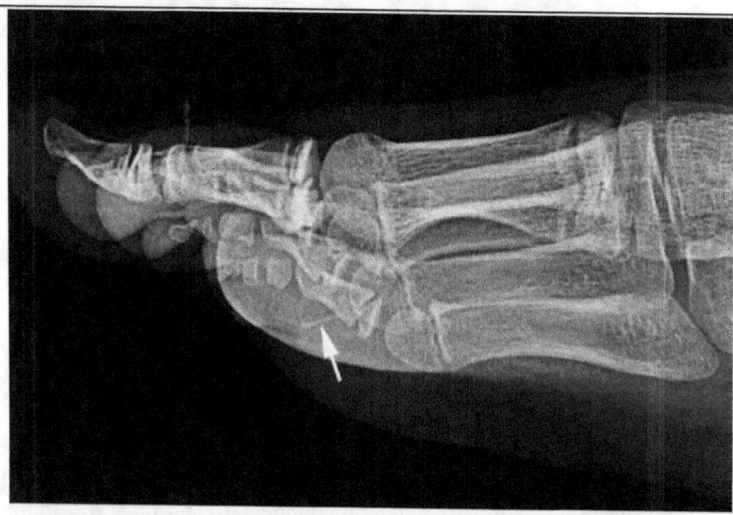

Lateral radiograph of the left foot shows a linear radiopaque foreign body deep to the skin defect in the plantar soft tissues of the forefoot.

Radiography is the most appropriate initial imaging study when there is suspicion for a radiopaque foreign body (e.g., gravel, glass or metal). Ultrasound is the initial imaging modality of choice when there is suspicion for a foreign body that is not radiopaque (e.g., wood or plastic).

## Case 13-10

A 55-year-old woman presents with a possible retained foreign body in her right foot. Last week, while snorkeling in Hawaii, she took off her flippers when she got near the shore and stepped on what seemed to be a sharp piece of coral or glass. She reports it went in quite deeply. Right foot radiographs are negative. Which imaging test is the most appropriate next study?

This scenario concerns the next imaging study for an adult or child over 5-years-old with acute injury to the foot; physical examination is concerning for penetrating trauma with a foreign body in the soft tissues. Initial radiographs of the foot are negative.

Sensible recommendation: US, region of interest

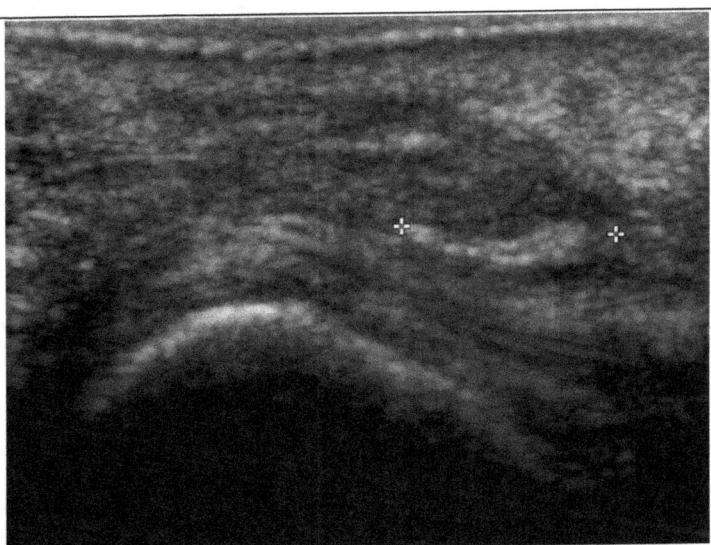

Sagittal US image of right plantar soft tissues at level of foreign body penetration (fifth metatarsal head). There is a curvilinear foreign body in the soft tissues demarcated by the calipers.

Ultrasound is the imaging modality of choice when there is suspicion for a foreign body that is not radiopaque (e.g., wood or plastic). The depiction of foreign bodies on CT scan is dependent on the attenuation value of the foreign body. While on MRI, the detection of foreign bodies is facilitated by the presence of susceptibility artifacts. One study reported low sensitivity and high specificity of radiography, CT and MRI for detection of a variety of foreign bodies (fresh wood, dry wood, glass, porcelain and plastic fragments) randomly placed in the plantar soft tissues of the sole and forefoot.

# References

1. American College of Radiology. ACR Appropriateness Criteria: Acute Trauma to the Foot. American College of Radiology, revised 2019. https://acsearch.acr.org/docs/70546/Narrative/ (accessed April 24, 2021).
2. Bancroft LW, Kransdorf MJ, Adler R, Appel M, Beaman FD, Bernard SA, Bruno MA, Dempsey ME, Fries IB, Khoury V, Khurana B, Mosher TJ, Roberts CC, Tuite MJ, Ward RJ, Zoga AC, Weissman BN. ACR Appropriateness Criteria Acute Trauma to the Foot. J Am Coll Radiol. 2015 Jun;12(6):575-81. doi: 10.1016/j.jacr.2015.02.018. Epub 2015 Apr 29. Review. PMID: 25935824.

# Chapter 14. Acute Chest Wall Trauma

Felix S. Chew, MD

Radiography is the best initial exam for isolated acute chest wall trauma, but CT should be obtained when the patient presentation or trauma mechanism suggest internal injuries. The radionuclide bone scan has a limited role.

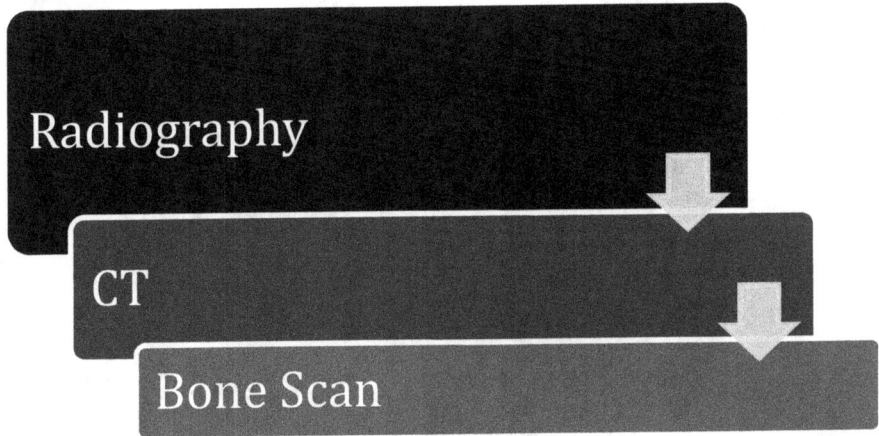

# Case 14-1

86-year-old woman with right rib and upper chest pain for a week after falling and hitting her chest in the bathtub. She denies shortness of breath or dyspnea. She denies loss of consciousness at the time of the fall. What is the best initial imaging study to evaluate her chest pain?

This scenario concerns the imaging evaluation of an adult with suspected rib fractures from minor blunt trauma (injury confined to ribs).

Sensible recommendation: XR CHEST 1 VIEW and XR RIBS, side(s) of interest

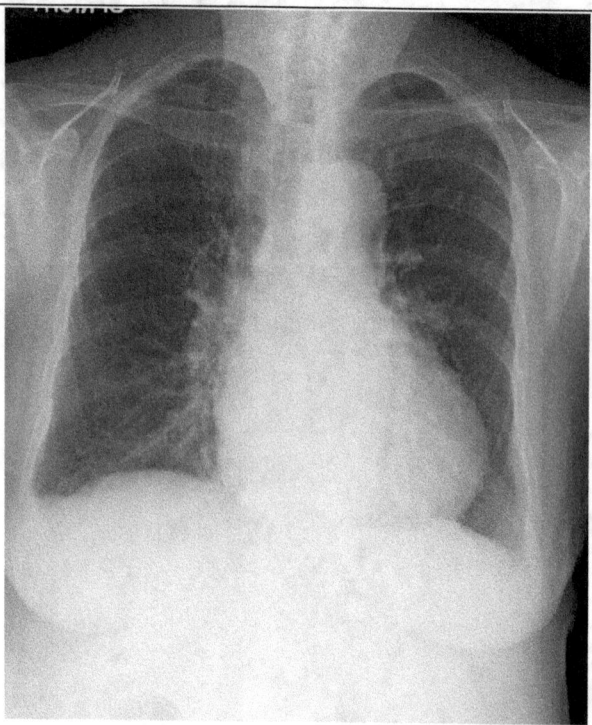

(A) The PA chest radiograph shows clear lungs and cardiomegaly, but no rib fractures.

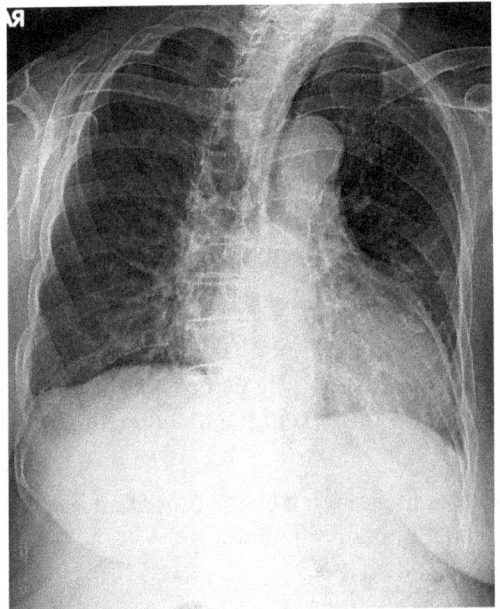

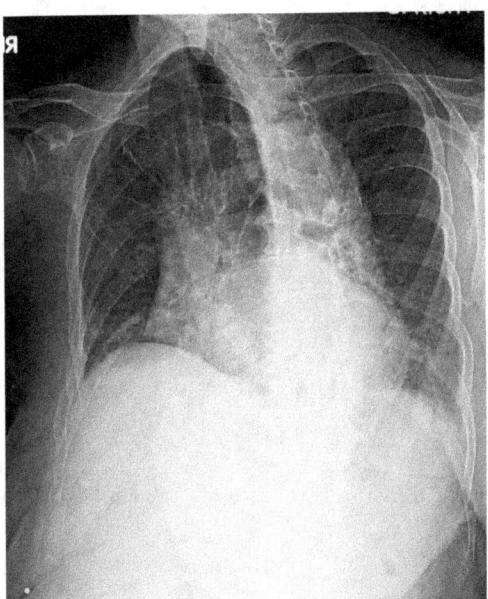

(B-C) Oblique radiographs of the ribs demonstrate multiple fractures involving the anterolateral aspects of the right sixth through ninth ribs, and a fracture of the left ninth rib. The age of this patient and the persistence of pain for a week would increase the likelihood that fractures are present, compared with a younger patient with a shorter history.

For the initial screening for rib fractures from low-energy blunt trauma, radiography is most appropriate. The PA chest radiograph can exclude urgent complications such as lung injury, pneumothorax or hemothorax, but many rib fractures will not be evident, depending on location and displacement. The radiographic rib series will be more accurate in detecting rib fractures than the chest radiograph. Cross-sectional and nuclear imaging would not be appropriate in this setting.

## Case 14-2

28-year-old man with chest pain and difficulty breathing for a week after being struck by a car as a pedestrian. He denies loss of consciousness at the time of the injury. What is the best initial imaging study to evaluate his chest pain?

This scenario concerns the imaging evaluation of an adult with suspected rib fractures from severe blunt polytrauma.

Sensible recommendation: XR CHEST 1 VIEW

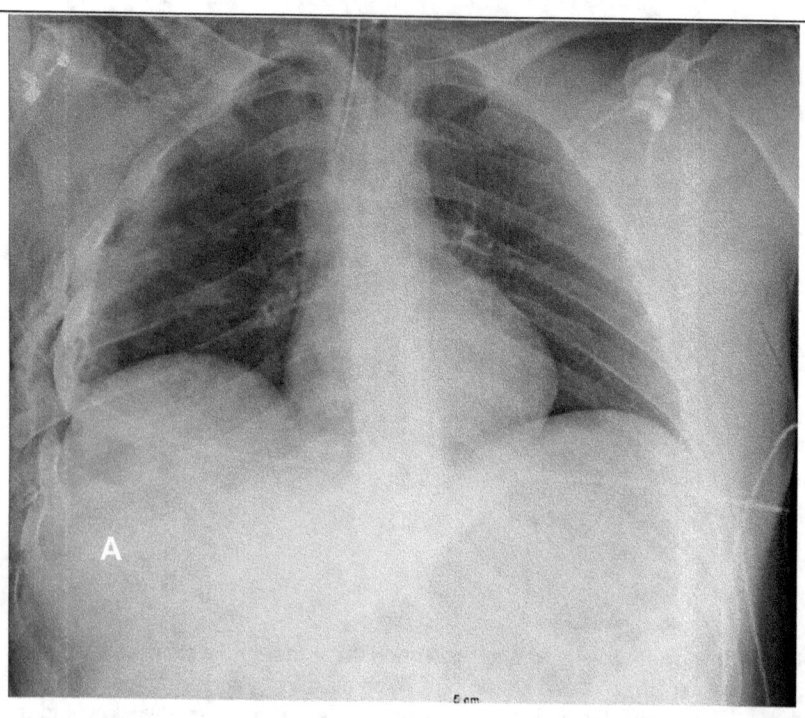

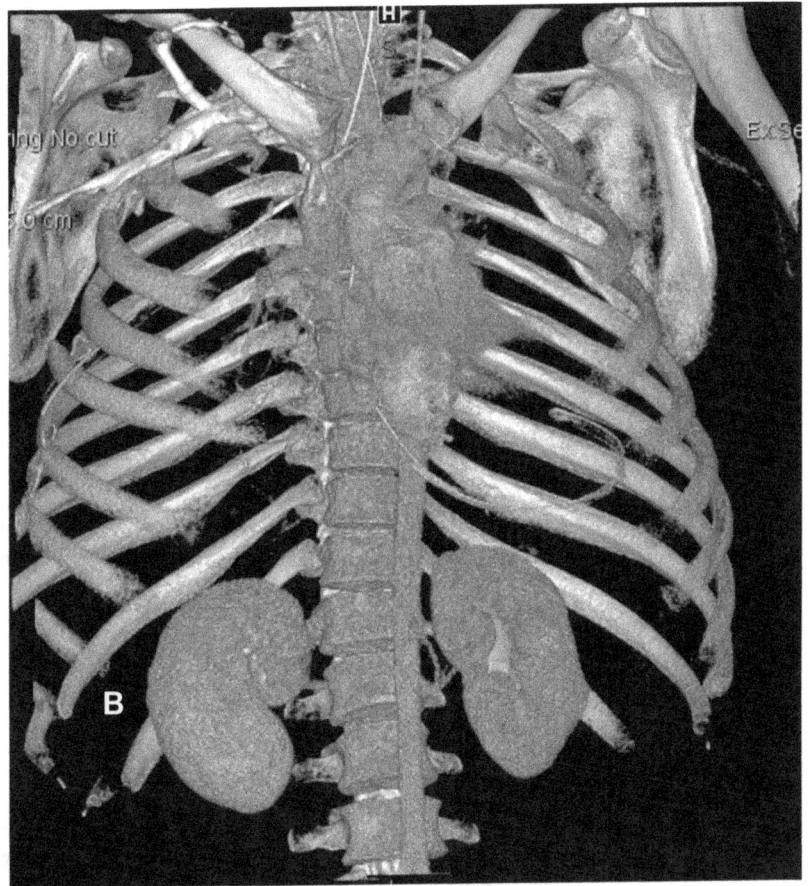

(A) The PA chest radiograph shows multiple right-sided rib fractures. There is a right pneumothorax and subcutaneous emphysema over the rib fractures. (B) 3D CT reconstruction of the rib cage showed segmental fractures of ribs 3-9 and posterior fractures of ribs 10-11.

For the initial screening for rib fractures from high-energy blunt trauma, radiography is most appropriate. The PA chest radiograph can also identify urgent complications such as lung injury, pneumothorax or hemothorax. Further evaluation with CT is warranted for any abnormalities found or suspected on the chest radiograph, including both skeletal and non-skeletal structures, and 3D reconstructions may be helpful in identifying fractures and planning treatment. Flail chest is of particular importance to identify.

# Case 14-3

58-year-old man who complained of chest wall pain after cardiopulmonary resuscitation (CPR). His cardiovascular status had been stabilized. What is the most appropriate first imaging step to evaluate his chest wall pain?

This scenario concerns the imaging evaluation of an adult with suspected rib fractures after successful CPR.

Sensible recommendation: XR CHEST 1 VIEW and XR RIBS, side(s) of interest

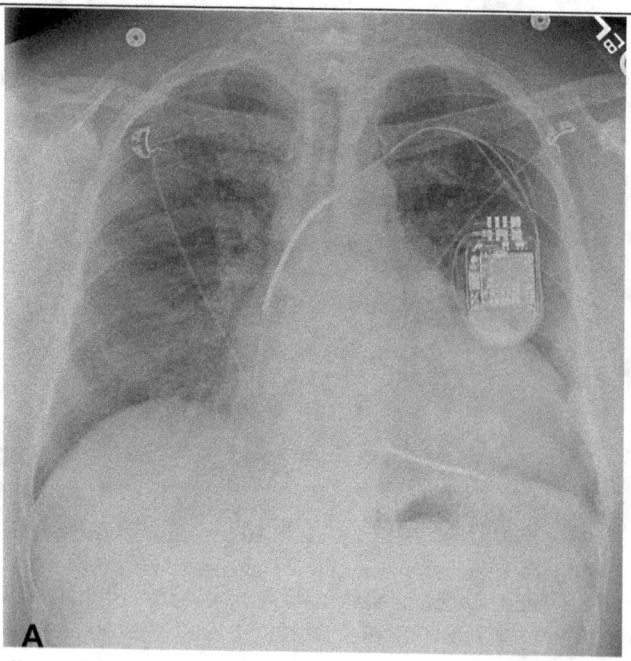

(A) Chest radiograph shows implanted cardioverter-defibrillator. The heart is enlarged but the lungs are clear.

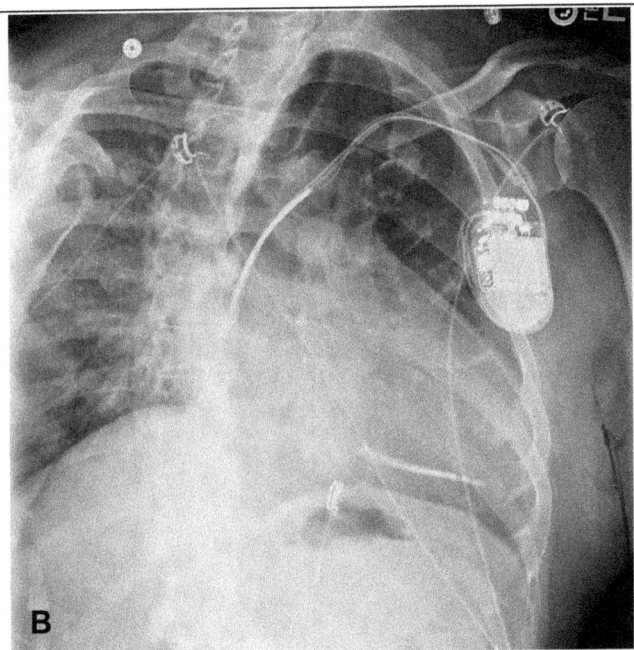

(B) Rib radiograph shows mildly displaced fractures through the calcified costo-chondral portions of the left third, fifth, and sixth ribs.

Skeletal chest wall injuries following CPR are common. A recent autopsy study of non-survivors of cardiac arrest who received CPR showed a prevalence of 86% in men and 91% in women, including rib fractures, sternal fractures, and sternocostal separations. The prevalence shown by imaging-based studies of survivors is much lower. Rib fractures may complicate the post-resuscitation recovery of CPR survivors.

## Case 14-4

19-year-old female crew athlete who complains of posterior medial rib discomfort on the right side and suspicion for stress fracture. She has had symptoms for several weeks. What is the most appropriate first imaging exam?

This scenario concerns the imaging evaluation of a patient with rib pain and a suspected stress fracture.

Sensible recommendation: XR CHEST 1 VIEW and XR RIBS, side(s) of interest

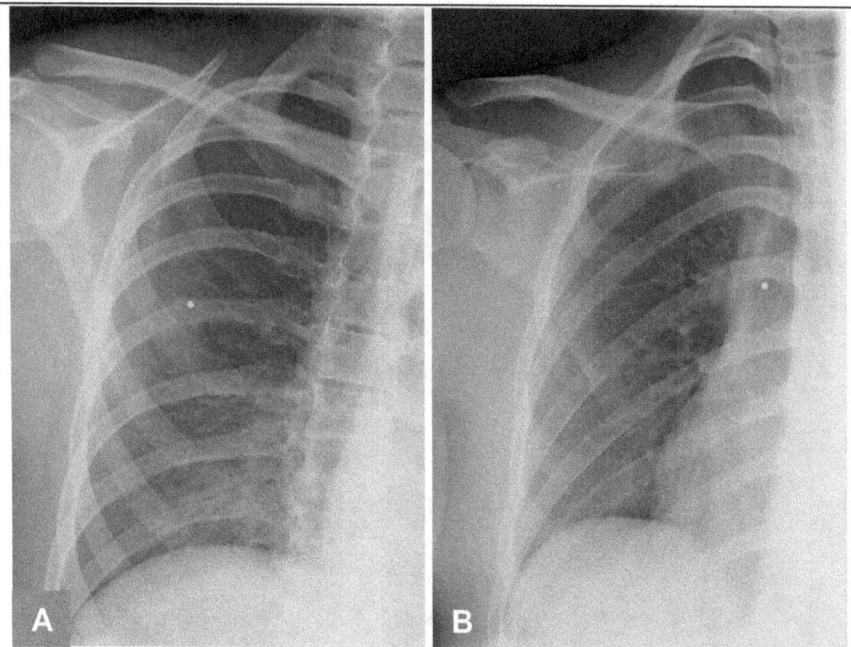

The chest radiograph was normal. (A-B) Right rib radiographs show periosteal reaction with irregular cortical margins of the posterior right sixth rib, corresponding to the location of the external skin marker that had been placed at the site of maximal pain. The diagnosis of healing stress fracture was made.

Stress fractures involving ribs may occur in patients with chronic coughing as well as in participants in a variety of activities, especially rowing, but also swimming, baseball and softball, golfing, backpacking, and others. For initial imaging evaluation, chest and rib radiographs are appropriate, and for most patients, the evaluation ends there if negative. For select patients, such as elite athletes for whom the timing of return to sport is critical, additional modalities such as CT, radionuclide bone scan, or MRI may be appropriate.

## Case 14-5

71-year-old man on hormonal therapy for metastatic prostate cancer with cough and new onset of rib pain. What is the most appropriate first imaging exam to evaluate his rib pain?

This scenario concerns the imaging evaluation of an adult with suspected pathologic rib fracture.

Sensible recommendation: XR CHEST 1 VIEW, CT CHEST WO CONTRAST, or Tc-99m BONE SCAN

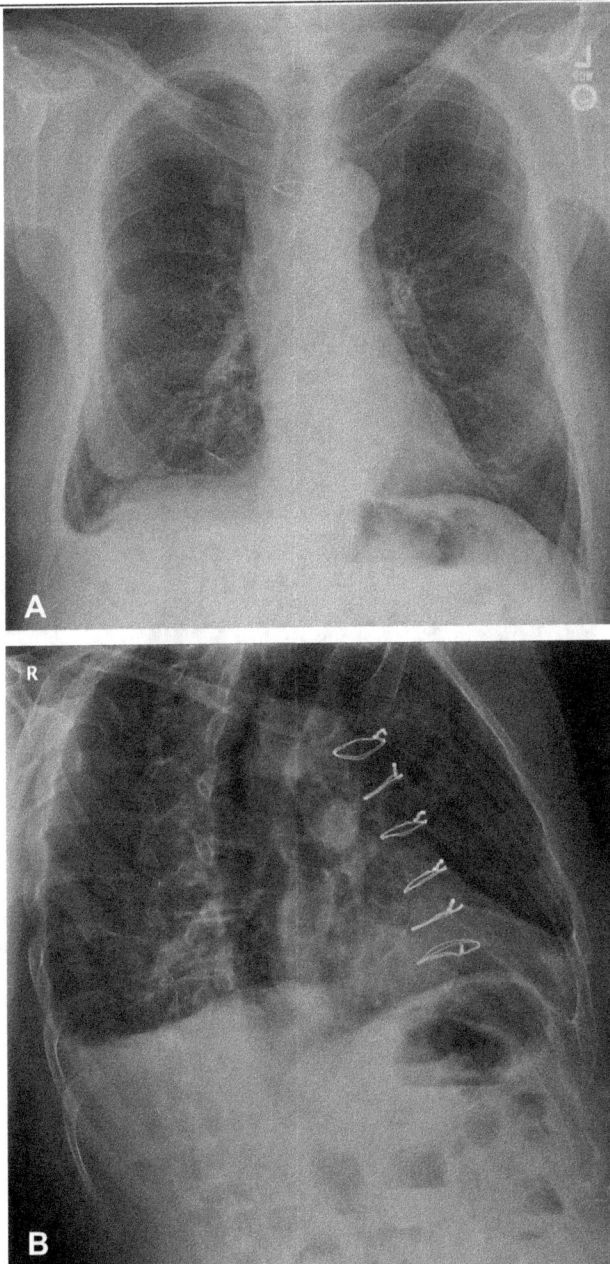

(A-B), the chest and rib radiographs show a fracture of the anterolateral right eighth rib. The lungs are clear and the heart size is normal. There has been previous median sternotomy. There is a small right pleural effusion.

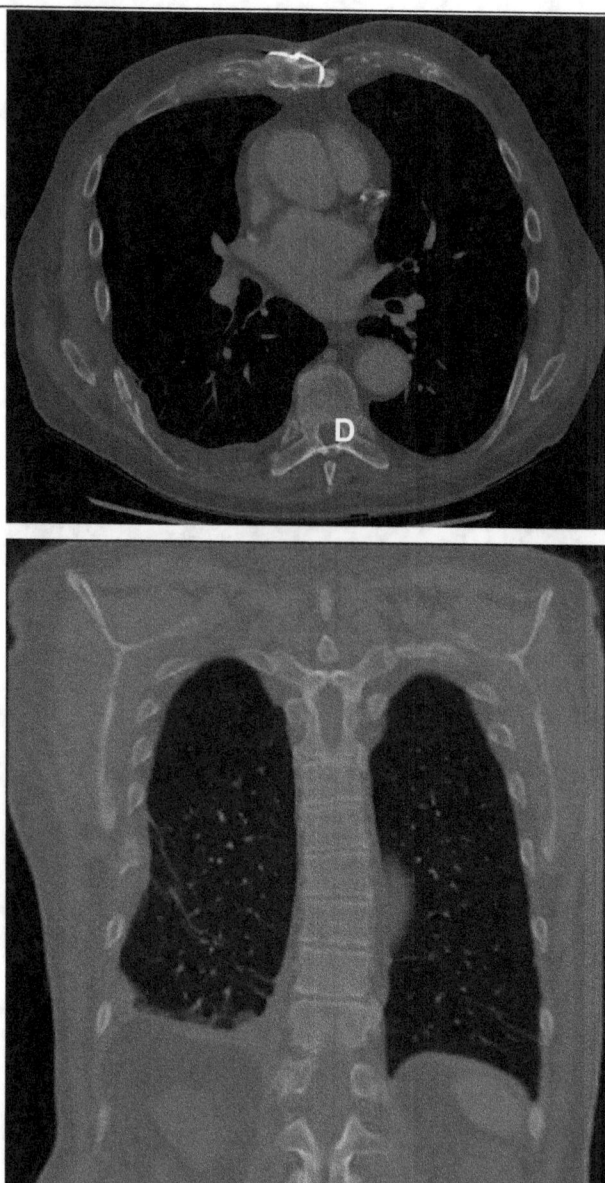

(C-D), axial and coronal CT images show the minimally displaced right eighth rib pathologic fracture.

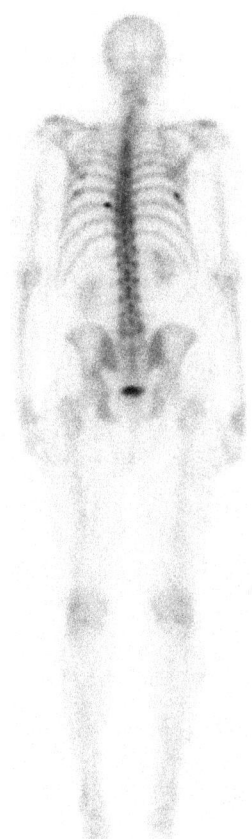

**E**

(E), radionuclide bone scan shows multiple skeletal lesions in the ribs and elsewhere, including the right eighth rib. Comparison with previous imaging (not shown here) confirmed progressive metastatic disease.

Pathologic rib fractures may be suspected in the setting of known metastatic disease as well as in patients with no known reason to have rib fractures. In additional to metastatic disease, benign and malignant primary bone lesions, benign and malignant hematologic conditions, various metabolic and systemic conditions, and direct extension from intrathoracic lesions may cause pathologic rib fractures. Once the presence of a pathologic fracture has been established, history and other clinical features should guide further steps in determining the underlying cause.

## Case 14-6

27-year-old man with persistent anterior chest pain after a severe crushing injury of the back with a hyperflexion T6 burst fracture and multiple adjacent spinous process avulsion fractures. The thoracic spine injury was

141

stabilized with posterior instrumentation and attention is now focused on his chest pain. A fracture of the sternum is suspected. What is the best initial study to evaluate his chest pain?

This scenario concerns the imaging evaluation of an adult with suspected sternal fracture from severe trauma.

Sensible recommendation: CT CHEST WO CONTRAST

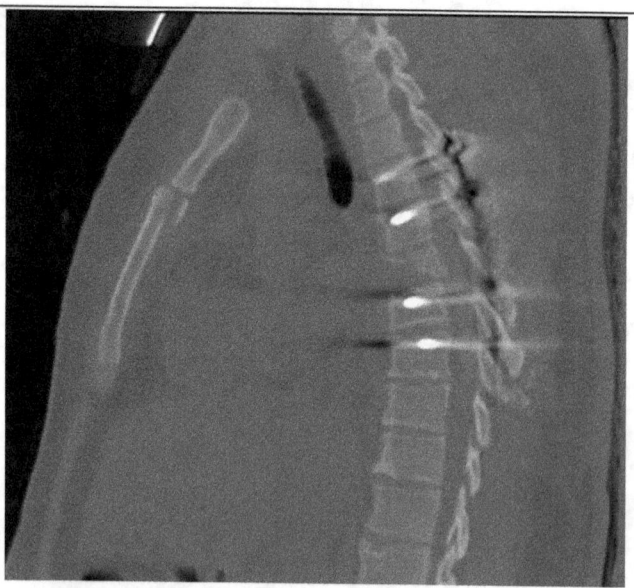

Sagittal CT through the sternum shows a partially reduced sternomanubrial dislocation with fracture of the posterior cortex of the sternum. The post-surgical T6 fracture is visible.

Sternal fractures may sometimes be seen on lateral radiographs, but generally not seen on other radiograph views; the oblique sternal view that may be available in sophisticated radiology departments is generally not useful in this regard. In the setting of high-energy trauma, chest CT is usually necessary. Sternal injuries are most conspicuous on sagittal CT.

# References

1.  American College of Radiology. ACR Appropriateness Criteria: Rib Fractures. American College of Radiology, revised 2018. https://acsearch.acr.org/docs/69450/Narrative/ (accessed April 24, 2021).
2.  Expert Panel on Thoracic Imaging, Henry TS, Kirsch J, Kanne JP, Chung JH, Donnelly EF, Ginsburg ME, Heitkamp DE, Kazerooni EA, Ketai LH, McComb BL, Parker JA, Ravenel JG, Restrepo CS, Saleh AG, Shah RD, Steiner RM, Suh RD, Mohammed TL; American College of Radiology. ACR

Appropriateness Criteria® rib fractures. J Thorac Imaging. 2014 Nov;29(6):364-6. doi: 10.1097/RTI.0000000000000113. PMID: 25340388.

3. Kralj E, Podbregar M, Kejžar N, Balažic J. Frequency and number of resuscitation related rib and sternum fractures are higher than generally considered. Resuscitation. 2015 Aug;93:136-41. doi:10.1016/j.resuscitation.2015.02.034. Epub 2015 Mar 12. PMID: 25771500.

# Chapter 15. Stress and Insufficiency Fractures

Vijaya Kosaraju, MD, Majid Chalian, MD

Radiography is the initial exam for stress fractures. However, radiographs are often normal in the early phase of injury. For high-risk areas such as femoral neck, MRI study may be performed if initial radiographs are negative or as an initial study to avoid risk of delayed diagnosis and progression. A prophylactic treatment plan for stress fracture followed by repeat radiographs in 10 to 14 days is a reasonable alternative for low-risk areas. CT and radionuclide bone scan may have role in selective scenarios but are associated with higher radiation than radiographs.

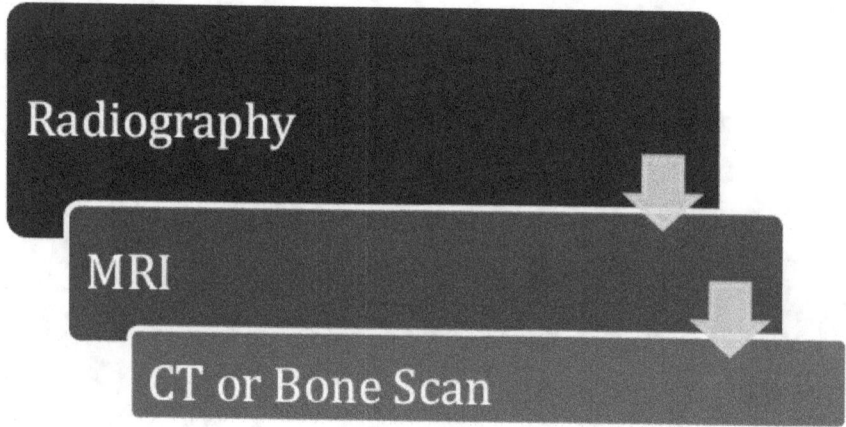

Radiography

MRI

CT or Bone Scan

# Case 15-1

24-year-old female runner presented with gradual onset leg pain that started while training for marathon. The patient reports worsening pain with activity that subsides with rest. What is the best initial study?

This scenario concerns the best initial imaging study for a patient with suspected fatigue fracture.

Sensible recommendation: XR, region of interest.

Imaging of the patient with suspected fatigue type insufficiency fracture should begin with a standard radiographic examination. Conventional radiographs are inexpensive and readily available. Initial radiographs are often normal with poor sensitivity, but positive findings can manifest as focal sclerosis or periosteal reaction. If the radiographs demonstrate findings of stress fracture, no additional imaging is usually needed. Patients should however be informed that majority of stress fractures may not be identified on radiographs and that additional imaging may be necessary based on the location of pain or if the symptoms are persistent despite conservative initial management.

# Case 15-2

A 22-year-old male runner with insidious onset hip pain while increasing his activity level. Patient had to stop his daily runs due to this. Initial screening radiographs were negative. What is the next best imaging study?

This scenario concerns the best next imaging study for a young patient with suspected fatigue type stress fracture of the hip following negative initial radiographs.

Sensible recommendation: MRI HIP WO CONTRAST

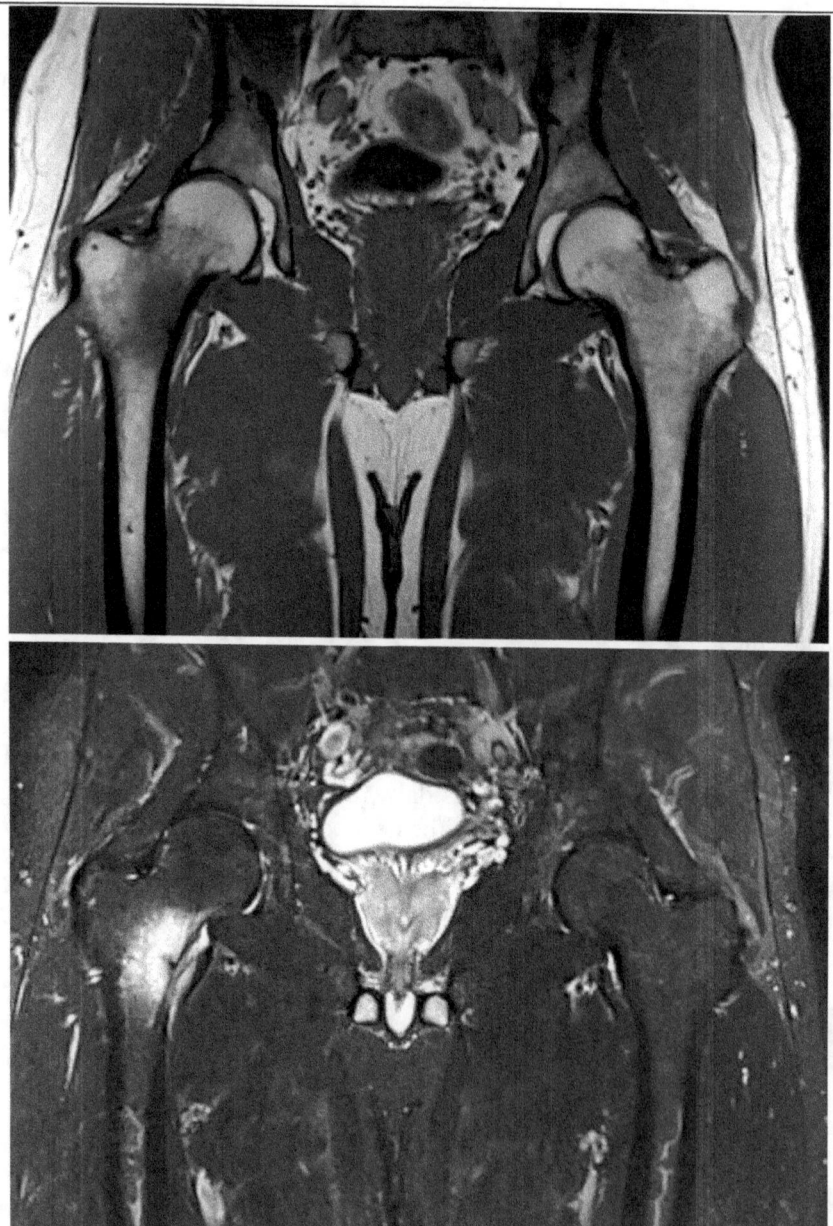

Coronal T1 (A) and coronal STIR (B) images of the pelvis demonstrate low signal fracture line in the medial inter-trochanteric region (compressive side) of the right femur with marked surrounding edema, consistent with stress fracture.

Femoral neck is a common location for stress fracture. Stress fractures of the lateral femoral neck (tensile side) have high risk of progression and stress fractures of the femoral head have association with avascular necrosis and premature development of osteoporosis. Hence, these need to be promptly recognized without delay. MRI has high sensitivity for identification of stress fractures in early phase and are recommended as next best imaging study following initial negative radiographs. Follow-up radiographs in 10 to 14 days have higher sensitivity than the initial radiographs, but however are less sensitive than MRI and additionally, delayed diagnosis is not desirable in high risk locations such as proximal femur. Bone scintigraphy, although has high sensitivity, has limited specificity and precise atomic localization can be difficult.

# Case 15-3

A 27-year-old high school soccer player presents with pain in the anterior leg. He is in the middle of intense practice sessions during fall season and could not continue his season due to this. Initial radiographs are negative. What is the best follow-up study?

This scenario concerns the best initial imaging study for a young patient with suspected fatigue type stress fracture following negative initial radiographs.

Sensible recommendation: MRI WO CONTRAST, region of interest

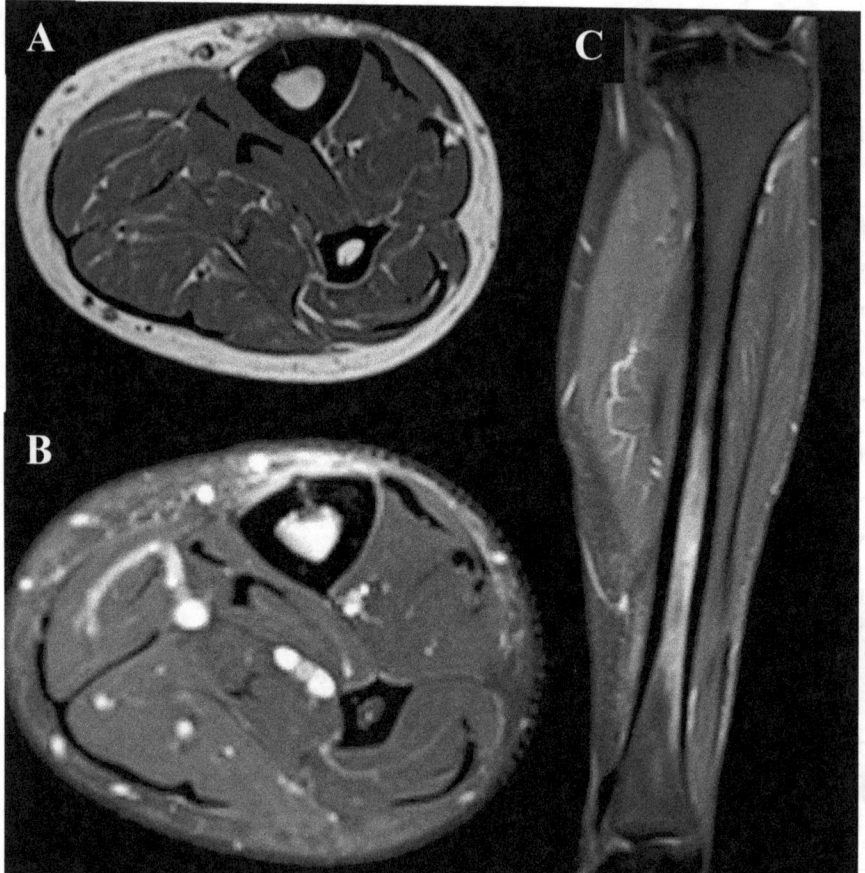

Axial T1 (A) and axial T2 fat saturated (B) images of the tibia demonstrate stress fracture in the anteromedial tibial cortex with surrounding periosteal reaction and intramedullary marrow edema. Coronal STIR image (C) shows craniocaudal extension of the reactive marrow edema.

If the suspected location of stress fracture is in high-risk areas such as femoral neck, anterior tibia, tarsal navicular, patella, or fifth metatarsal where there is a risk for progression to complete fracture or nonunion, an MRI study is recommended to avoid risk of delayed diagnosis and progression. However, if the suspected location is in low-risk areas such as femoral shaft, fibula, or calcaneus, a prophylactic treatment plan for stress fracture followed by repeat radiographs in 10 to 14 days is a reasonable alternative.

## Case 15-4

A 22-year-old college basketball player presents with severe heel pain that started during practice. His jumping activity is markedly limited due to this. Initial radiographs are negative. The team coach wants to determine the cause of pain in a timely fashion as the season is about to start and he must decide of whether to rest the player for few weeks or not.

This scenario concerns the best initial imaging study for an athlete with immediate need to know diagnosis due to risk for progression to more serious injury.

Sensible recommendation: MRI WO CONTRAST, region of interest

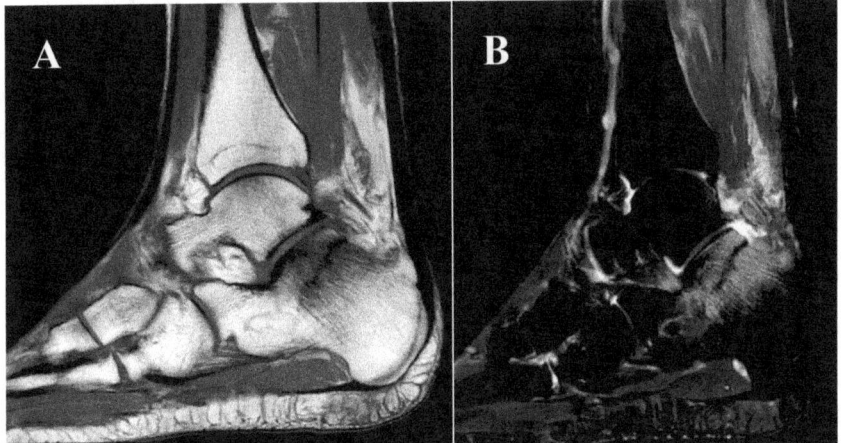

Sagittal T1 (A) and sagittal STIR (B) images of the ankle demonstrate low signal fracture line in the superior calcaneus perpendicular to the orientation of the trabecula with surrounding edema, consistent with stress fracture.

In scenario such as this where immediate diagnosis needs to be made facilitating immediate decision-making and treatment plan, MRI of the region of interest is recommended. Based on MRI findings, decision to immobilize and potential surgical treatment can be planned without delay.

## Case 15-5

A 19-year-old high school soccer player presented with persistent leg pain despite rest and treatment with anti-inflammatory medication. Patient participated in intense daily practice sessions in the preceding 3 months before onset of symptoms. Initial radiographs revealed periosteal reaction concerning for stress fracture. Patient is interested in returning to sport during the current season if situation permits and further imaging is requested to assess the severity of injury.

This scenario concerns athlete with confirmed stress fracture on radiographs in whom, additional imaging is requested to make a return to play decision.

Sensible recommendation: MRI WO CONTRAST, region of interest

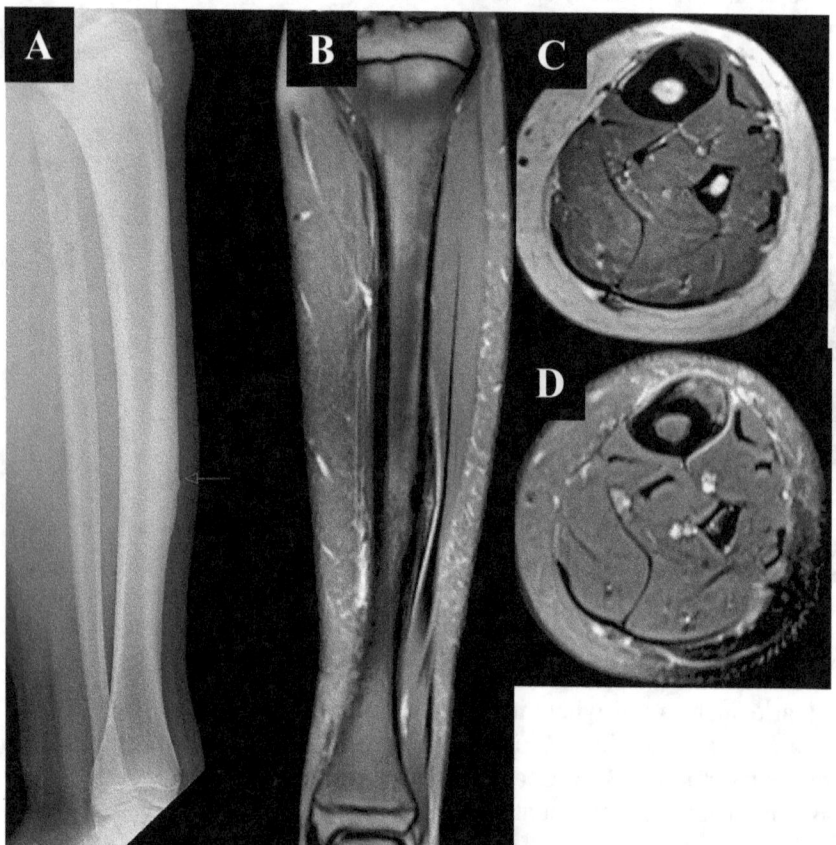

Lateral radiograph (A) demonstrates cortical thickening and periosteal reaction. Sagittal STIR image (B) confirms cortical thickening and subtle incomplete fracture line. Axial T1-weighted (C) and axial T2 fat saturated (D) images of the tibia demonstrate marked cortical thickening and intracortical signal abnormality of the anterolateral tibia consistent with stress fracture.

Previous studies have demonstrated that MRI-based grading of stress fracture, location of the fracture (cortical versus trabecular), and bone mineral density were associated with predicting time to recovery. Assessment of the grade of injury may help plan treatment and predict time to recovery for return to sport.

# Case 15-6

An 86-year-old woman presents with vague lower back pain for the past several weeks. She has history of osteoporosis. She denies history of falls or trauma. Her pain worsens with daily activities and is relieved by rest. She was initially managed by her primary practice physician with over-the-counter pain medication; however, the pain is persistent and hence she presents for additional evaluation.

This scenario concerns the initial imaging exam for patient with suspected insufficiency type stress fracture of the pelvis or hip due to existing risk factors.

Sensible recommendation: XR PELVIS AND HIP

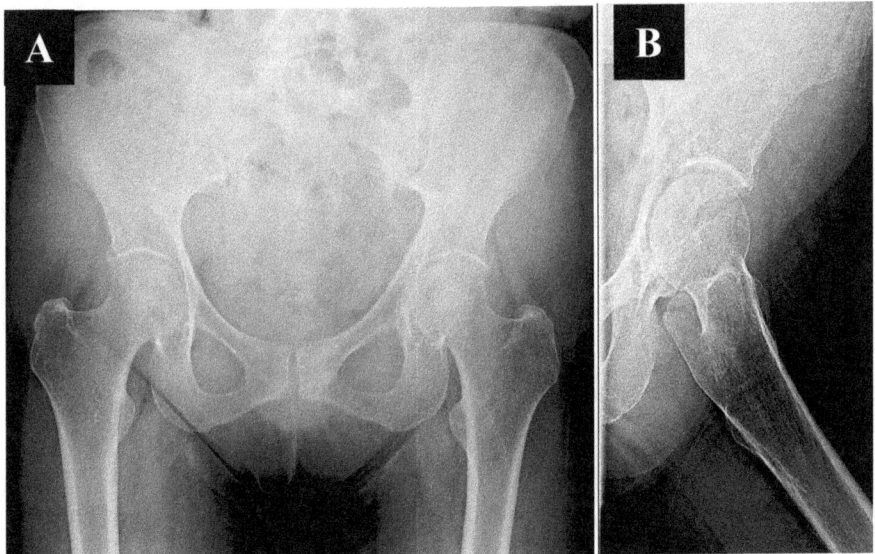

AP radiograph the pelvis (A) and frog leg lateral (B) radiographs of the left hip are negative for acute fracture or malalignment.

Common locations for insufficiency fractures include sacrum, pubic rami, supra-acetabular ilium, and femoral neck, and risk factors include age, female sex, anorexia, and steroid use. Despite the fact that radiographs are relatively insensitive for stress fractures occurring in the pelvis due to overlying bowel gas and osteopenia, they are often utilized as the initial imaging study. Radiographs are more sensitive in subacute or chronic phases and findings include linear sclerosis perpendicular to the long axis of the bone. They are relatively inexpensive, quick, and enable timely management in positive cases and no further imaging may be necessary.

# Case 15-7

A 75-year-old female patients present to the primary care clinic for continued pelvic pain. Patient initially presented a week prior with similar symptoms. Radiographs were obtained at initial presentation and were negative for fractures, however demonstrated bilateral hip degenerative changes and osteopenia. Patient was given instructions to limit weight bearing and recommended to use over-the-counter pain medications for symptom relief. However, due to lack of symptom relief, patient presents again for repeat evaluation.

Sensible recommendation: MRI WO CONTRAST, region of interest

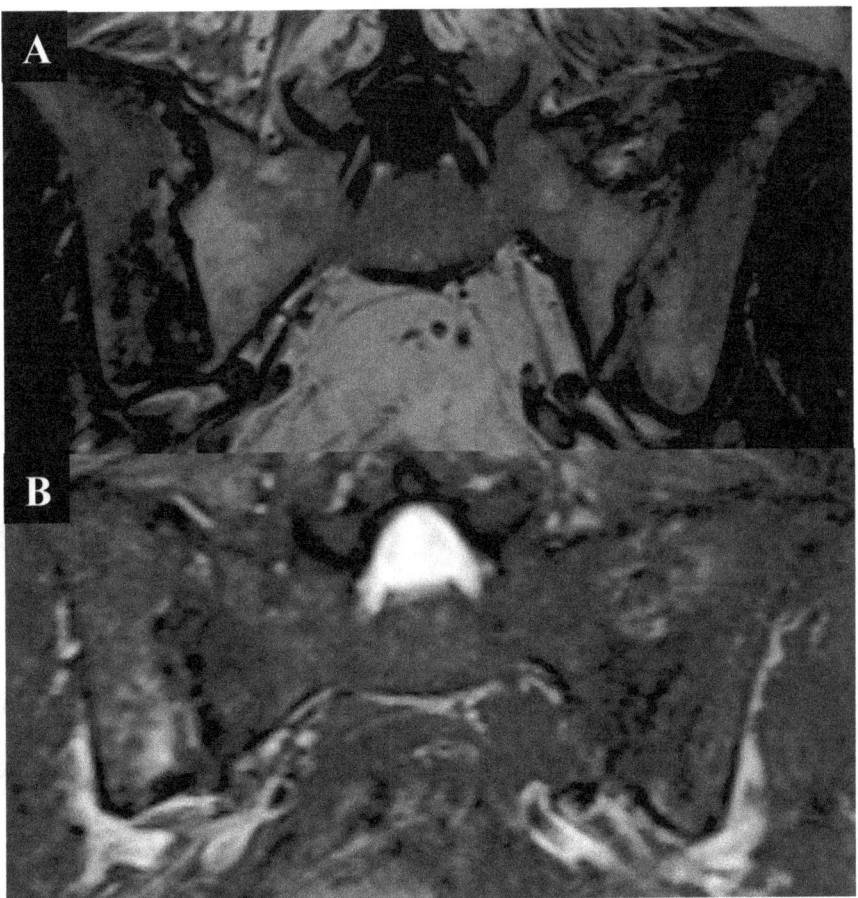

Coronal T1 (A) and STIR (B) images of the pelvis demonstrate low signal fracture line with surrounding edema in the inferior medial aspect of right ilium subjacent to sacroiliac joint, consistent with insufficiency type stress fracture.

The scenario concerns suspected insufficiency type stress fracture in a patient with negative initial radiographs. In this scenario, the follow-up imaging options include CT, bone scintigraphy, and repeat radiographs. MRI or CT of the pelvis/hips including the images of sacrum are recommended to categorize the risk level of fracture and determine appropriate treatment plan. Although bone scintigraphy has high sensitivity for detection of fractures, it is less specific than cross-sectional studies and often requires additional cross-sectional images for anatomic localization and may be time-consuming.

# Case 15-8

A 60-year-old physically active male presents for evaluation of leg pain that started a week ago. He has no history of trauma. Pain localized to anterior lower leg, worsens with daily morning walks and is relieved with rest. What is the best imaging study?

This scenario concerns suspected insufficiency type stress fracture in a late middle-aged patient.

Sensible recommendation: XR TIBIA-FIBULA 2 VIEW

Although radiographs have limited sensitivity for evaluation of stress fractures of extremities, it is often the first imaging study due to easy availability, and low cost. It can be of value in ruling out differentials such as to overt fracture, infection, or tumor. Positive radiographic findings include linear sclerosis perpendicular to the trabeculae, callus formation, and periosteal reaction. If radiographs are positive, no further imaging may be necessary. In this case, the radiographs were normal (not shown).

# Case 15-9

A 60-year-old physically active male presents for evaluation of leg pain that started a week ago. He has no history of trauma. Pain localized to anterior lower leg, worsens with daily morning walks and is relieved with rest. Initial radiographs are negative. What is the next preferred imaging study?

This scenario concerns suspected insufficiency type stress fracture in the late middle-aged patient with negative initial radiographs.

Sensible recommendation: MRI WO CONTRAST, region of interest

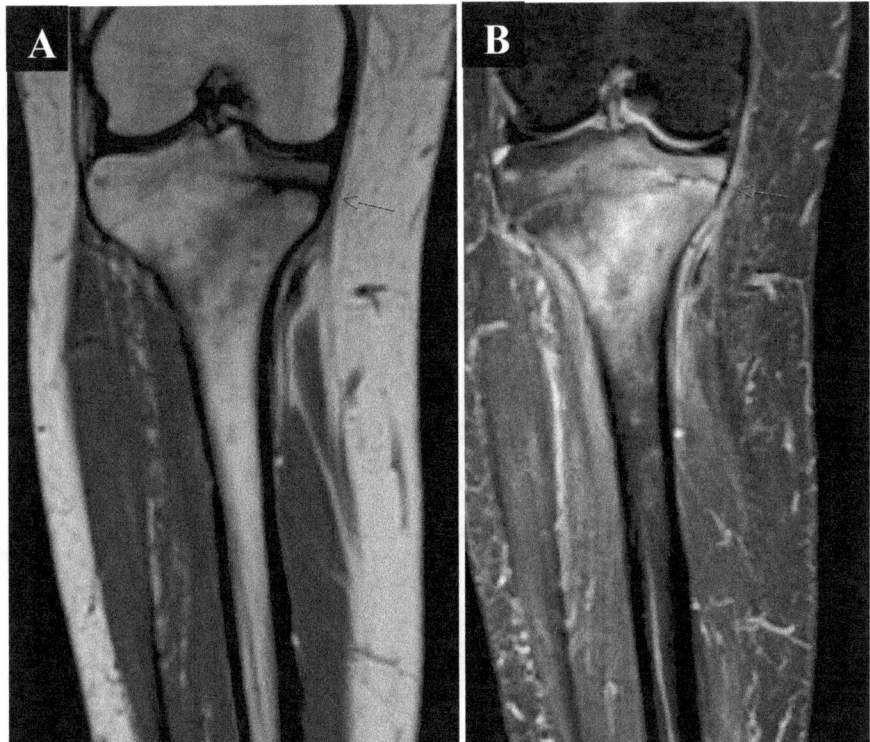

Coronal T1 (A) and STIR (B) images of the tibia demonstrate low signal fracture line with surrounding edema in the medial aspect of proximal tibial epiphysis.

In a patient with suspected insufficiency fracture with initial negative radiographs, MRI or repeat radiographs in 10 to 14 days after rest are the next best imaging studies. MRI has high-sensitivity and enables detection in early phase of injury. Findings on MRI include low signal fracture line and marrow edema as well periosteal and surrounding soft tissue edema. If there is high clinical suspicion initially even after negative radiographs, a reasonable alternative would be repeating radiographs in 10 to 14 days after resting the patient with non-weight -bearing instructions. Repeat radiographs may demonstrate changes of healing with linear sclerosis and periosteal reaction. Follow-up radiographs are more sensitive and specific than the initial radiographs for stress fractures.

## Case 15-10

A 56-year-old female with history of breast cancer underwent bone scan for detection of osseous metastasis after she reported severe knee pain. Bone scan revealed focal update in the region of the right proximal femur. What is the next best imaging study?

This scenario concerns follow-up of incidental focal update on bone scintigraphy, with differential considerations including stress fractures among other etiologies.

Sensible recommendation: MRI WO CONTRAST, region of interest

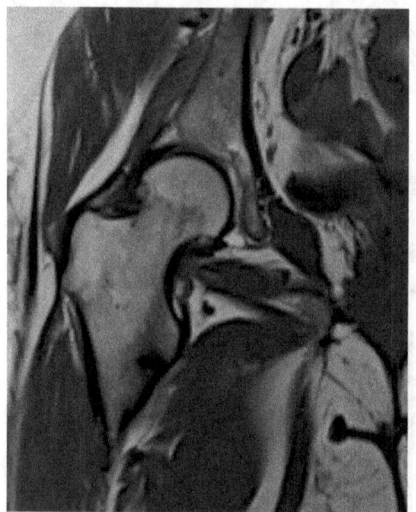 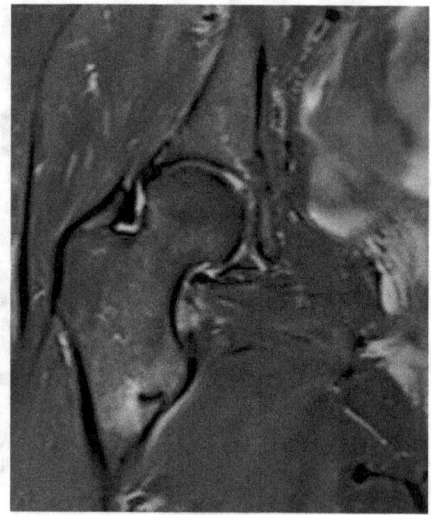

Coronal T1 (A) and STIR (B) images of the pelvis demonstrate low signal fracture line with surrounding edema in the medial aspect of proximal femur along lesser trochanter.

Nuclear medicine studies are very sensitive for detection of osseous injury and fractures, however, lack specificity. Bone scintigraphy detects bone turnover which can occur in tumor, arthritis, fracture, osteonecrosis, infection, or surrounding inflammatory changes. Multifocal involvement is usually suggestive of metastatic disease. However, unifocal involvement, involvement near a large joint, or an atypical location pose diagnostic dilemmas. Radiographs are inexpensive, readily available and show classic manifestations of stress fracture (linear sclerosis, callus, periosteal reaction), osteoarthritis (joint space narrowing and osteophytosis), osseous lesions (margins, matrix, periosteal reaction, and cortical break through), infection (erosion, cortical indistinctness) and overt fractures. If a diagnosis can confidently be made on radiographs, no further imaging is usually necessary although follow-up radiographs to document stability may be recommended in a subset of cases. In cases where more precise anatomic localization and characterization is deemed necessary, an MRI study of the region of interest may be performed with optional utilization of intravenous contrast in cases where neoplastic involvement or infectious process is suspected.

# References

1. Expert Panel on Musculoskeletal I, Bencardino JT, Stone TJ, Roberts CC, Appel M, Baccei SJ, et al. ACR Appropriateness Criteria((R)) Stress (Fatigue/Insufficiency) Fracture, Including Sacrum, Excluding Other Vertebrae. J Am Coll Radiol. 2017;14(5S):S293-S306. Epub 2017/05/06. doi: 10.1016/j.jacr.2017.02.035. PubMed PMID: 28473086.

2. Nattiv A, Kennedy G, Barrack MT, Abdelkerim A, Goolsby MA, Arends JC, et al. Correlation of MRI Grading of Bone Stress Injuries With Clinical Risk Factors and Return to Play. The American Journal of Sports Medicine. 2013;41(8):1930-41. doi: 10.1177/0363546513490645.

3. Agrawal A, Purandare N, Shah S, Rangarajan V. Metastatic mimics on bone scan: "All that glitters is not metastatic". Indian J Nucl Med. 2016;31(3):185-90. Epub 2016/07/08. doi: 10.4103/0972-3919.183605. PubMed PMID: 27385887; PubMed Central PMCID: PMCPMC4918480.

# Part III. Chronic or Nontraumatic Pain

Patients complaining of chronic musculoskeletal-related pain (6 weeks or more) represent a broad range of potential diseases. Radiography is usually the first imaging study, if only to eliminate certain diagnoses or to document the baseline condition. The next imaging recommendation is often MRI, but depending on specific circumstances, sometimes US, nuclear imaging, or CT are better choices.

# Chapter 16. Chronic or Nontraumatic Hand Pain

Felix S. Chew, MD, Hyojeong Lee, MD.

Radiography is the initial exam for nontraumatic hand pain. MRI, US, or CT may be helpful for further evaluation, and the bone scan may have a problem-solving role.

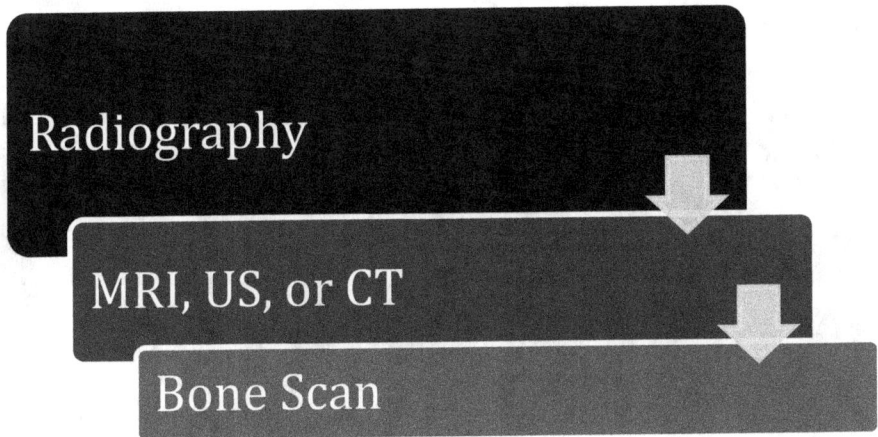

# Case 16-1

62-year-old woman who presented with chronic bilateral hand pain of gradual onset that was worse in the fingers. She denied trauma. What is the best initial study to further evaluate the etiology of her pain?

This scenario concerns the most appropriate imaging study for a patient with chronic hand pain of no particular etiology.

Sensible recommendation: XR HANDS 3 VIEW

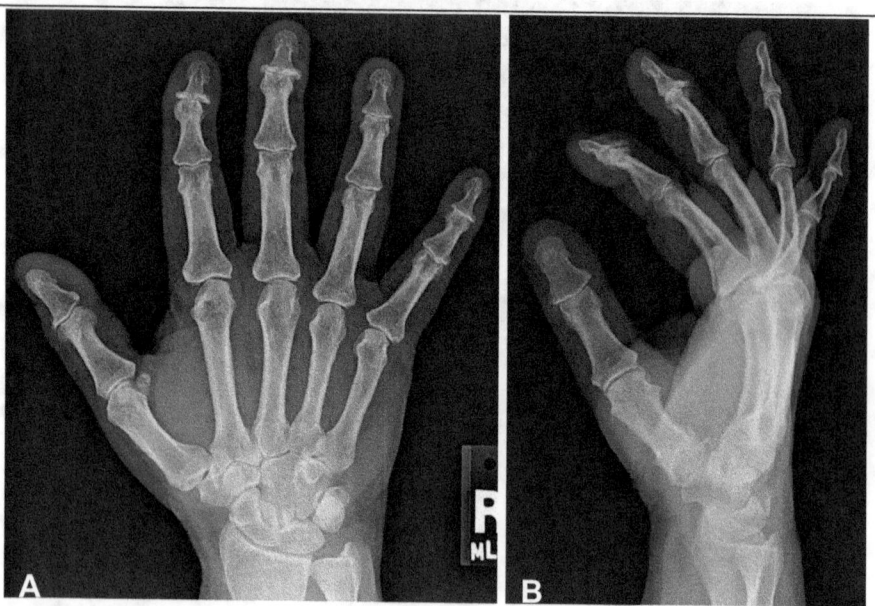

PA (A) and lateral radiographs (B) of the right hand show features of osteoarthritis at the DIP joints of the fingers. Radiographs of the left hand (not shown) had similar findings.

Radiography should be the initial imaging exam for patients with chronic hand pain. In this case, the findings and the distribution of disease, when combined with clinical findings, should be sufficient to provide the diagnosis. Routine radiography of the hand often consists of PA, oblique, and lateral views. The lateral view is particularly valuable in identifying osteophytes in the interphalangeal joints, a hallmark of osteoarthritis.

# Case 16-2

59-year-old woman with chronic bilateral hand pain and a diagnosis of rheumatoid arthritis. Her pain and disabilities have been worsening despite medical therapy. What is the best initial imaging study to evaluate her disease?

This scenario concerns the most appropriate imaging study for a patient with known arthritis.

Sensible recommendation: XR HANDS 3 VIEW

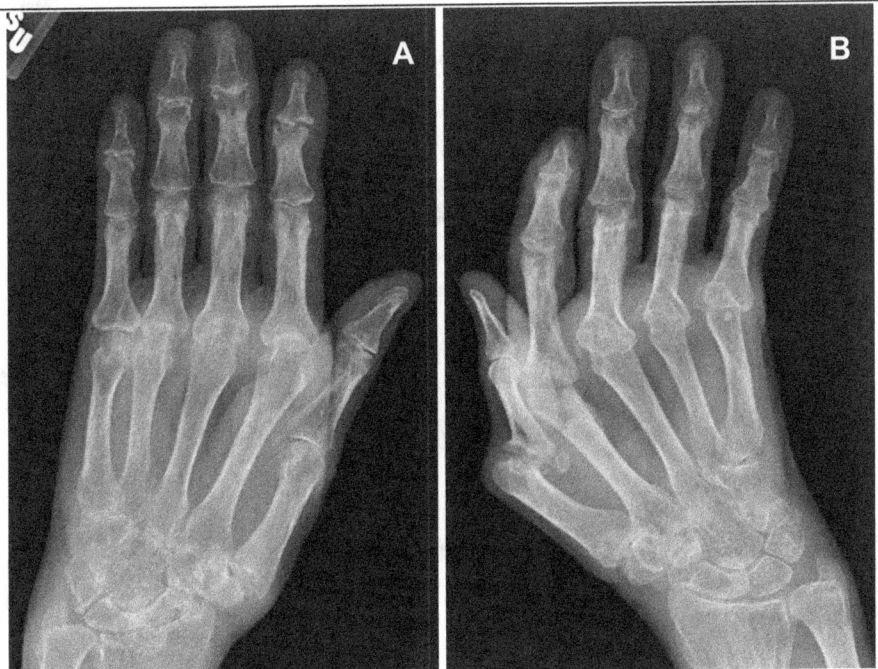

PA radiographs of the left (A) and right (B) hands show marked osteopenia, deformties, and erosions, worst at the MCP joints.

Radiography is the procedure of choice for initial evaluation of arthritis of the hand. Further evaluation for synovitis could be performed with MRI HANDS WOW CONTRAST or, if the local expertise is available, ultrasound.

## Case 16-3

A 45-year-old man with a history of psoriasis presents with diffuse hand pain. The patient also has severe morning stiffness and has diffuse psoriatic lesions over his body and severe nail disease. What is the best initial imaging study to evaluate her disease?

This scenario concerns the most appropriate imaging study for a patient with chronic hand pain. Suspect seronegative spondyloarthropathy.

Sensible recommendation: XR HANDS 3 VIEW

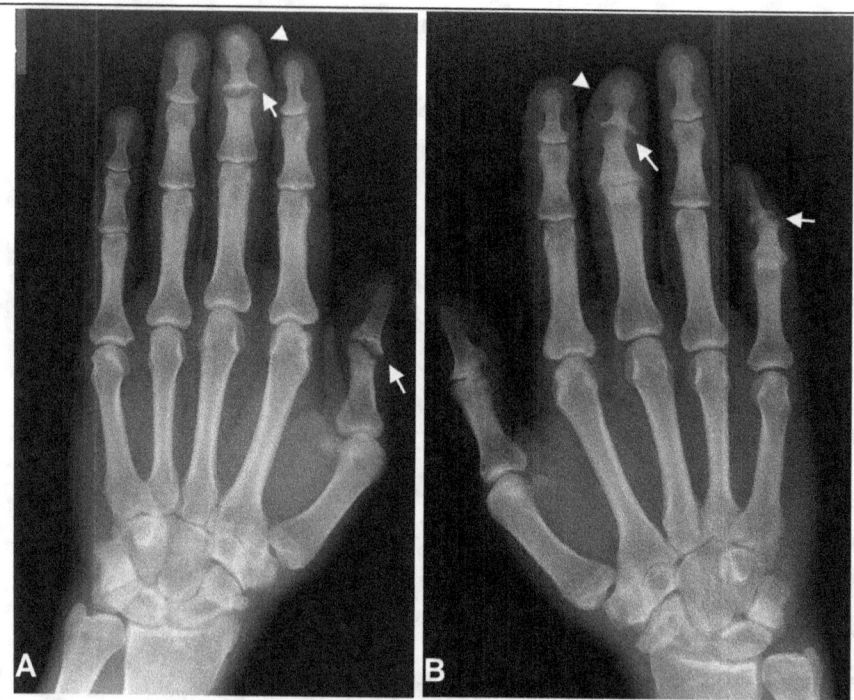

PA radiographs of the left (A) and right (B) hands show pencil-in-cup erosions involving DIP joints of middle finger and thumb on the left (white arrows in A), and DIP joints of middle and small fingers (white arrows in B). There is soft tissue swelling involving middle fingers in both hands (white arrowheads in A and B).

Imaging assessment for the seronegative spondyloarthropathies, which include psoriatic arthritis, reactive arthritis, ankylosing spondylitis, and arthritis associated with inflammatory bowel disease, includes the synovial spaces, entheses, and osseous surfaces of the extremities. The radiographic findings of spondyloarthropathy related to erosions, enthesitis, and bone proliferation are well characterized by radiography. Bone proliferation, in the form of periostitis and enthesitis, is a hallmark of the spondyloarthropathies and may occur at any cortical bone, including both tendon and ligament attachments.

# Case 16-4

73-year-old man with previously diagnosed with gout, presenting with bilateral prominent nodules on his hands. Reports that over the last 2 day he has started having some pain in his middle fingers, left greater than the right, with motion. What is the best initial imaging study to evaluate his disease?

This scenario concerns the most appropriate imaging study for a patient with chronic hand pain. Suspect gout.

Sensible recommendation: XR HANDS 3 VIEW

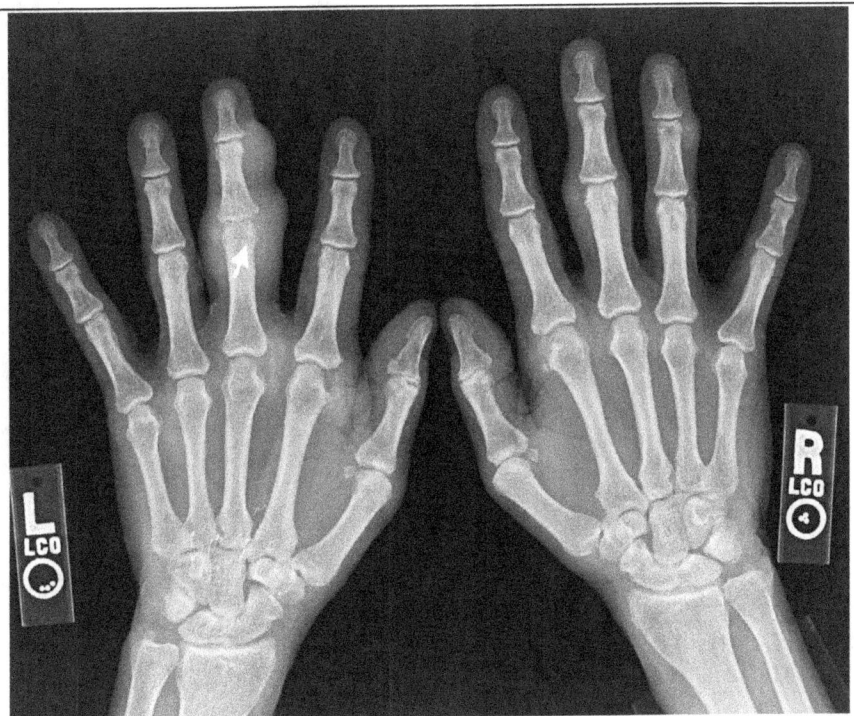

PA radiographs of bilateral hands show multifocal nodular soft tissue tophi in both hands with amorphous soft tissue density. A subtle bony erosion is noted in the PIP joint of left middle finger.

Gout can involve the synovial spaces, showing joint distention due to effusion and synovial hypertrophy. Soft tissue tophi, if not calcified, may appear nonspecific as focal increased opacity on radiography; however, adjacent characteristic erosions may be identified. Identification of erosions may prove difficult when located where osseous structures overlap.

## Case 16-5

92-year-old man presents chronic bilateral hand pain and swelling of MCP joints of right middle finger. Patient doesn't have any prior injury, and also denies any history of arthritis. The clinician is concerned about pseudogout. What is the best initial imaging study to evaluate his disease?

This scenario concerns the most appropriate imaging study for a patient with chronic hand pain. Suspect calcium pyrophosphate dihydrate disease (pseudogout).

Sensible recommendation: XR HANDS 3 VIEW

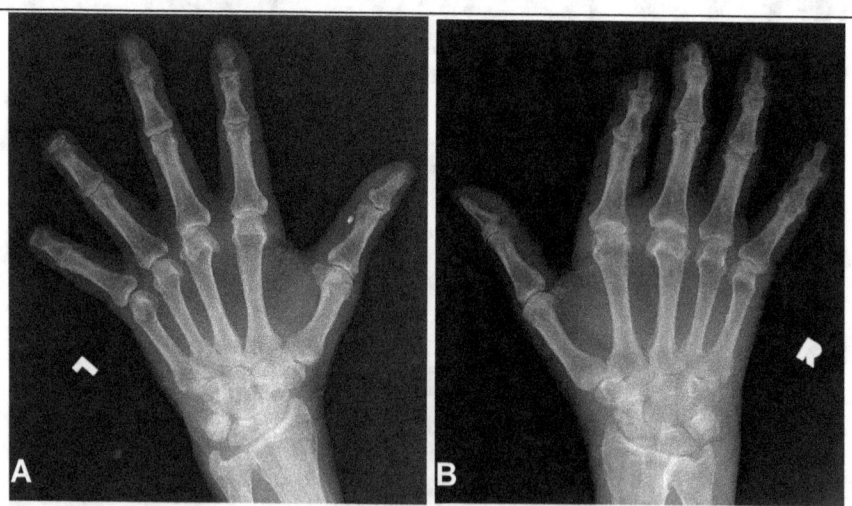

PA radiographs of left (A) and right hand (B) show joint space narrowing and hook-like osteophytosis in MCP joints of both middle fingers. There is chondrocalcinosis of triangular fibrocartilage in left hand (A), and a large subchondral cyst in right distal radius (B). Also, there is joint space narrowing involving the radiocarpal joints. Amputated distal phalanges are noted at left ring and small fingers.

The radiographic hallmark of pseudogout is soft tissue calcification in the form of chondrocalcinosis, as well as tendon, ligament, and capsular calcification. Radiography can be effective in demonstrating such calcifications in the extremities. Target sites to evaluate for fibrocartilage chondrocalcinosis include the triangular fibrocartilage of the wrists, the menisci of the knees, and the symphysis pubis and labrum at the pelvis, whereas involvement of the hyaline cartilage may occur at any joint. The osseous changes from associated arthropathy characteristically involve the radiocarpal, metacarpophalangeal, and patellofemoral joints and are well demonstrated by radiography.

## Case 16-6

A 69-year-old man presents with pain and swelling in the bilateral hands that has been ongoing for more than five years. Patient denies any history of trauma or injury to the hand. He states that he has noticed an increase in stiffness over the past few years. He occasionally takes anti-inflammatories for pain but has not been limited in activities by the pain. Pain is aggravated by activity and cold. What is the best initial imaging study to evaluate his disease?

This scenario concerns the most appropriate imaging study for a patient with chronic hand pain. Suspect erosive osteoarthritis.

Sensible recommendation: XR HANDS 3 VIEW

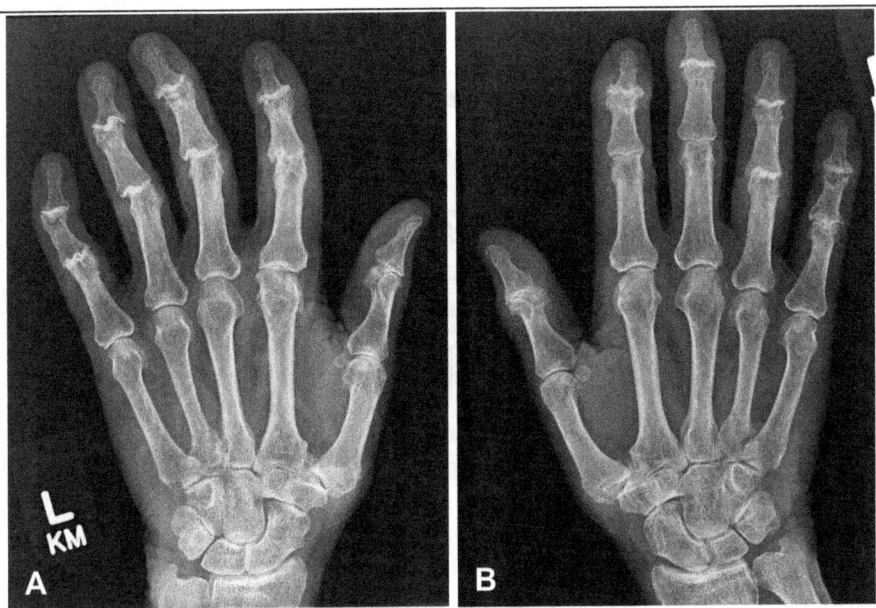

PA radiographs of the left (A) and right (B) hands show advanced joint space narrowing involving interphalangeal joints, distal greater than the proximal, associated with subchondral erosions, mainly along the distal interphalangeal joints.

In addition to joint space narrowing, the osseous abnormalities of arthritis that are assessed include erosions and bone proliferation. Erosions, which appear as cortical discontinuity, may be seen at the margins of synovial joints (rheumatoid arthritis and spondyloarthropathies), periarticular (gout), central (erosive osteoarthritis), and at the enthesis (spondyloarthropathies). Imaging of osseous abnormalities typically begins with radiography]. Although specific, radiography has somewhat low sensitivity given the degree of overlap of the osseous structures. Multiple radiographic views of a joint are often needed to improve erosion identification, such as the hands (posteroanterior, oblique, lateral, semisupinated). The characteristic central erosions of erosive osteoarthritis involving the interphalangeal joints are well demonstrated by radiography.

# Case 16-7

48-year-old man with chronic thumb pain. His pain and disabilities have been worsening despite medical therapy. Radiographs of the hand are normal. What is the next study to evaluate his condition?

This scenario concerns the most appropriate imaging study for a patient with suspected De Quervain disease.

Sensible recommendation: MRI WRIST WO CONTRAST

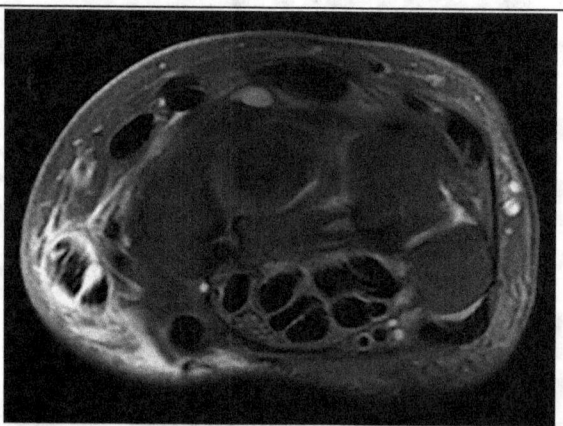

De Quervain tenosynovitis. Axial T2 FS MRI of the left wrist shows T2 hyperintensity adjacent to the extensor pollicis brevis and abductor pollicis longus compatible with inflammation. There is tendinosis of both tendons, with evidence of split tears.

MRI is the procedure of choice for initial evaluation of tenosynovitis of the hand. Further evaluation for synovitis could be performed with MRI wo/w contrast or ultrasound. US may also be used to evaluate tendons and tenosynovitis, but its effectiveness depends on the local expertise.

# References

1.  Jacobson JA, Roberts CC, Bencardino JT, Appel M, Arnold E, Baccei SJ, Cassidy RC, Chang EY, Fox MG, Greenspan BS, Gyftopoulos S, Hochman MG, Mintz DN, Newman JS, Rosenberg ZS, Shah NA, Small KM, Weissman BN. ACR Appropriateness Criteria(®) Chronic Extremity Joint Pain-Suspected Inflammatory Arthritis. J Am Coll Radiol. 2017 May;14(5S):S81-S89. doi: 10.1016/j.jacr.2017.02.006. Review. PMID: 28473097.
2.  American College of Radiology. ACR Appropriateness Criteria: Chronic Extremity Joint Pain- Suspected Inflammatory Arthritis, 2016. https://acsearch.acr.org/docs/3097211/Narrative/ (accessed April 24, 2021).

# Chapter 17. Chronic or Nontraumatic Wrist Pain

Jack Porrino, MD, Erin Flaherty, MD, Jennifer Favinger, MD

Radiography is the initial exam for nontraumatic or chronic wrist pain. MRI, US, or CT may be helpful for further evaluation, and the bone scan may have a problem-solving role.

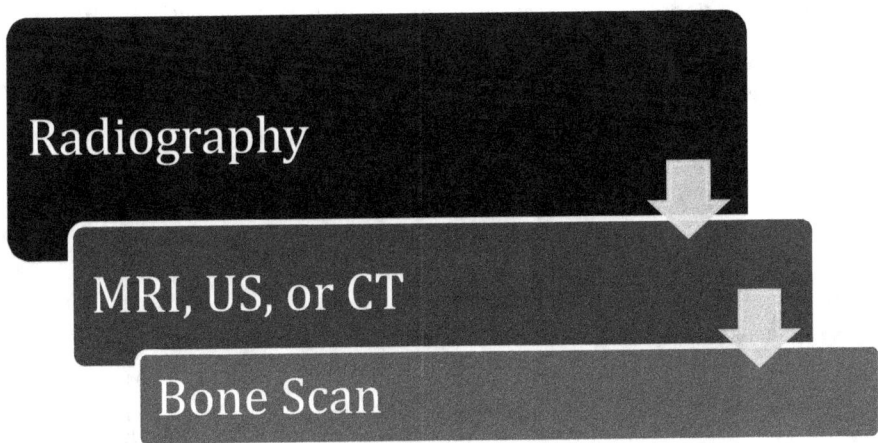

# Case 17-1

22-year-old man with chronic right wrist pain that began approximately 2 years prior when he twisted his wrist while being arrested. The patient reports weakness and limited extension of the right wrist, and intermittent episodes of pain. What is the best initial study?

This scenario concerns the best initial imaging study for a patient with chronic wrist pain, with or without prior injury.

Sensible recommendation: XR WRIST 3 VIEW

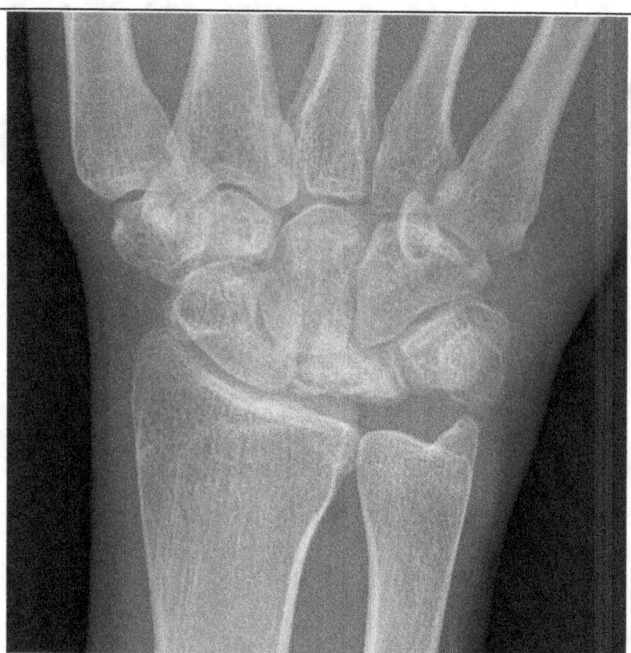

PA radiograph of the right wrist demonstrates irregular sclerosis and collapse of the lunate bone related to avascular necrosis of the lunate.

Imaging of the patient with chronic wrist pain should begin with a standard radiographic examination. This provides a simple and inexpensive means to diagnose a variety of potential pain generators such as arthritis, complications of prior injury, infection, musculoskeletal tumors, impaction syndromes, and static wrist instability. Radiographs can also be used to assess ulnar variance.

## Case 17-2

36-year-old woman with 1.5-year history of dorsal central left wrist pain worse with extension. Two prior radiographic series spanning a 15-month time frame were normal. What is the most appropriate next study?

This scenario concerns the next imaging study for a patient with chronic wrist pain where routine radiographs are normal or nonspecific and symptoms are persistent.

Sensible recommendation: MRI WRIST WO CONTRAST

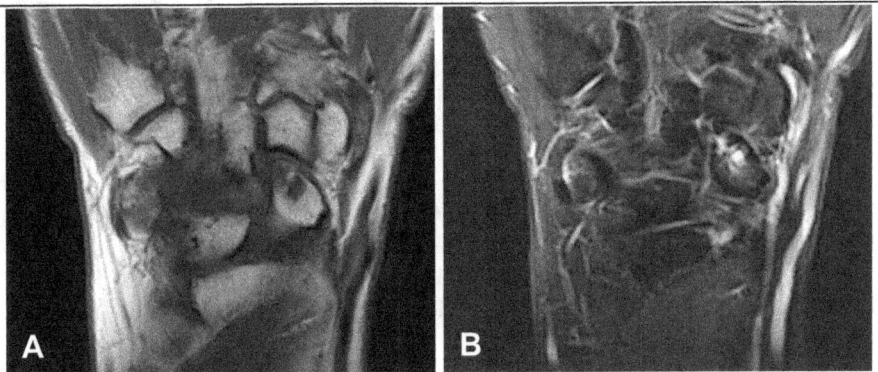

Coronal T1 (A) and T2 FS (A) MRI of the left wrist demonstrate subchondral cystic change within the distal pole of the scaphoid related to osteoarthritis of the triscaphe joint.

In those with chronic wrist pain, and a normal routine radiographic series, MRI of the wrist is the study of choice capable of identifying the cause of pain from a variety of etiologies. MRI of the wrist accurately demonstrates abnormalities of the bone marrow, articular cartilage, intrinsic and extrinsic ligaments, triangular fibrocartilage complex (TFCC), synovium, tendons, and neurovascular structures.

## Case 17-3

76-year-old man with normal radiographs of the right wrist, but with clinical suspicion for inflammatory arthritis involving the wrist. Next study?

This scenario concerns the next imaging study for a patient with chronic wrist pain where routine radiographs are normal or nonspecific and the clinician suspects inflammatory arthritis.

Sensible recommendation: MRI WRIST WO/W CONTRAST

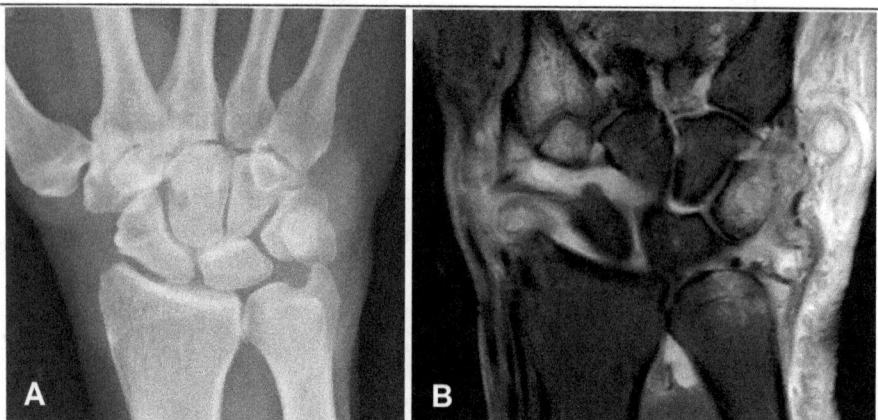

Frontal radiograph (A) of the right wrist and coronal T2 FS MRI (B), the latter with extensive joint effusion, synovitis, and reactive marrow changes suggesting inflammatory arthritis.

For those with suspected inflammatory arthritis, and a normal routine radiographic series of the wrist, MRI with intravenous gadolinium may be helpful to stage disease and guide therapy. In those with inflammatory arthritis, intravenous contrast helps to identify active synovitis as well as inflammatory tenosynovitis, allowing for early diagnosis, prognostication, and treatment guidance. MRI is more sensitive than radiographs and ultrasound in the detection of erosions. MRI can also identify enhancing bone marrow edema, or osteitis, a predictor of future disease progression and functional deterioration.

## Case 17-4

45-year-old woman with a history of intravenous drug use, prior left wrist infection with debridement, and prior proximal row carpectomy for post-infectious arthritis presents with left wrist pain and swelling with chills. There is clinical concern for septic arthritis involving the wrist, however no significant change in appearance of the wrist on radiographs acquired upon admission when compared to the previous studies. What is the most appropriate next study to obtain to establish the diagnosis of septic arthritis?

This scenario concerns the next imaging study for a patient with chronic wrist pain where routine radiographs are normal or show nonspecific arthritis, and infection is suspected.

Sensible recommendation: XR JOINT ASPIRATION WRIST

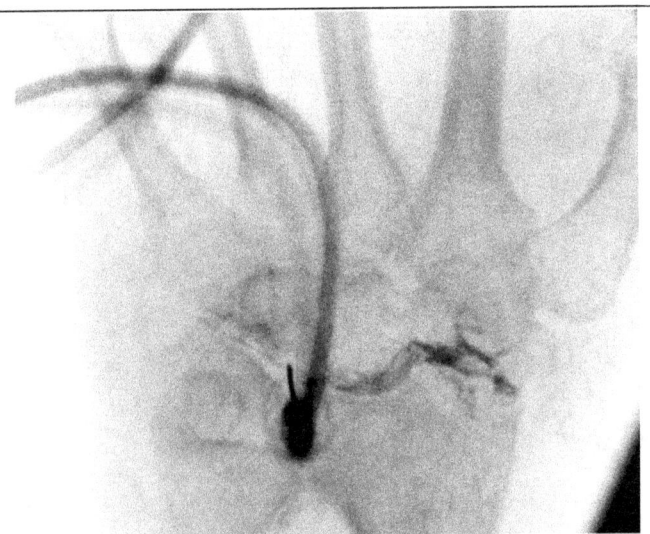

A single fluoroscopic image of the left wrist acquired during image-guided arthrocentesis for suspected septic arthritis. Contrast confirms intra-articular location of the needle, and there are post-operative changes of proximal row carpectomy.

When radiographs are normal, or demonstrate nonspecific arthritis, and infection is of clinical concern, arthrocentesis of the wrist should be performed. Neither Tc-99m bone scan, ultrasound, CT wo/w contrast, and MRI wo/w contrast are considered appropriate to establish the diagnosis of infection in this clinical context. Image guidance may be necessary.

# Case 17-5

A 26-year-old woman reports chronic left ulnar-sided wrist pain with a history of remote trauma to the affected area. She reports no improvement with non-steroidal anti-inflammatory drugs or splinting, and her radiographs were interpreted as normal. What is the next most appropriate study to obtain?

This scenario concerns the next imaging study for a patient with chronic ulnar-sided wrist pain and routine radiographs are normal or nonspecific.

Sensible recommendation: MRI WRIST WO CONTRAST

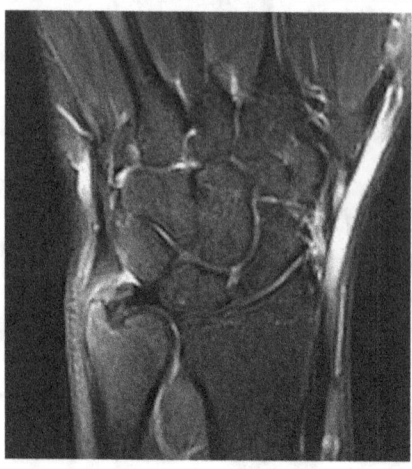

Coronal T2 FS MRI of the left wrist demonstrates edema within the ulnar styloid and partial tear of the peripheral triangular fibrocartilage.

Ulnar-sided wrist pain is often related to ulnocarpal impaction, TFCC lesions, and/or lunotriquetral ligament tears. High-resolution MRI is an effective examination in these patients, with the caveat being a relatively low sensitivity for the identification of lesions involving the distal and ulnar attachments of the TFCC. MR arthrography improves diagnosis for TFCC lesions.

# Case 17-6

58-year-old woman reports progressive radial-sided wrist pain and swelling. Her right wrist radiographic series was interpreted as normal. What is the next most appropriate study to establish a diagnosis?

This scenario concerns the next imaging study for a patient with chronic radial-sided wrist pain and radiographs are normal or nonspecific.

Sensible recommendation: MRI WRIST WO CONTRAST

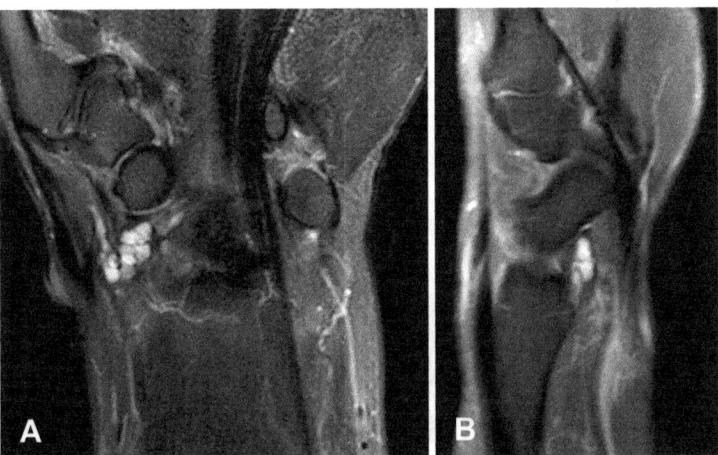

Coronal T2 FS (A) and sagittal PD FS (B) MRI demonstrate a large ganglion cyst along the volar surface of the radial wrist.

MRI is the preferred examination in those with chronic radial-sided wrist pain, with the ability to diagnose bone, tendon, tendon sheath, ligament, and synovial abnormalities. Direct MR arthrography increases the accuracy for the detection of scapholunate ligament tears. When there is strong clinical suspicion that the cause of pain may be a ganglion cyst or de Quervain disease, US may be a better choice than MRI as a screening test, recognizing that a second study (typically MRI) may be necessary if the US is normal or demonstrates a non-specific solid mass

## Case 17-7

29-year-old woman with chronic left-sided wrist pain obtains a routine radiographic series of the left wrist demonstrating minimal degenerative change at the basal joint of the thumb and vague sclerosis within the lunate suspicious for Kienbock disease but not conclusive. What is the next most appropriate study to confirm the diagnosis?

This scenario concerns the next imaging study for a patient with chronic wrist pain in whom Kienbock disease is suspected but radiographs are not definitive.

Sensible recommendation: MRI WRIST WO CONTRAST

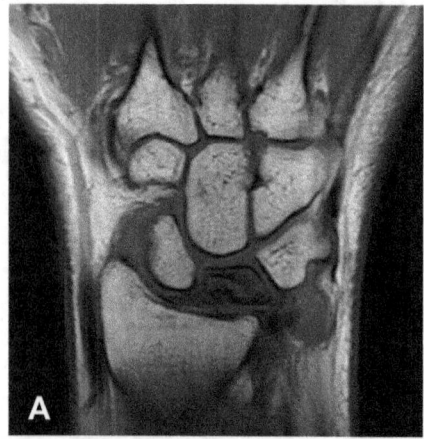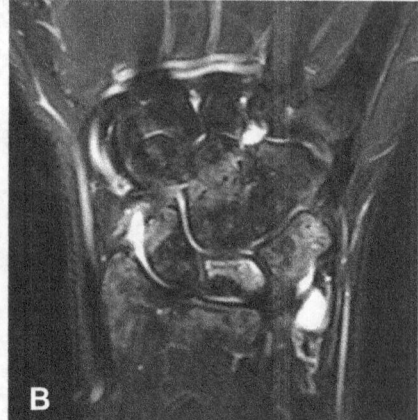

Coronal T1 (A) and T2 FS (B) MRI of the left wrist with abnormal bone marrow signal, fracture, and collapse of the lunate compatible with Kienbock disease.

MRI is more accurate than radiographs in the diagnosis of Kienbock disease. When there is strong clinical concern for osteonecrosis of the wrist, but with normal or nonspecific wrist radiographs, MRI is the most appropriate study to obtain. In general, MRI is considered the probable study of choice in patients without fractures who have suspected osteonecrosis of the wrist.

## Case 17-8

A 57-year-old woman with Kienbock disease diagnosed on clinical examination and radiographic findings is seeking operative intervention. If the surgeon is interested in pre-operative planning, specifically to assess the degree of lunate collapse and fragmentation/fracture, what would be the most appropriate next study?

This scenario concerns the next imaging study for a patient with chronic wrist pain and a radiographic diagnosis of Kienbock disease.

Sensible recommendation: CT WRIST WO CONTRAST

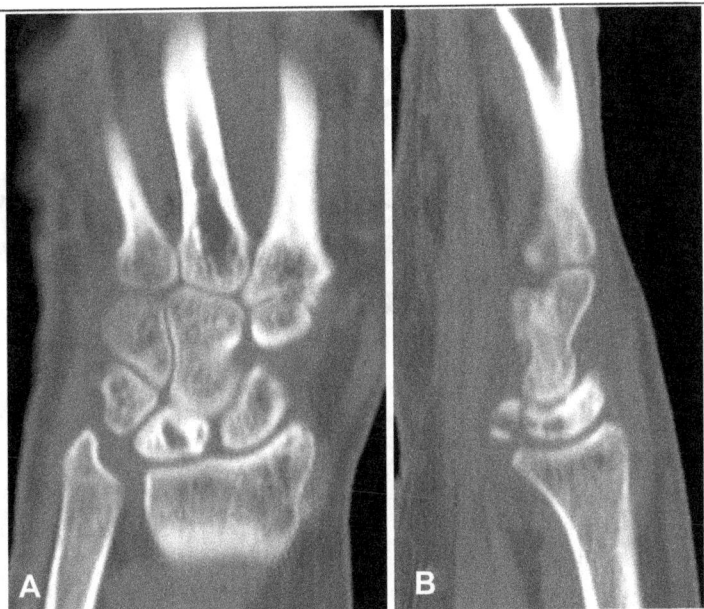

Coronal (A) and sagittal (B) CT images of the wrist demonstrate a mixed lucent and sclerotic appearance of the lunate with fragmentation/fracture compatible with Kienbock disease.

CT permits high-resolution imaging with much shorter acquisition time than MRI. When high-detail imaging of bone cortex or trabeculae is necessary for surgical planning, CT is the most appropriate study to obtain. Specifically, CT helps with assessing the degree of collapse and presence of associated fractures.

## Case 17-9

A 32-year-old man with ongoing right dorsal wrist pain for 2 years and with fluctuance in the area suspicious for an underlying ganglion cyst obtains a routine right wrist radiographic series with no apparent abnormality. What is the most appropriate next imaging step?

This scenario concerns the next imaging study for a patient with chronic wrist pain and palpable mass or suspected occult ganglion cyst; normal or nonspecific radiographs.

Sensible recommendation: US WRIST, MRI WRIST WO CONTRAST, or MRI WRIST WO/W CONTRAST

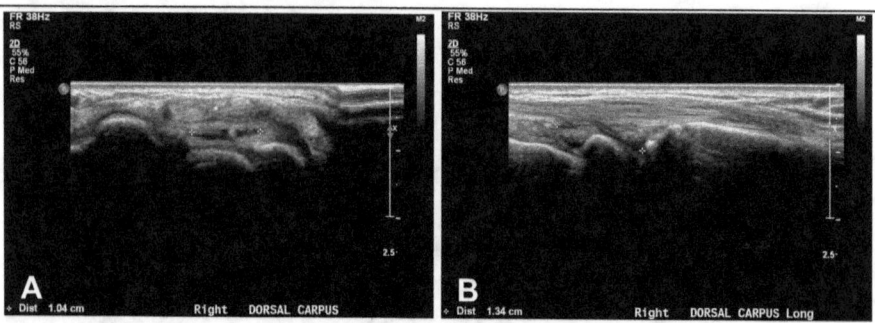

Transverse (A) and longitudinal (B) sonographic images of the right wrist demonstrate a thin, serpiginous ganglion cyst arising from the radiocarpal joint.

When there is clinical concern for a ganglion cyst, US, MRI WRIST WO/W CONTRAST, and MRI WRIST WO CONTRAST are all considered equally appropriate. MRI can be performed without contrast if a radiologist is available to check the initial images and administer contrast if these images are inconclusive. The use of intravenous contrast with MRI may also be helpful in distinguishing ganglia from synovitis or solid tumors. US is often the most cost-effective initial examination, recognizing that a second study (typically MRI) may be needed if the initial US is normal or shows a non-specific solid mass.

## Case 17-10

A 25-year-old woman who recently fell and landed onto an outstretched right wrist reports persistent pain despite a normal radiographic series acquired approximately 3.5 weeks prior. Her most likely diagnosis is a radiographically occult fracture of the wrist. What is the most appropriate next study to confirm the diagnosis?

This scenario concerns the next imaging study for a patient with chronic wrist pain for more than 3 weeks in whom there is suspicion for radiographically occult fracture or stress fracture because initial radiographs were negative.

Sensible recommendation: MRI WRIST WO CONTRAST or CT WRIST WO CONTRAST

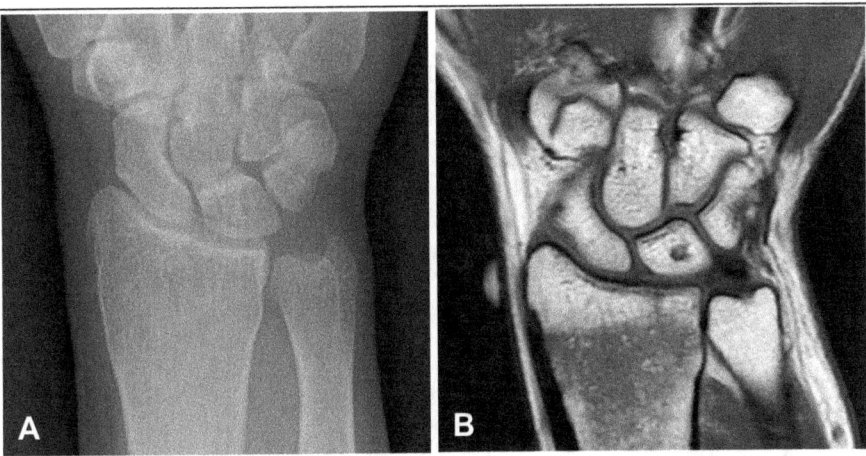

Initial frontal radiograph (A) was normal. (B) Follow-up T1 MRI performed 3.5 weeks later shows distal radius fracture and triquetral contusion.

For the diagnosis of radiographically occult fractures responsible for chronic wrist pain, both MRI and CT have a role in specific circumstances. MRI can be used as an alternative to presumptive casting and repeat radiographs. MRI is also sensitive to stress fractures of the physes.

## Case 17-11

A 70-year-old woman presents with chronic limited range of motion involving her right wrist following a volleyball injury that occurred approximately 20 years prior, managed non-operatively and without imaging. Two months before presentation, she sustained a fall while hiking at which time she landed on an outstretched hand, resulting in pain. Upon presentation, radiographs demonstrate a chronic appearing fracture through the waist of the scaphoid. The clinician is interested in evaluating the vascular status of the scaphoid and would like to know the most appropriate imaging modality.

This scenario concerns the next imaging study for a patient with chronic wrist pain where initial radiographs show an old scaphoid fracture. Imaging is needed to assess for nonunion, malunion, osteonecrosis, and/or post-traumatic osteoarthritis.

Sensible recommendation: MRI WRIST WO CONTRAST

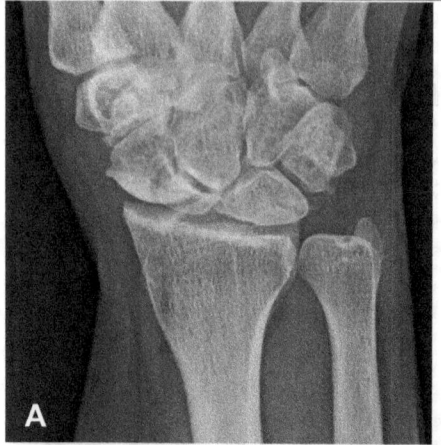

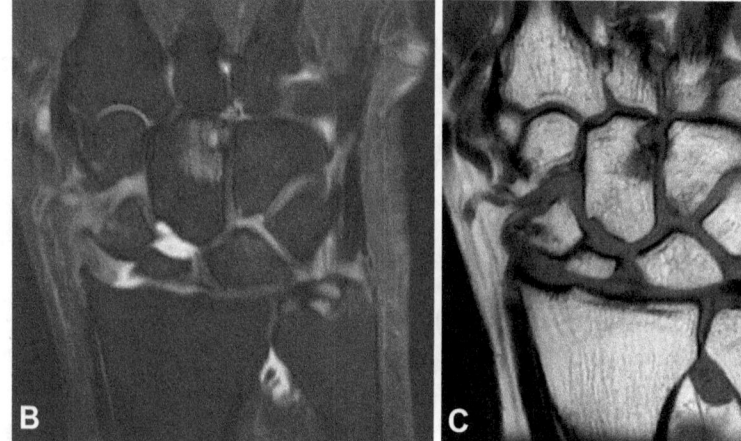

PA radiograph of the right wrist (A) demonstrates chronic scaphoid fracture non-union with radiocarpal osteoarthritis. Coronal T2 FS MRI (B) and T1 MRI (C) exhibit normal, viable bone marrow signal within the proximal and distal pole of the scaphoid.

MRI has a moderate sensitivity and specificity for predicting osteonecrosis of the proximal pole of the scaphoid following fracture. The routine use of intravenous contrast for this indication is controversial, despite improved accuracy for determining osteonecrosis and predicting graft healing, as enhancement can be seen in both viable and nonviable fragments.

## Case 17-12

A 56-year-old woman with paresthesias along the distribution of her first through third digits of her left hand presents to clinic with a presumptive diagnosis of carpal tunnel syndrome. She is diagnosed with rheumatoid arthritis. What is the most appropriate study to order during the initial work-up?

This scenario concerns the initial imaging study for a patient with chronic wrist pain and suspected carpal tunnel syndrome.

Sensible recommendation: MRI WRIST WO CONTRAST or US WRIST

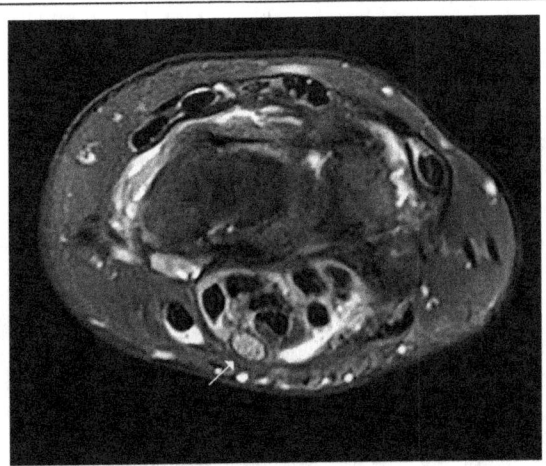

Axial T2 FS MRI of the left wrist demonstrates enlarged median nerve in the carpal tunnel with increased signal intensity (white arrow). There is fluid along the flexor and extensor tendon sheath in keeping with tenosynovitis.

The diagnosis of carpal tunnel syndrome is typically established by clinical signs and symptoms, combined with electrodiagnostic studies. While both MRI and US findings correlate with the diagnosis and severity of carpal tunnel syndrome, they are typically not necessary. MRI may have value in rare cases where a mass is thought to be responsible for medial nerve dysfunction.

# References

1. Rubin DA, Roberts CC, Bencardino JT, Bell AM, Cassidy RC, Chang EY, Gyftopoulos S, Metter DF, Morrison WB, Subhas N, Tambar S, Towers JD, Yu JS, Kransdorf MJ. ACR Appropriateness Criteria(®) Chronic Wrist Pain. J Am Coll Radiol. 2018 May;15(5S):S39-S55. doi: 10.1016/j.jacr.2018.03.021. PMID: 29724426.
2. American College of Radiology. ACR Appropriateness Criteria: Chronic Wrist Pain. American College of Radiology, revised 2017. https://acsearch.acr.org/docs/69427/Narrative/ (accessed April 24, 2021).
3. Dalinka MK, Alazraki N, Berquist TH, Daffner RH, DeSmet AA, el-Khoury GY, Goergen TG, Keats TE, Manaster BJ, Newberg A, Pavlov H, Schweitzer ME, Haralson RH 3rd, McCabe JB. Chronic wrist pain. American College of Radiology. ACR Appropriateness Criteria. Radiology. 2000 Jun;215 Suppl:333-8. PMID: 11037445.

# Chapter 18. Chronic or Nontraumatic Elbow Pain

Lindsay Stratchko, DO, Eric Walker, MD, Jonelle Petscavage-Thomas, MD, Hyojeong Lee, MD.

Radiography is the initial exam for chronic or nontraumatic elbow pain. MRI, US, or CT may be helpful for further evaluation, and the bone scan may have a problem-solving role.

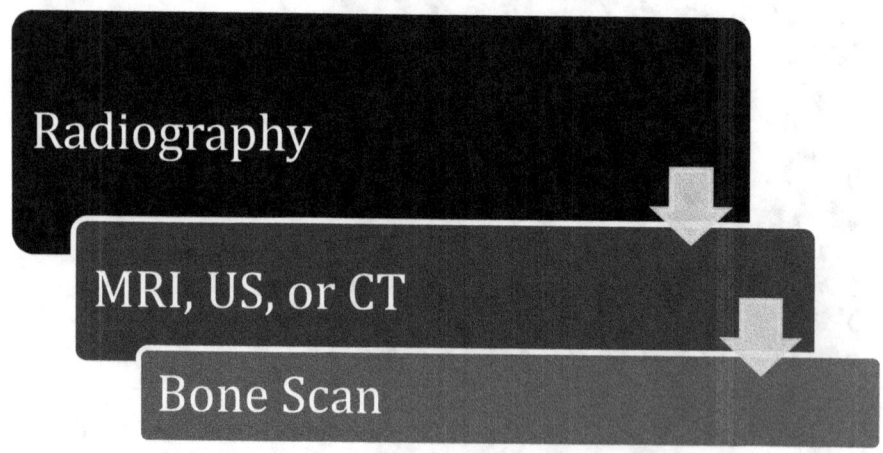

# Case 18-1

A 53-year-old right-handed woman presents to her primary care physician with a 3-month history of right elbow pain. She is able to perform her activities of daily living and continues to work as an administrative assistant. She denies a history of preceding trauma. Which imaging test should be the first study ordered?

This scenario concerns the first imaging evaluation of chronic elbow pain.

Sensible recommendation: XR ELBOW 2 VIEW

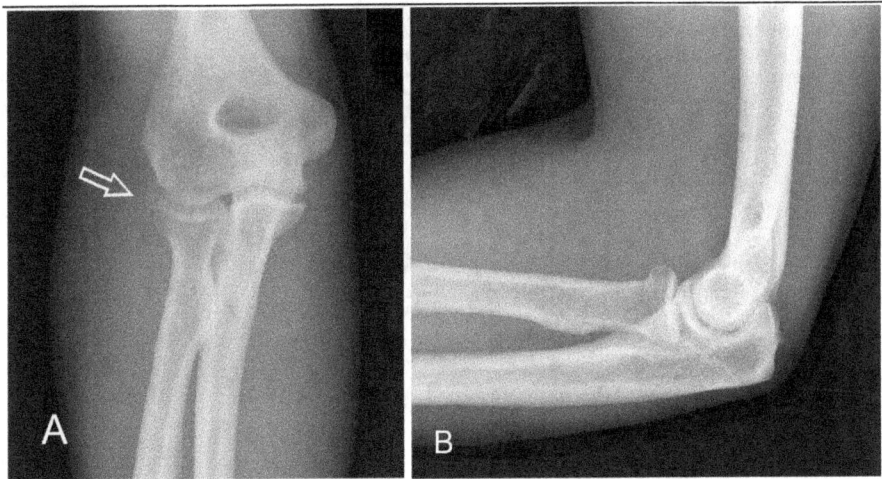

AP (A) and lateral (B) right elbow radiographs demonstrate amorphous calcifications along the lateral aspect of the elbow joint in the region of the extensor tendons. These findings reflect hydroxyapatite deposition (HADD) within the extensor tendons, which is commonly seen in the setting of calcific tendinitis.

Radiographs are the initial diagnostic test of choice in the assessment of non-traumatic chronic elbow pain. An etiology of the patient's symptoms may be established via radiography, allowing appropriate treatment without the need for more expensive imaging studies. Findings of osteophytes or intra-articular/peri-articular calcifications can be readily seen on radiographs, suggesting common diagnoses such as osteoarthritis, heterotopic ossification, calcific tendinitis, and chondrocalcinosis. Radiography also plays an initial role in identifying pathology that requires surgical intervention, particularly in the setting of intra-articular osteocartilaginous fragments. Additional imaging may be indicated for surgical planning, or if pain persists and radiographs are negative or equivocal.

# Case 18-2

44-year-old right-hand-dominant tennis player presents with right elbow pain. A couple of months she noticed that her elbow was sore with clicking and locking. She has no instability. Radiographs of elbow were negative. What is the most appropriate next imaging study?

This scenario concerns patients with mechanical symptoms (locking, clicking, limited motion); suspect intra-articular osteocartilaginous body or synovial abnormality; radiographs nondiagnostic.

Sensible recommendation: MRI ELBOW WO CONTRAST or MRI ARTHROGRAPHY ELBOW

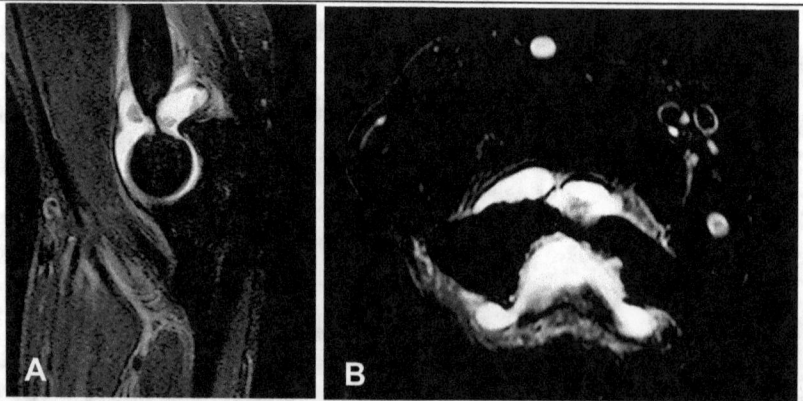

MR arthrography of elbow sagittal (A) and axial (B) T2 weighted FS images demonstrate cartilaginous intra-articular bodies and synovial thickening consistent with synovitis.

Radiographs are the initial diagnostic test of choice in the assessment of non-traumatic chronic elbow pain. An etiology of the patient's symptoms may be established via radiography, allowing appropriate treatment without the need for more expensive imaging studies. Findings of osteophytes or intra-articular/peri-articular calcifications can be readily seen on radiographs, suggesting common diagnoses such as osteoarthritis, heterotopic ossification, calcific tendinitis, and chondrocalcinosis. Radiography also plays an initial role in identifying pathology that requires surgical intervention, particularly in the setting of intra-articular osteocartilaginous fragments. Additional imaging may be indicated for surgical planning, or if pain persists and radiographs are negative or equivocal.

## Case 18-3

40-year-old man who has been a tennis and a volleyball player for a long period of time presents with chronic pain to the medial aspect of his right elbow, denies neurologic symptoms. The pain is associated with loss of extension of about 5 degrees and no signs of instability. He also has pain with overhead activities and increased stiffness after the volleyball game. Radiographs of elbow were negative. What is the most appropriate next imaging study?

This scenario concerns about a patient with chronic elbow pain. Suspect occult fracture or other bone abnormality; radiographs nondiagnostic.

Sensible recommendation: MRI ELBOW WO CONTRAST

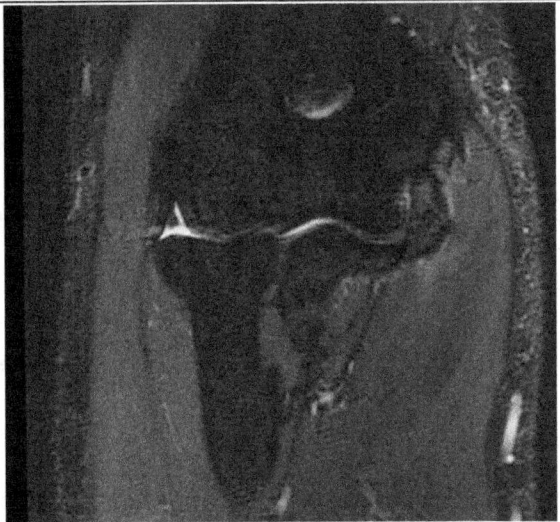

Coronal T2 MRI demonstrates fracture of the coronoid osteophyte.

Initial evaluation should begin with radiography, but if the radiographs are nondiagnostic, both traumatic and stress fractures may be identified with MRI and 3-phase bone scan. CT may have utility in detection and further evaluation of acute traumatic elbow fractures, as well as limited usefulness in identifying stress fractures at the elbow. US is helpful in demonstrating lipohemarthrosis in cases of occult elbow fractures in children. Additional imaging may be indicated for surgical planning, or if pain persists and radiographs are negative or equivocal.

## Case 18-4

14-year-old girl who is a gymnast presents with chronic right elbow pain.

On radiographs of elbow an osteochondral lesion is suspected. What is the most appropriate next imaging study?

This scenario concerns about a patient with chronic elbow pain. Assess stability of osteochondral injury; radiographs nondiagnostic.

Sensible recommendation: MRI ELBOW WO CONTRAST or MRI ARTHROGRAPHY ELBOW

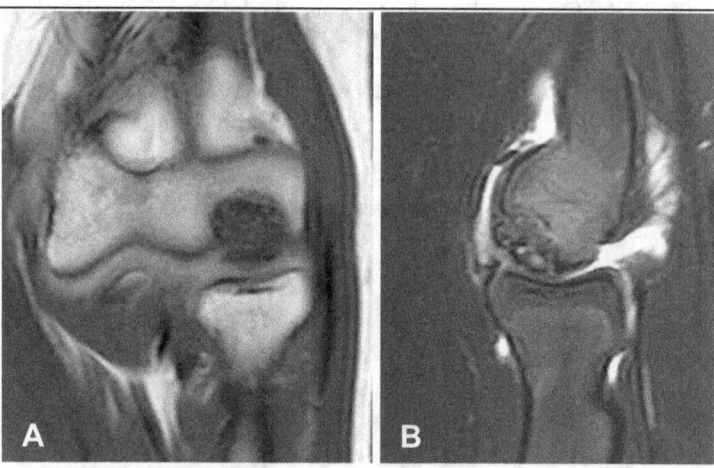

Coronal T1-weighted (A), and sagittal T2-weighted fat saturated image (B) demonstrate an osteochondral lesion in the capitellum. There are multiple cysts around the osteochondral lesion (B).

Some authors advocate MRI as the initial study for suspected osteochondral fracture. Intra-articular contrast has some limited usefulness in the diagnosis of chondral injuries on MRI. Both CT and MRI can assess for osteochondral fragment stability. MRI following direct intra-articular contrast administration (MR arthrography) can play a role in improving evaluation of stability of an osteochondral lesion. Similarly, CT arthrography provides more diagnostic information than standard CT in this setting.

## Case 18-5

64-year-old woman presents for evaluation of a mass in her left elbow. She noticed this a couple of months ago. It has not been painful. The mass gradually increased in size. Her elbow radiographs were non-diagnostic. What is the most appropriate next imaging study?

This scenario concerns about a patient with a palpable soft tissue mass; radiographs nondiagnostic.

Sensible recommendation: MRI ELBOW WO/W CONTRAST

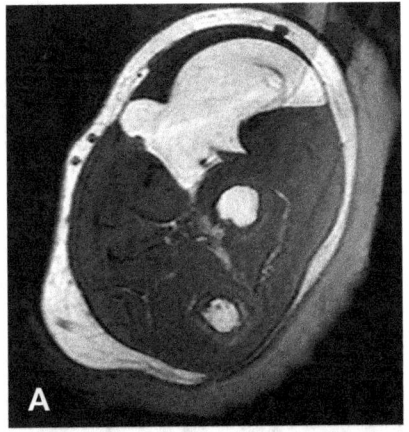

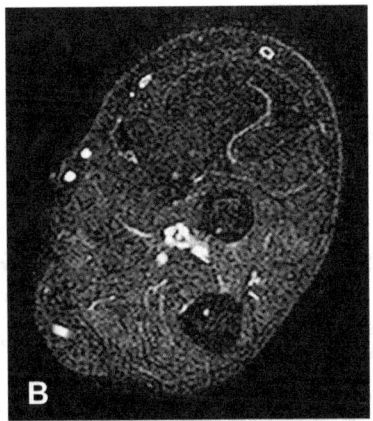

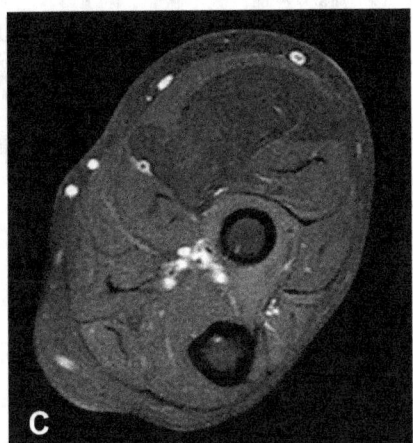

Axial MR images of elbow. Axial T1-weighted (A), T2-weighted fat saturated (B) and post-contrast T1-weighted fat saturated (C) images demonstrate an intra-muscular mass which demonstrates fat signal intensity on all sequences. There is single linear septal enhancement (C). An intra-muscular lipoma.

Both MRI and US effectively evaluate suspected soft tissue masses around the elbow. IV contrast is needed for MR evaluation of some, but not all, soft tissue masses. CT can be used as an alternative procedure, particularly for patients who have a contraindication to MRI, but is a second-tier imaging study. As with MRI, IV contrast can be a useful adjunct for diagnosis but is not necessary in all cases. Since palpable soft tissue masses are typically located outside the joint, arthrography is not appropriate for initial evaluation of a mass.

## Case 18-6

A 46-year-old left-handed male presents with left lateral elbow pain for the past three weeks. He works as an electrician and notes his elbow pain worsens throughout the week and improves somewhat when he is not working. He has been taking nonsteroidal anti-inflammatory (NSAIDS) medications, resting and using ice on a regular basis, which does not improve his pain. Radiographs were normal; however, the patient is concerned that the pain has not completely resolved. What is the most appropriate next imaging examination to perform?

This scenario concerns the further imaging evaluation of a patient with chronic elbow pain and suspected lateral epicondylitis; negative diagnostic radiographs and failed conservative treatment.

Sensible recommendation: MRI ELBOW WO CONTRAST

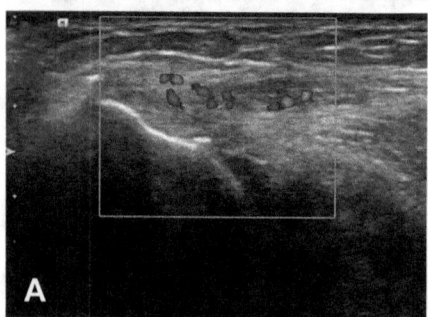
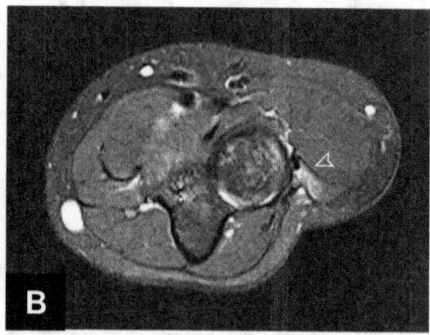
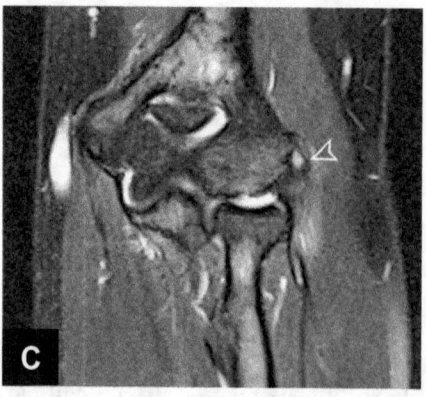

Longitudinal ultrasound image at the level of the lateral epicondyle (A) reveals thickening, hypoechoic areas, and hypervascularity of the common extensor tendons, which is seen in lateral epicondylitis. Axial (B) and coronal (C) T2 FS MRI confirms edema of the common extensor tendon origin (arrowheads) along the lateral epicondyle extending to the level of the radial head.

Medial and lateral epicondylitis are common degenerative tendinopathies involving the common flexor and extensor tendons, respectively. Typically, epicondylitis is diagnosed clinically and managed conservatively, however, persistent pain warrants further evaluation with radiography. In the setting of negative elbow radiographs, ultrasound or MRI can be used to confirm the diagnosis when pain persists and to evaluate for tendinopathy and tendon/ligament tears. Intravenous and intra-articular contrast typically do not aid in the diagnosis. Tissue contrast is limited with CT, making this option less appropriate.

## Case 18-7

34-year-old right-handed woman presents with chronic medial right elbow pain and tingling in her fourth and fifth fingers for the past 4 months. On physical examination, she has asymmetrically reduced grip strength on the right and decreased sensation in her hypothenar eminence as well as her fourth and fifth digits. Elbow radiographs were normal. What is the most appropriate imaging test to further evaluate the patient's ulnar nerve symptoms?

This scenario concerns patients with elbow pain with suspected nerve abnormality and negative radiographs.

Sensible recommendation: MRI ELBOW WO CONTRAST

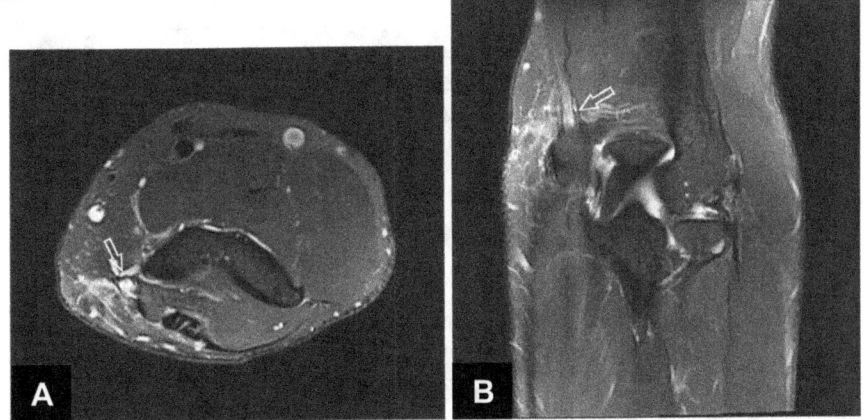

Axial (A) and coronal (B) T2 FS MRI show enlargement of the ulnar nerve just proximal to the cubital tunnel (arrows). There is associated increased T2 signal of the ulnar nerve and adjacent subcutaneous fat. Findings are compatible with cubital tunnel syndrome.

The ulnar nerve is particularly susceptible to trauma or compression at the level of the cubital tunnel. Multiple pathologies can result in thickening and hypervascularity of the ulnar nerve in the setting of neuritis. MRI provides detailed evaluation of the nerves and soft tissues of the elbow. If there is concern for ulnar nerve dislocation, MRI can be performed in elbow flexion and extension, however, real time dynamic evaluation of the ulnar nerve with ultrasound is ideal for assessment of nerve dislocation or subluxation.

CT and nuclear medicine bone scan are of limited utility due to their suboptimal soft tissue detail.

# Case 18-8

A 66-year-old man presents with chronic left elbow pain and limited range of motion. The patient has a remote history of left distal humerus fracture at the age of 24, which was treated with casting. The patient denies recent trauma or surgery. Physical examination reveals non-localizable left elbow discomfort and decreased range of motion in elbow flexion. Elbow radiographs show heterotopic ossification of the elbow without acute fracture. What is the most appropriate examination to further evaluate the patient's elbow pain?

This scenario concerns the further imaging evaluation of chronic elbow pain and stiffness with concern for heterotopic ossification and osteophytosis on radiographs.

Sensible recommendation: CT ELBOW WO CONTRAST

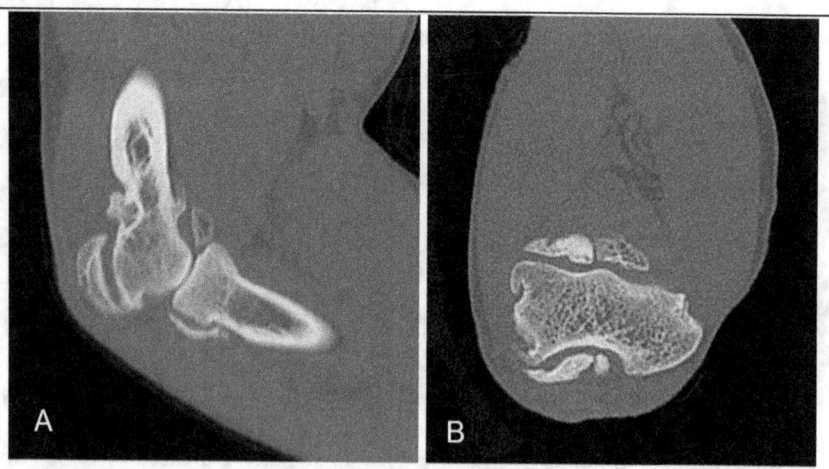

Sagittal (A) and axial (B) CT images of the left elbow show severe osteoarthritis with marginal osteophytes and several well-corticated foci of heterotopic ossification with a mature peripheral cortex and central, fat-containing marrow elements along the dorsal and volar aspect of the radiocapitellar joint adjacent to the coronoid process.

Elbow pain with concern for heterotopic ossification, osteochondral bodies, or osteophytosis on initial radiographs can be further evaluated with CT due to its superior osseous detail. CT may be beneficial for surgical planning. MRI can be useful in evaluation of inflammation associated with myositis ossificans, however, the degree of bony detail is less compared to CT. Intra-articular contrast does not aid in the diagnosis and is usually not necessary. Some authors advocate using functional imaging with Tc-99m bone scan for preoperative planning in hopes to decrease intraoperative complications and postoperative recurrence. Ultrasound does not play a role in evaluation of heterotopic ossification or osteophytosis secondary to shadowing from the ossification, which limits visualization.

## Case 18-9

A 58-year-old woman presents with right elbow mass associated with pain. She is diagnosed with seropopositive rheumatoid arthritis 10 years ago. She noticed the mass about a year ago. There was no injury. Elbow radiographs were non-diagnostic. What is the most appropriate next imaging study?

This scenario concerns the further imaging evaluation of a patient with chronic elbow pain suspecting inflammatory arthritis or bursitis; radiographs obtained.

Sensible recommendation: MRI ELBOW WO/W CONTRAST

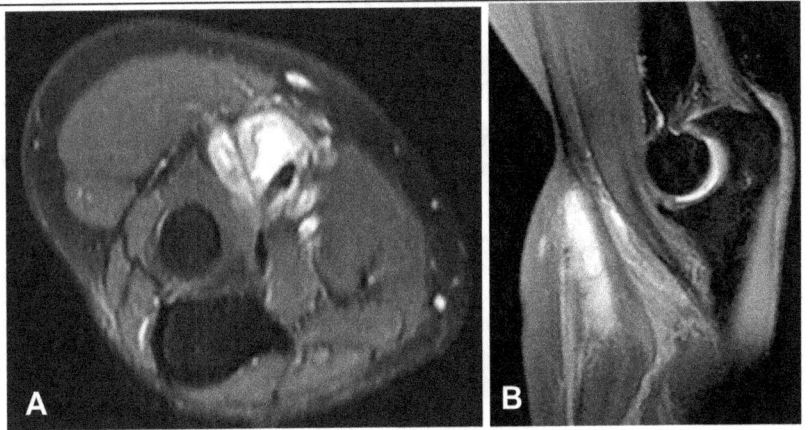

Axial (A) and sagittal (B) T2-weighted fat saturated MR images of the right elbow show a large bicipitoradial bursitis.

Chronic elbow pain can also be caused by a number of joint-related processes, such as inflammatory arthritis and synovial proliferative disorders. Evaluation begins with radiography to assess for joint distention and erosions. MRI can also show erosions and is effective in characterizing synovitis (a low signal suggests hemosiderin) and the extent and activity of disease. In the setting of rheumatoid arthritis, US can also be used to detect joint effusion, synovitis, and erosions. Bicipitoradial and interosseous bursitis around the distal biceps tendon is a source of elbow pain that can be assessed with MRI or US. MRI also demonstrates the effects of the bursa on adjacent structures, including the posterior interosseous and median nerves. Inflammatory arthritis or bursitis can be detected by the early phases of a 3-phase bone scan, as well as on the delayed images, by increased uptake.

# References

1.  American College of Radiology. ACR Appropriateness Criteria: Chronic Elbow Pain. American College of Radiology, reviewed 2015. https://acsearch.acr.org/docs/69423/Narrative/ (accessed April 24, 2021).
2.  Kijowski R, De Smet AA. MRI findings of osteochondritis dissecans of the capitellum with surgical correlation. AJR Am J Roentgenol. 2005 Dec;185(6):1453-9.
3.  American College of Radiology. ACR Appropriateness Criteria: Soft tissue Masses. American College of Radiology, 2013. https://acsearch.acr.org/docs/69434/Narrative/ (accessed Jun 11, 2018).
4.  Walz DM, Newman JS, Konin GP et-al. Epicondylitis: pathogenesis, imaging, and treatment. Radiographics. 2010;30 (1): 167-84.
5.  Levin D, Nazarian LN, Miller TT et-al. Lateral epicondylitis of the elbow: US findings. Radiology. 2005;237 (1): 230-4.
6.  Chew ML, Giuffre BM. Disorders of the Distal Biceps Brachii Tendon. Radiographics. 2005;25 (5): 1227-37.
7.  Shehab D, Elgazzar AH, Collier BD. Heterotopic ossification. J Nucl Med. 2002;43(3):346-353.

# Chapter 19. Chronic or Nontraumatic Shoulder Pain

Jack Porrino, MD, Erin Flaherty, MD, Jennifer Favinger, MD

Radiography is the initial exam for chronic or nontraumatic shoulder pain. MRI, US, or CT may be helpful for further evaluation, and the bone scan may have a problem-solving role.

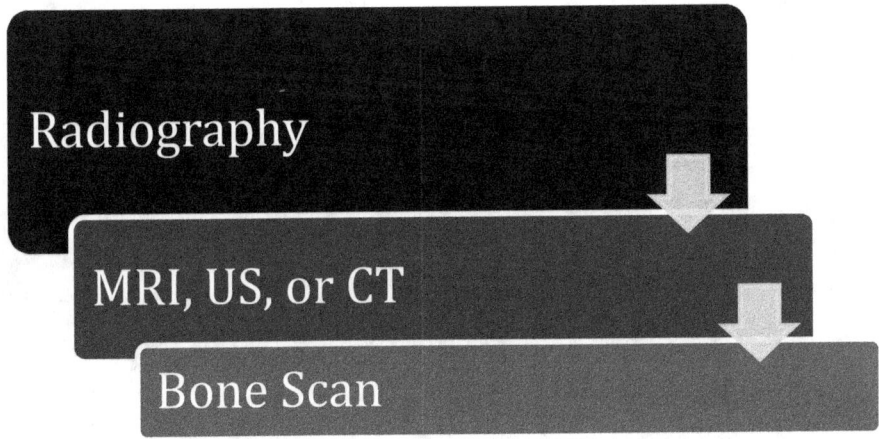

## Case 19-1

45-year-old woman who presented with left shoulder pain after starting an exercise regimen that included swimming. She was returning to physical activity following a 10-month hiatus. Radiographs were interpreted as normal. What is the best study to further evaluate the etiology of her pain?

This scenario concerns the most appropriate next imaging study for a patient with acute shoulder pain of no particular etiology. The initial radiographs were negative.

Sensible recommendation: MRI SHOULDER WO CONTRAST

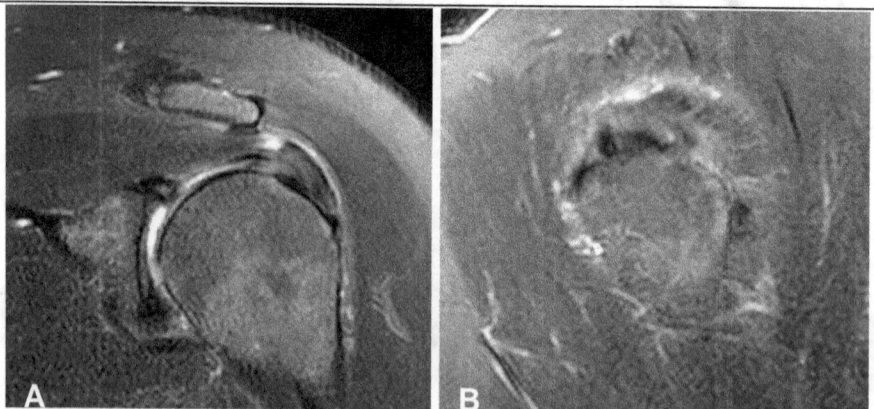

Coronal (A) and sagittal (B) T2 FS MRI of the left shoulder demonstrate a partial thickness bursal surface tear of the supraspinatus tendon.

In those with persistent significant shoulder pain and a non-contributory radiographic series, MRI is the most appropriate next study. MRI can aid in detecting osseous and soft tissue abnormalities. Tendon retraction, muscle atrophy, and fatty infiltration are important findings associated with rotator cuff tear that can influence decisions regarding management, and that are readily apparent on MRI. MR arthrography can help distinguish between full and partial-thickness rotator cuff tear when this is ambiguous otherwise.

## Case 19-2

30-year-old woman who works as a barista reports chronic aching shoulder pain while working with occasional sharp stabbing pains as well. She has attended physical therapy without noticeable improvement in her symptoms. She was noted to have a positive O'Brien's test on physical exam. Radiographs were interpreted as normal. What is the most appropriate next test to diagnose a suspected labral tear?

This scenario concerns the most appropriate next imaging study for a patient under 35 years of age with acute shoulder pain and suspected tear of the glenoid labrum, with possible glenohumeral instability. The initial radiographs were negative.

Sensible recommendation: MRI ARTHROGRAPHY SHOULDER

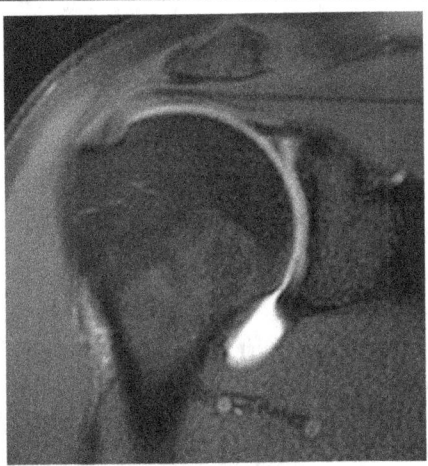

Coronal T1 FS MR arthrogram demonstrates abnormal linear fluid signal within the superior labrum, compatible with a type II SLAP tear.

The shoulder joint is the most unstable joint in the body. MRI permits direct visualization of many of the lesions related to instability, aiding in diagnosis, therapeutic planning, and follow-up. Direct MR arthrography with intra-articular injection of a dilute gadolinium solution distends the joint and outlines labral and capsular structures. MR arthrography is therefore generally recommended in those under 35 years of age with a question of instability; instability in older patients is predominately related to rotator cuff disease.

## Case 19-3

27-year-old man with acute on chronic shoulder pain. His job includes lifting 50 lb bags of cement several times per day. On physical exam, he was noted to have fullness inferior to his acromioclavicular joint, which was tender to palpation. Radiographs were normal. What is the modality of choice to establish the diagnosis of bursitis?

This scenario concerns the most appropriate next imaging study for a patient with acute shoulder pain possibly caused by bursitis or long head of biceps tenosynovitis, based on clinical findings. The initial radiographs were negative.

Sensible recommendation: MRI SHOULDER WO CONTRAST

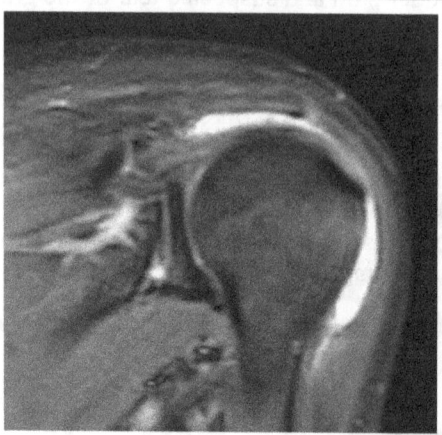

Coronal T2 FS MRI of the left shoulder demonstrates a moderate amount of fluid within the subacromial/subdeltoid bursa.

MRI is the procedure of choice for evaluation of occult fractures and the shoulder soft tissues, including the tendons, ligaments, muscles, and labrocapsular structures. Abnormalities involving the subacromial-subdeltoid bursa and the long head biceps tendon are well seen, and do not require the routine use of intra-articular contrast. Notably, MRI and US are considered equivalent in this evaluation if the necessary expertise is available locally.

## References

1.   American College of Radiology. ACR Appropriateness Criteria: Shoulder Pain-Atraumatic. American College of Radiology, 2018.
     https://acsearch.acr.org/docs/3101482/Narrative/ (accessed April 24, 2021).

# Chapter 20. Chronic or Nontraumatic Neck Pain

Barun Aryal, MD, Majid Chalian, MD

Radiography is the initial imaging exam for acute or chronic, nontraumatic pain or radiculopathy of the cervical spine. MRI and CT both are both employed for a more detailed assessment but may be used as initial imaging if the clinical context is appropriate. CT myelograms can be used specific clinical situations. There is a limited role for nuclear medicine imaging.

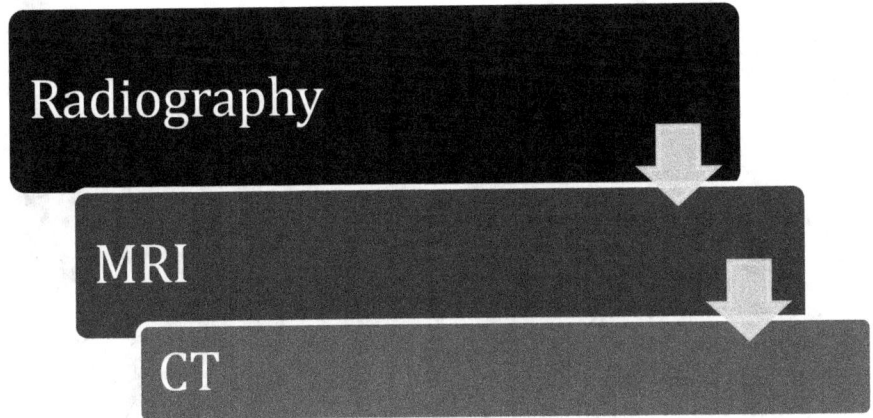

## Case 20-1

An 86-year-old man has neck pain that he rates as 7/10, which started about 10 days ago and is exacerbated by activity. The pain has not resolved despite massages, heating packs, and over the counter muscle creams. What is the best initial imaging for these symptoms?

This scenario concerns initial imaging for new or increasing nontraumatic cervical or neck pain without "red flag" symptoms.

Sensible recommendation: XR C-SPINE 2 VIEWS

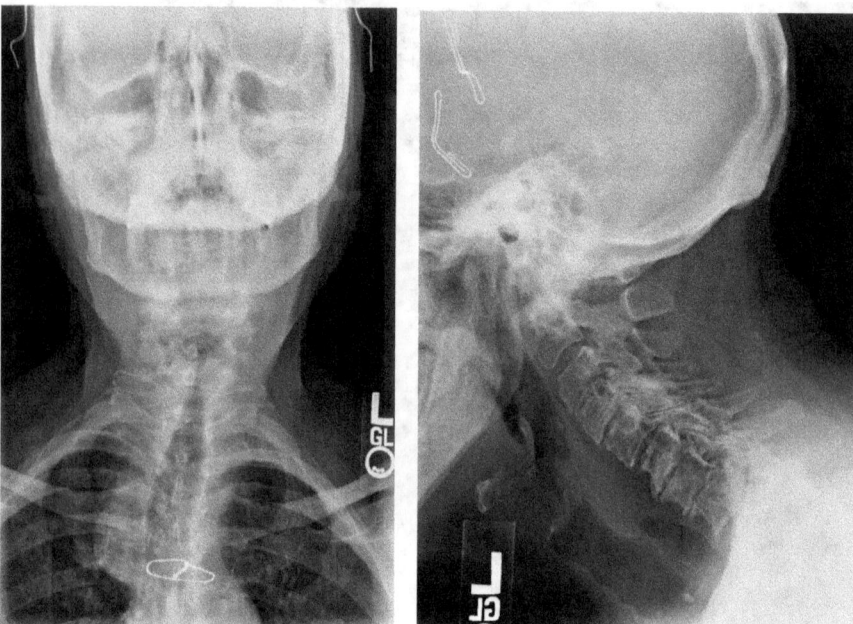

Frontal and lateral radiographs demonstrate multilevel degenerative disc disease with multilevel disc height loss, osteophytosis, and minimal anterolisthesis of C7 on T1.

Frontal and lateral cervical spine radiographs are appropriate for initial imaging in most patients with new cervical pain and no "red flag" symptoms (defined by the Bone and Joint Decade 2000-2010 Task Force on Neck Pain and Its Associated Disorders). Radiographs are easily obtained and adequate to demonstrate spondylosis, malalignment, or other degenerative changes. CT of the cervical spine offers more detail in assessing degenerative changes and therefore may be appropriate, but due to cost, availability, and the unclear comparative impact, is acceptable but less recommended than radiograph. Cervical MRI is most sensitive for soft tissue abnormalities of the neck but has a high rate of abnormal findings in asymptomatic patients and is therefore not recommended for acute or uncomplicated neck pain. Nuclear imaging and CT myelogram have no role.

## Case 20-2

A 59-year-old female presents with right neck pain radiating to her right shoulder and forearm that started two months ago. The pain ranges up to 8/10 and is associated with numbness/tingling in her right hand. She denies changes in strength or coordination, or difficulty with balance, or bowel/bladder dysfunction. What is the best initial imaging evaluation for these symptoms?

This scenario concerns initial imaging for new or increasing cervical radiculopathy without "red flag" symptoms.

Sensible recommendation: MRI C SPINE WO CONTRAST

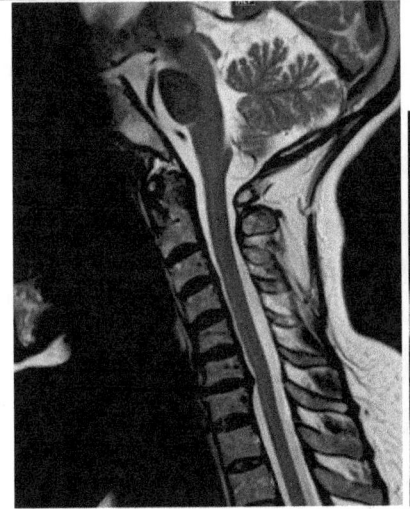 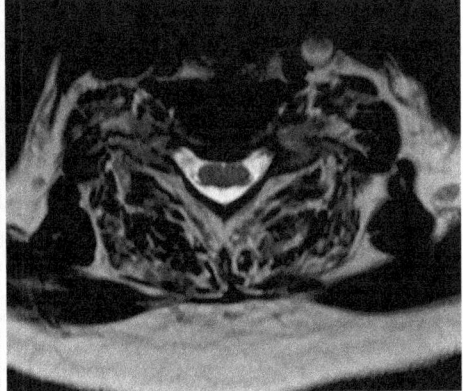

Sagittal (A) and axial (B) T2 MRI of the cervical spine demonstrates mild degenerative disc disease, including a small disc protrusion at C6-C7 level, with mild central canal narrowing. There is no mass effect on the spinal cord, and the bilateral neuroforamina are patent.

Cervical radiculopathy is less common than cervical pain, and can result from physical compression on nerves, sometimes seen with facet or uncovertebral arthropathy, neuroforaminal narrowing, or vertebral disc bulges. These anatomic changes are best evaluated by cervical spine MRI, which is therefore the best imaging to pursue. However, multiple research studies have demonstrated limited correlation between physical exam findings and MRI findings of nerve root compression. CT of the cervical spine offers excellent evaluation of osseous structures as well as the C6-C7 joint, which can be obscured on radiograph, but MRI remains more sensitive in evaluating for nerve compression. CT myelography is usually only considered for patients who have contraindications for MRI, or if MRI exam findings are equivocal. Nuclear imaging has no role.

## Case 20-3

A 64-year-old female with history of C5-7 Anterior Cervical Discectomy and Fusion (ACDF) performed nine years ago following a motor vehicle collision presents with chronic neck pain. The pain is in her posterior neck and radiates down her posterior arms, extending to the palms of her hands. These symptoms are exacerbated by physical activity such as yard, or kitchen work. What is the best initial imaging?

This scenario concerns initial imaging for new or increasing nontraumatic cervical or neck pain or radiculopathy in patients with prior cervical spine surgery.

Sensible recommendation: XR C-SPINE 2-4 VIEWS

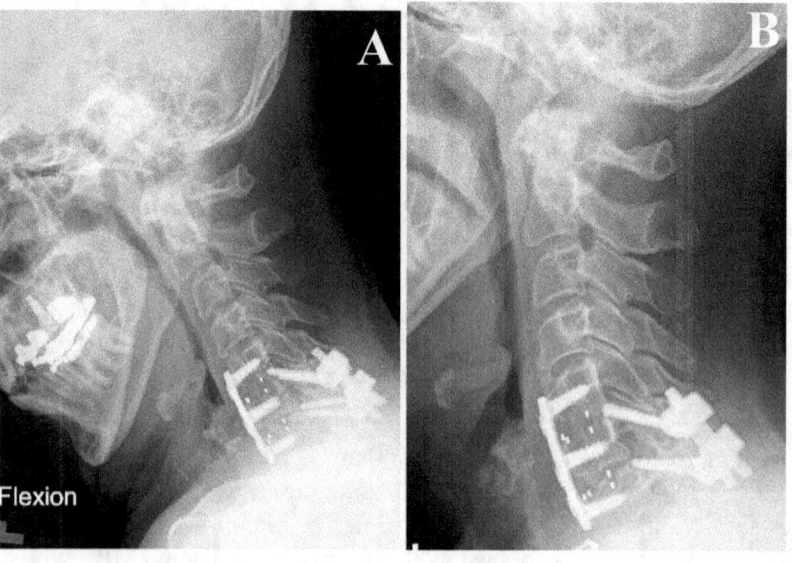

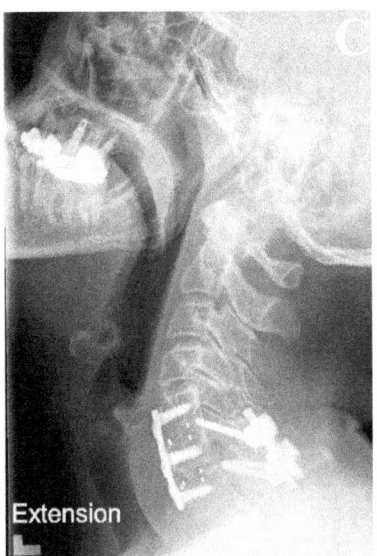

Flexion (A), neutral (B), and extension (C) lateral cervical radiographs demonstrate C5-C7 Anterior Cervical Discectomy and Fusion (ACDF), and C6-C7 posterior surgical instrumentation and fixation. Hardware is intact. There is comparative accelerated degeneration at C4-C5 consistent with a transfer lesion superimposed on a background of mild degenerative disc disease. There is complete osseous fusion across the C5-C6 disc spaces, and partial fusion across C6-C7.

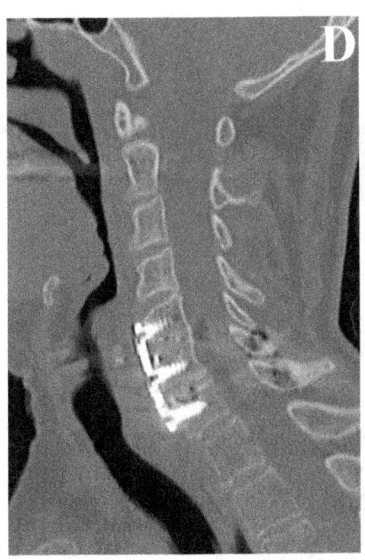

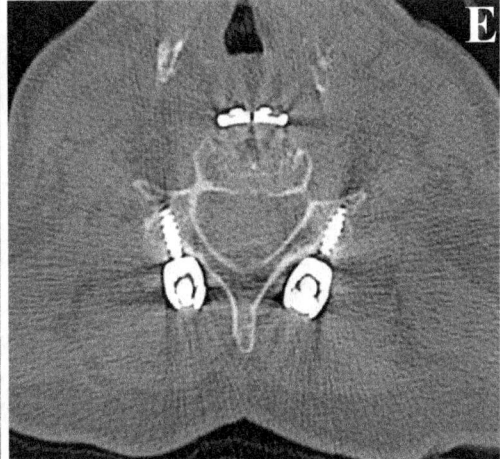

These findings are corroborated in selected sagittal (D) and axial (E) CT imaging of the cervical spine.

Anterior Cervical Discectomy and Fusion (ACDF) is a common treatment for radiculopathy and myelopathy related to cervical disc disease. Clinically impactful imaging findings include evidence of hardware complications, pseudoarthrosis, and adjacent accelerated degeneration, all of which can be seen well by radiography. Additionally, flexion and extension views can be obtained for more sensitive evaluation of pseudoarthrosis or vertebral body nonunion. CT is the most sensitive and specific imaging tool to evaluate for fusion and adjacent accelerated degeneration and is equally efficacious.

MRI is not a preferred method of imaging because of limiting artifact inherent with metallic hardware. CT myelography is not the first-line test for this set of patients and symptoms; however, it can be considered in patients with radiculopathy. Nuclear imaging has no role.

# Case 20-4

A 30-year-old woman presents with five days of worsening neck and shoulder pain in the context of ongoing intravenous drug use, specifically methamphetamine in her groin. Her muscle strength is normal and symmetric bilaterally. What is the best initial imaging study?

This scenario concerns initial imaging for new or increasing nontraumatic cervical or neck pain or radiculopathy in the setting of suspected infection.

Sensible recommendation: MRI C-SPINE WO/W CONTRAST

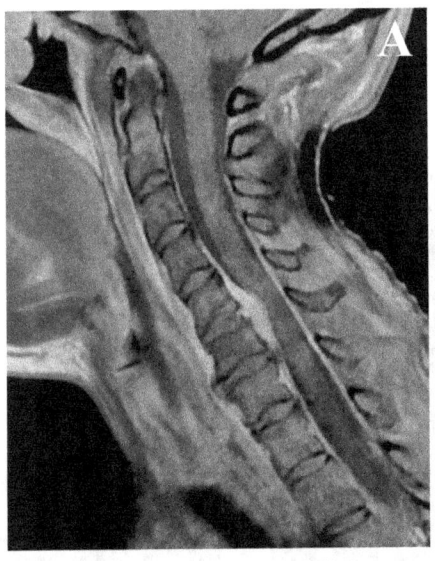
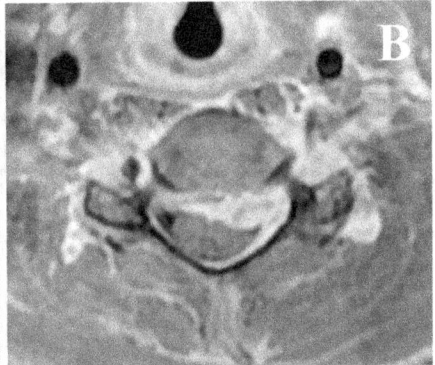

Sagittal T1 weighted post gadolinium contrast enhanced MRI (A) image demonstrates an enhancing epidural collection spanning from the C3-C4 level, to the C7-T1 level. Axial T1 weighted post gadolinium MRI at the C5-C6 level (B) demonstrates the largest portion of the epidural abscess, which causes moderate spinal canal stenosis at this level.

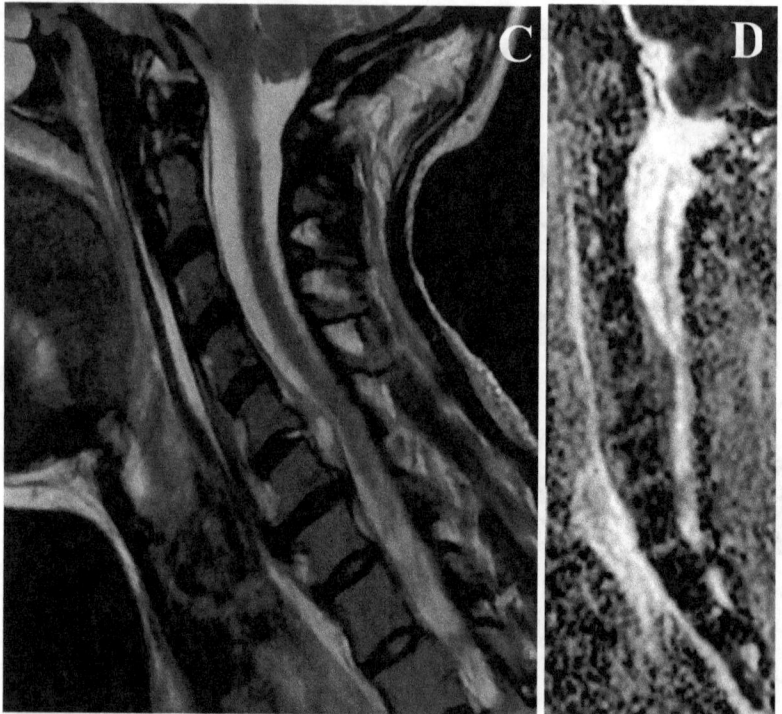

Sagittal T2 weighted imaging (C) shows the focal epidural T2 hyperintense fluid collection, which demonstrates signal drop on sagittal ADC sequence (D), consistent with epidural abscess superimposed on a background of discitis/osteomyelitis. Additionally, the prevertebral spaces also demonstrate enhancement and thickening, favored to represent pyomyositis.

Fever, leukocytosis, elevated erythrocyte sedimentation rate, or C-reactive protein levels in a patient with appropriate history, such as immunosuppression, diabetes, long term steroid use, renal failure, liver failure, or drug use, should prompt suspicion for an infectious process. MRI with and without contrast is the best modality to evaluate for spinal infection because of its high sensitivity and specificity, as well as its ability to characterize extent of leptomeningeal or epidural involvement. CT with contrast can be performed as a complimentary exam but remains second to contrast enhanced MRI. If there is contraindication to gadolinium-based contrast, an MRI without contrast can be obtained. Radiography is much less sensitive and specific than CT with contrast, let alone MRI, and is therefore not the most helpful imaging tool. Three phase Tc-99m BMP scintigraphy is sensitive, but not specific for cervical osteomyelitis, and although specificity can be increased by using a complimentary Gallium-67 whole body scan, again MRI remains superior. CT myelogram is inappropriate for initial evaluation.

# Case 20-5

A 78-year-old male has a history of recently diagnosed small cell lung cancer three months ago. His prior PET CT demonstrated osseous disease including metastatic lesions at the right iliac crest, C4, T2, and T3 vertebral bodies. He has since started chemotherapy, but now presents with worsening severe right shoulder and neck pain. What is the best next imaging evaluation?

This scenario concerns initial imaging for new or increasing nontraumatic cervical or neck pain or radiculopathy in the setting of known malignancy.

Sensible recommendation: MRI C-SPINE WO/W CONTRAST

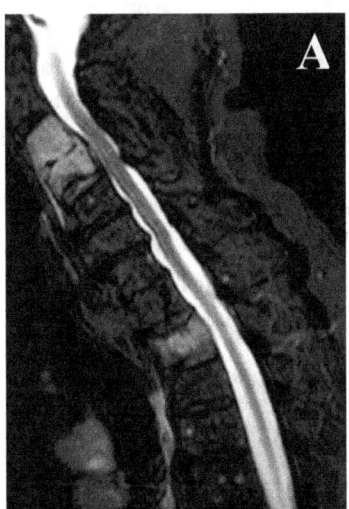 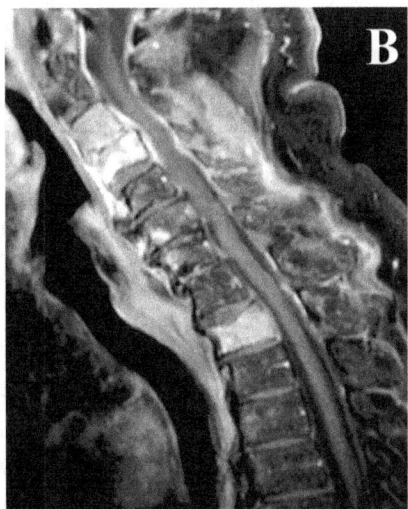

Sagittal T2 weighted (A) and T1 weighted post gadolinium contrast enhanced (B) images of the cervical spine demonstrate multiple vertebral bodies with signal abnormality consistent with osseous metastases. There is epidural extension of an enhancing soft tissue lesion at the C3-C4 level, mildly increased compared to prior PET scan (not depicted).

Approximately 10% of cancer patients develop osseous metastatic disease, which is best diagnosed with cross sectional imaging. In addition to identifying lesions, evaluating the extent of malignancy, such as evidence of cord or nerve root impingement, is clinically significant. Cervical spine MRI with and without contrast is the best exam to both identify and characterize spinal metastases. Radiographs can identify cortical bone changes, but CT is much more sensitive for these lesions and has better evaluation of osseous structures. However, MRI with contrast remains the optimal exam because CT fails to easily identify deep marrow lesions. While PET CT makes up for this shortcoming, it does not delineate nearly the same detail as MRI in terms of spinal cord and nerve root impingement or involvement. Tc-99m bone scan is the most common imaging study for detecting osseous metastases but is limited by a high false positive rate as the labeled MDP highlights osseous turnover, which can occur in benign processes such as degenerative osteoarthrosis. CT myelogram has no role in initial imaging.

## Case 20-6

A 58-year-old woman presents with severe daily left-sided frontotemporal headaches, associated with lacrimation, retroorbital pain, and rhinorrhea, as well as sharp left-sided cervicalgia. These episodes last from 5 minutes, up to 15 minutes, and can occur up to 30 times per day. Prolonged flexion, extension, or pressure in the back of her neck triggers similar headaches. The pain is non-radiating and has no associated numbness, tingling, or weakness. Physical therapy and cervical traction have not provided any relief. A prior left C3-C4 facet block with bupivacaine and dexamethasone relieved the pain up to 50% for several weeks but her pain returned after engaging in physical activity. What is the best initial imaging study?

This scenario concerns initial imaging for new or increasing nontraumatic cervical or neck pain in the setting of cervicogenic headache, without neurologic deficit.

Sensible recommendation: XR C-SPINE 2-4 VIEWS

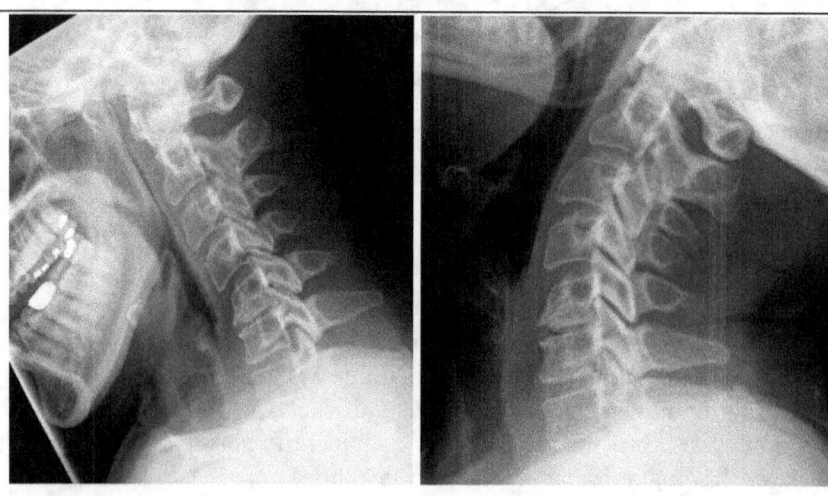

Trace anterolisthesis of C4 on C5 on lateral flexion view (A), without evidence of dynamic instability on lateral extension (B) view. Mild multilevel degenerative disc disease, most prominent at C5-C6.

---

Cervicogenic headaches can be attributed to degenerative disease of the cervical spine. Potential culprit joints include the atlanto-axial, and C2-C3 facet joints, or intervertebral discs. These degenerative changes are evaluated well by cervical spine radiographs. Although CT of the cervical spine provides a more thorough evaluation of the osseous structures, there is no evidence that medical imaging is diagnostic for etiologies of cervicogenic headaches. MRI examinations are similarly not recommended as initial imaging because of the lack of correlation between findings and reported symptoms. The international Classification of Headache Disorders states that headaches abolished by blockade of a cervical structure or nerve supply can be diagnostic of a cervicogenic headache; however, it is not necessary to make the diagnosis and is not the first line routine test. The use of Tc-99m bone scan is very limited, although some authors have advocated its use to identify a possible pain source. There is no role for CT myelography in the absence of radiographic abnormality, or neurologic symptoms.

# Case 20-7

A 50-year-old female has a history of bilateral hand pain and weakness that has been on and off for at least nine months. What is the best initial imaging study?

This scenario concerns initial imaging for chronic cervical or neck pain.

Sensible recommendation: XR C-SPINE 2 VIEWS

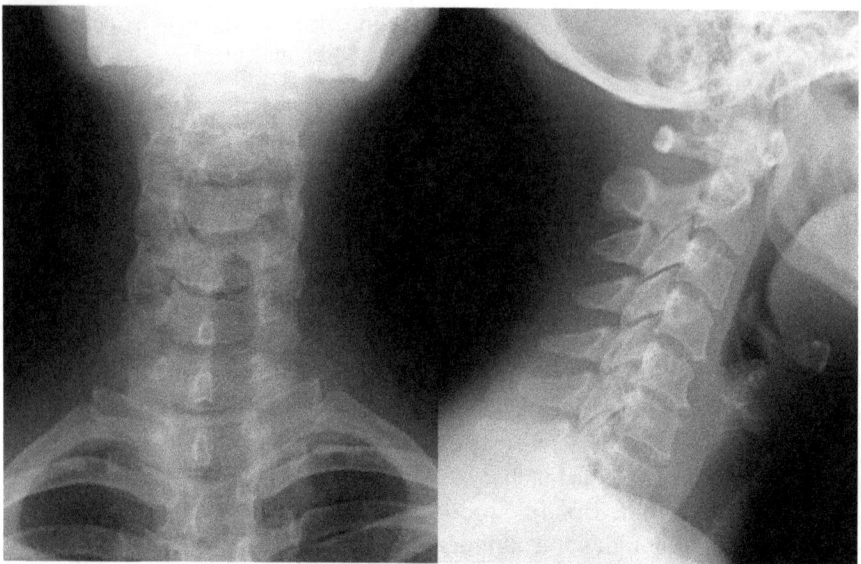

Frontal and lateral radiographs demonstrate mild degenerative changes, such as osteophytosis and intervertebral disc space narrowing, most prominent at C5-C6, and to a lesser extent at C4-C5. There is no evidence of acute fracture or traumatic subluxation.

Many patients have persistent neck pain with recurrent episodes continuing for up to one year. Radiography is the best initial imaging to efficiently evaluate for cervical spondylosis, versus a mechanical, inflammatory, or metabolic process. MRI and CT will show more anatomic detail but are unnecessary for the initial evaluation in most patients with chronic neck pain. Furthermore, imaging findings do not always correlate with symptoms. There may be a limited role for Tc-99m MDP bone scan, which can be coupled with SPECT to help identify a pain source; however, it is not an appropriate first line imaging tool. CT myelography has no role.

## Case 20-8

A 73-year-old male presents with sharp left neck pain, which is worsened with chin tuck, and is associated with tightness in his shoulder girdle and ear, as well as headache. He initially presented with neck pain three months ago and had difficulty turning his head for three weeks. Cervical radiographs at that time showed moderate degenerative disc disease, and no acute fracture or lytic bone lesions. His symptoms have improved but his cervical pain worsens with physical therapy. What is the next best imaging exam for further evaluation?

This scenario concerns next step imaging for a patient with degenerative changes on prior radiograph and chronic neck or cervical pain without neurologic deficit.

Sensible recommendation: MRI C-SPINE WO CONTRAST

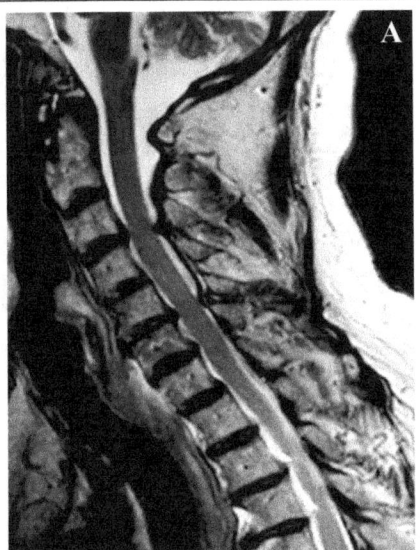

Sagittal (A) T2 weighted MRI of the cervical spine demonstrates multilevel degenerative disc disease.

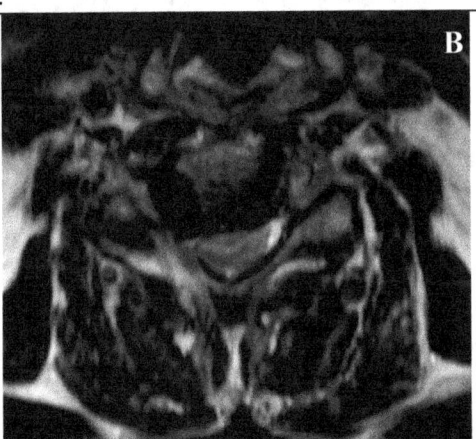

An axial section through the C5-C6 disc space (B) shows an asymmetric right paracentral posterior disc osteophyte complex, in addition to ligamentum flavum hypertrophy that cause moderate central canal narrowing and right greater than left ventral cord flattening. There is severe right and mild to moderate left neuroforaminal narrowing secondary to uncovertebral and facet arthropathy. At C3-C4 a posterior disc osteophyte complex and ligamentum flavum thickening cause mild to moderate central narrowing with cord effacement, and at C6-C7 there is a disc osteophyte complex that causes mild central canal narrowing.

Degenerative changes of the cervical spine are common on radiographs, especially as patients age. Cross sectional imaging may be unnecessary in patients with chronic, unchanged cervical neck pain. The poor correlation of spondylotic changes with patient symptoms further complicates evaluation. Regardless, MRI of the cervical spine is the most sensitive tool to evaluate degenerative changes. Patients with developing symptoms more frequently demonstrate progressed degenerative changes including foraminal stenosis, disc space narrowing, posterior disc protrusion, and/or compression of the dura or spinal cord. CT of the cervical spine may be utilized because it offers a more detailed evaluation of osseous structures compared to radiograph, but MRI remains preferred. There may be a limited role for Tc-99m MDP bone scan, which can be coupled with SPECT to help identify a pain source; however, it is not an appropriate first line imaging tool. CT myelography is not appropriate in the absence of radicular or myelopathic symptoms.

# Case 20-9

A 53-year-old female presents for evaluation of gradually worsening neck pain accompanied by numbness and weakness that began roughly a year ago. Her weakness has moderately exacerbated over the past month, and she has had multiple falls more recently due to an unsteady gait, which she describes as "feeling drunk," and an inability to control her movements. She started using a walker about 9 months ago. She has occasional loss of bladder and bowel control, which has been going on for the past six months. She also notes difficulty with writing. Prior radiograph demonstrates calcification along anterior aspect of the spinal canal, which suggests ossification of the posterior longitudinal ligament. What is the next best next imaging study for further evaluation?

This scenario concerns next imaging for a patient with prior radiograph showing ossification in the posterior longitudinal ligament (OPLL), with chronic cervical or neck pain with or without radiculopathy.

Sensible recommendation: CT C-SPINE WO CONTRAST

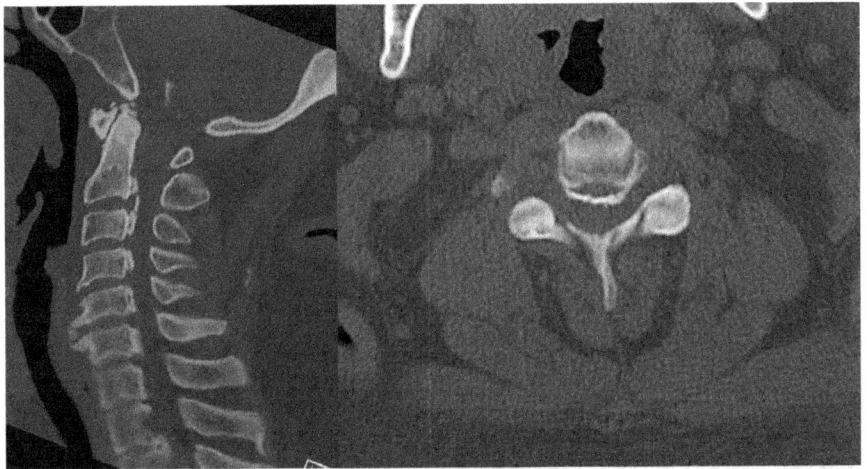

Sagittal (A) and axial (B) CT images of the cervical spine demonstrate discontinuous ossification of the posterior longitudinal ligament, which causes moderate spinal canal stenosis that spans from the C2-C5 vertebral body levels and is most prominent at the C3 level.

Ossification of the posterior longitudinal ligament (OPLL) occurs most commonly in patients 50-70 years old. Although the finding can be made by cervical radiograph alone, CT is more reliable and offers more information on the length and thickness of the ossification, as well as any associated spinal canal or neuroforaminal narrowing. The use of MRI and CT myelography is controversial but may be appropriate for further imaging in this patient population. Nuclear imaging has no role.

# References

1.   American College of Radiology. ACR Appropriateness Criteria: Cervical Neck Pain or Cervical Radiculopathy. American College of Radiology. Last review date: 2018. https://acsearch.acr.org/docs/69426/Narrative/ (accessed on April 24, 2021).

# Chapter 21. Low Back Pain

Tanner Clark, MD, Carolyn Clark, MD, Majid Chalian, MD

Radiography is often the initial exam for uncomplicated low back pain. However, MRI or CT have important roles as initial imaging in certain clinical scenarios. A focused history and physical exam are paramount when selecting the appropriate initial imaging exam. Bone scans can be helpful for evaluation of osteoblastic bone metastases or for problem solving.

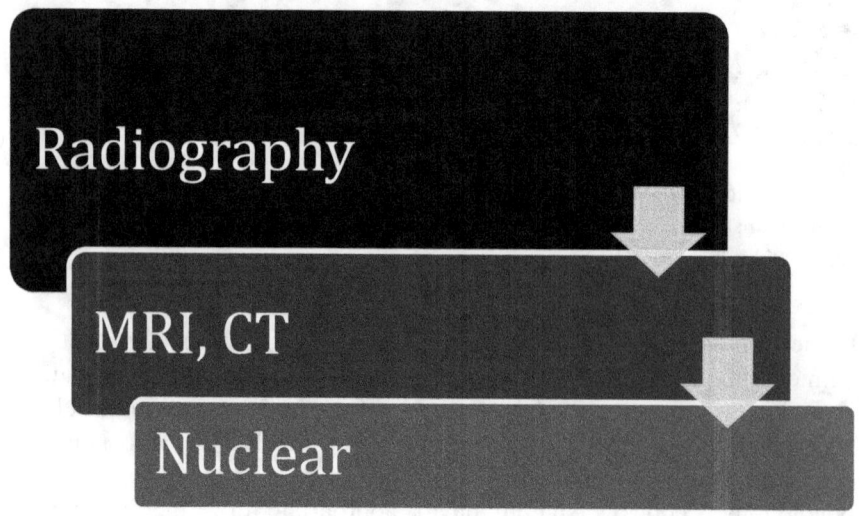

# Case 21-1

Acute, subacute, or chronic uncomplicated low back pain or radiculopathy. No red flags. No prior management.

25-year-old male previously healthy presents with localized low back pain near his lumbosacral junction. Patient notes that the pain is sharp and aggravated by bending forward but denies any radiculopathy type symptoms.

This scenario illustrates acute, subacute, or chronic uncomplicated low back pain without red flags.

Sensible recommendation: NO IMAGING

No imaging is necessary for a healthy patient without any red flag symptoms (Table 1). With a lifetime prevalence of 80-85%, low back pain is the leading cause of disability and is the second most common reason for a physician visit. Reassurance along with physical therapy and/or home exercises will often help resolve nonspecific low back pain symptoms.

Table 1. Red Flags: Indications of a more complicated status include back pain/radiculopathy.

| Red Flags | Potential Underlying Condition as Cause of LBP |
|---|---|
| • History of cancer<br>• Unexplained weight loss<br>• Immunosuppression<br>• Urinary infection<br>• Intravenous drug use<br>• Prolonged use of corticosteroids<br>• Back pain not improved with conservative management | • Cancer or infection |
| • History of significant trauma<br>• Minor fall or heavy lift in a potentially osteoporotic or elderly individual<br>• Prolonged use of steroids | • Spinal fracture |
| • Acute onset of urinary retention or overflow incontinence<br>• Loss of anal sphincter tone or fecal incontinence | • Cauda equina syndrome or severe neurologic compromise |

| | |
|---|---|
| • Saddle anesthesia<br>• Global or progressive motor weakness in the lower limbs | |

## Case 21-2

Acute, subacute, or chronic uncomplicated low back pain or radiculopathy. One or more of the following: low velocity trauma, osteoporosis, elderly individual, or chronic steroid use.

35-year-old female with history of Crohn's disease presents with localized low back pain after falling onto buttocks after tripping while hiking. She notes the pain is sharp and rates pain 5 out of 10 but denies any neurologic symptoms. Regarding her Crohn's disease, she is currently in remission, but notes that she recently had a flare and for which she took glucocorticoids for a month. She also notes that she has taken steroids on multiple occasions in past for prior flares.

This scenario illustrates uncomplicated low back pain but with a history of low velocity trauma and chronic steroid use.

Sensible recommendation: XR LUMBAR SPINE

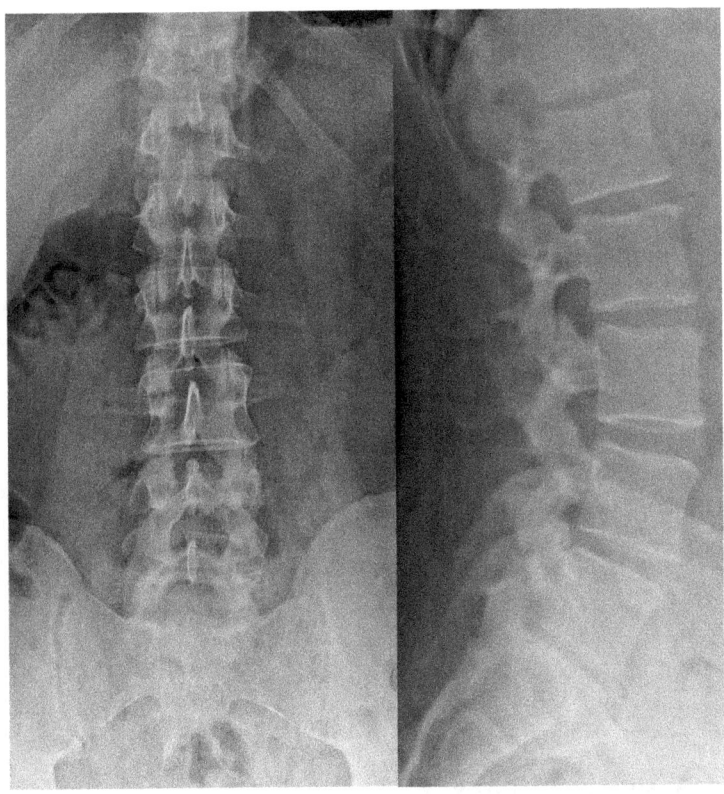

AP and sagittal lumbar spine radiograph without fracture or subluxation

Lumbar spine radiograph is usually the best initial imaging choice and is often normal, as shown above. Of note, there are incidental 6 non-rib bearing lumbar type vertebral bodies that are likely related to hypoplastic T12 ribs. This is a normal variant, but important to report if the patient is to undergo surgical intervention to ensure correct level surgery is performed. In a patient with increased risk for low bone mineral density, but with normal radiographs, caution should be exercised because subtle compression fractures can be radiographically occult on initial radiographs and be present on CT and MRI. Therefore, if clinical suspicion persists then further imaging should be obtained in high-risk populations. MRI can be useful to evaluate for ligamentous injury or worsening neurologic deficit, but CT would be the preferred exam prior to obtaining MRI to assess for fracture.

## Case 21-3

Acute, subacute, or chronic low back pain or radiculopathy. One or more of the following: suspicion of cancer, infection, or immunosuppression

32-year-old previously healthy male presented to his primary care provider with bilateral lower extremity weakness, pain radiating into right buttocks, and night sweats. He denied intravenous drug use or other underlying health conditions. Further workup was performed and demonstrated a profound leukopenia and a subsequent HIV test was performed and was positive.

This scenario illustrates radiculopathy with immunosuppression and concern for infection.

Sensible recommendation: MRI LUMBAR SPINE WO/W CONTRAST

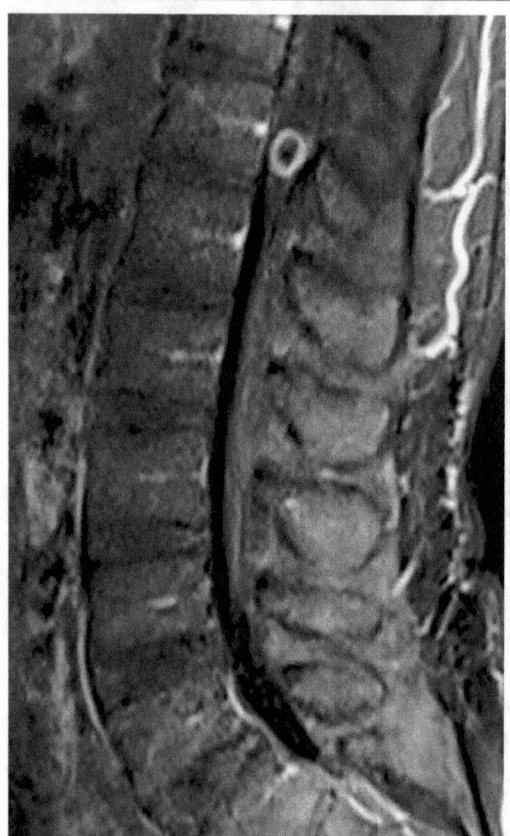

T1 weighted post contrast sagittal sequence of the lumbar spine demonstrates an intramedullary ring enhancing lesion in the distal spinal cord near the conus medullaris that was proven to be toxoplasmosis. Interestingly, this was a solitary lesion at time of diagnosis without evidence of intracranial disease.

When high risk populations present with low back pain, clinicians should be vigilant and have low threshold for further evaluation with imaging given high risk for underlying pathology. This clinical context is unique in that MRI is an initial imaging recommendation in contrary to the majority of other clinical scenarios. A spine radiograph would be unhelpful in this scenario and would only add cost and radiation exposure to patient. CT would also be less helpful given limited evaluation of intradural and intramedullary/cord pathologies.

# Case 21-4

Acute, subacute, or chronic low back pain or radiculopathy. Surgery or intervention candidate with persistent or progressive symptoms during or following 6 weeks of conservative management.

45-year-old male presents to his primary care provider for a 6-week follow-up appointment after initial presentation of low back pain with radiation to the left buttocks. He has performed physical therapy and taken nonsteroidal anti-inflammatories as prescribed, but without improvement. Otherwise, he is healthy and is an avid bicyclist that yearns to get back in the saddle.

This scenario illustrates low back pain with radiculopathy with persistent symptoms following 6-weeks of conservative management.

Sensible recommendation: MRI LUMBAR SPINE WO CONTRAST

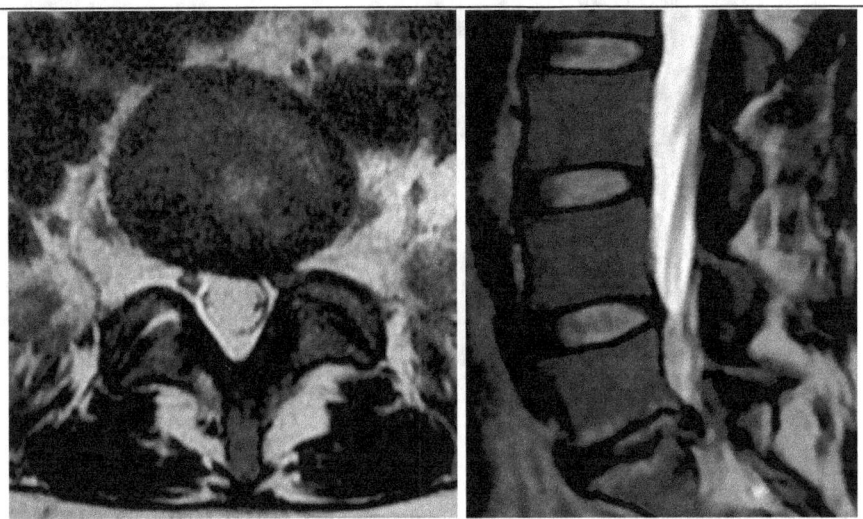

MRI axial T2 weighted and sagittal T2 weighted sequences of the lumbar spine demonstrates an asymmetric left posterolateral disc bulge resulting in narrowing of the lateral recess with mild compression and displacement of the S1 nerve root which corresponds with patient symptoms. There is also abutment of the right S1 nerve root.

Patients who have unresolving back pain with radiculopathy who have failed 4-6 weeks of conservative therapy warrant further imaging with lumbar spine MRI as the initial imaging study. Spine radiographs are typically unhelpful in this scenario but may be needed prior to surgical intervention for surgical planning.

## Case 21-5

Low back pain or radiculopathy. New or progressing symptoms or clinical findings with history of prior lumbar surgery.

57-year-old female presents with recurrent radiculopathy in the left L5 distribution. She had a L4-L5 microdiscectomy 1 year ago with resolution of her radiculopathy, but now has recurrent symptoms. She notes that it feels similar to her pre-procedural pain and discomfort.

This scenario illustrates recurrent radiculopathy with history of prior lumbar surgery.

Sensible recommendation: MRI LUMBAR SPINE WO/W CONTRAST

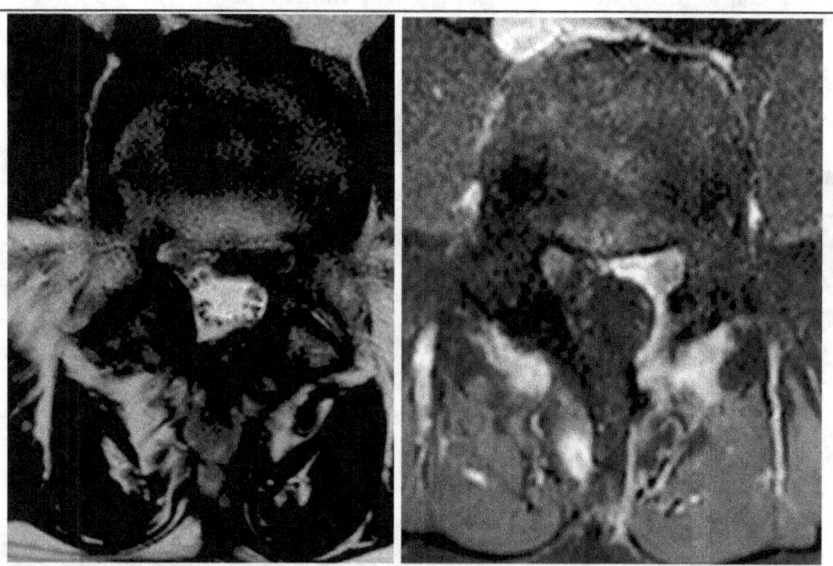

MRI axial T2 weighted (A) and T1 weighted post contrast sequences (B) through the lumbar spine demonstrates T2 hypointense granulation tissue/scar surrounding the left L5 nerve root, which avidly enhances on the T1 post contrast sequence. No evidence of recurrent disc herniation. Post-surgical changes of prior microdiscectomy are present.

In patients with prior lumbar surgery and new or progressing symptoms, MRI of the lumbar spine without and with IV contrast is a critical component of the evaluation. If patient has underlying fusion hardware, then a lumbar spine radiograph would be needed to evaluate the hardware. Contrast is helpful in the postsurgical context to help differentiate herniated disc versus granulation/scar tissue. CT myelography can be performed if patient has extensive spinal fusion or MRI is contraindicated.

# Case 21-6

Low back pain with suspected cauda equina syndrome or rapidly progressive neurologic deficit.

35-year-old female with acute progressive low back pain with new incontinence presents to urgent care for evaluation. Physical exam demonstrated perianal numbness/saddle anesthesia.

This clinical scenario illustrates low back pain with suspected cauda equina syndrome.

Sensible recommendation: URGENT MRI LUMBAR SPINE WO CONTRAST

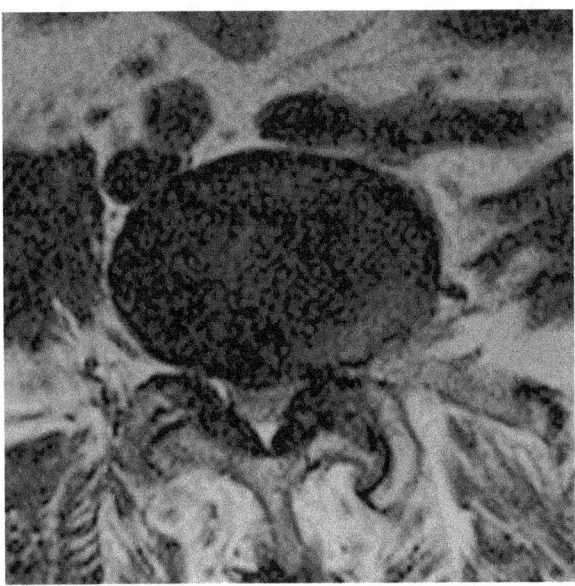

MRI axial T2 weighted sequence spine without IV contrast through the lumbar spine demonstrates L5-S1 severe dural sac compression, with complete effacement of CSF space and clumping of the nerve roots from combination of circumferential disc bulge with superimposed disc protrusion, facet hypertrophy, ligamentum flavum infolding/hypertrophy.

Cauda equina syndrome is an emergency and needs to be evaluated with imaging promptly to guide surgical intervention, if clinically indicated. This syndrome is a clinical diagnosis however, and imaging only reveals the underlying cause. Some institutions have abbreviated MRI protocols to help expedite the evaluation. IV contrast is generally not required but may be needed if patient has history of prior surgery or if there is concern for epidural abscess/infection. Radiographs are typically unhelpful for evaluating the underlying cause given limited intradural evaluation. If MRI is contraindicated or unable to be performed in a timely manner, CT or CT myelogram could be obtained, although CT alone may be indeterminate.

# References

1.  American College of Radiology. ACR Appropriateness Criteria: Low backpain. American College of Radiology. 2015. https://acsearch.acr.org/docs/69483/Narrative/ (Accessed April 24, 2021)
2.  Murray CJ, Lopez AD. Measuring the global burden of disease. N Engl J Med. 2013;369(5):448-457.

# Chapter 22. Suspected Sacroiliitis and Spondyloarthropathy

Maryam Soltanolkotabi, MD, Amanda M Crawford, MD, Megan K Mills, MD, Majid Chalian, MD

Radiography of the lumbar spine and pelvis is preferred in the initial investigation of suspected sacroiliitis and spondyloarthropathy (SpA). MRI of the sacroiliac joints is the next step in the absence of radiographic findings. If MRI is not possible, CT may be considered. Bone scintigraphy is occasionally part of the individualized approach to the diagnosis of axial SpA.

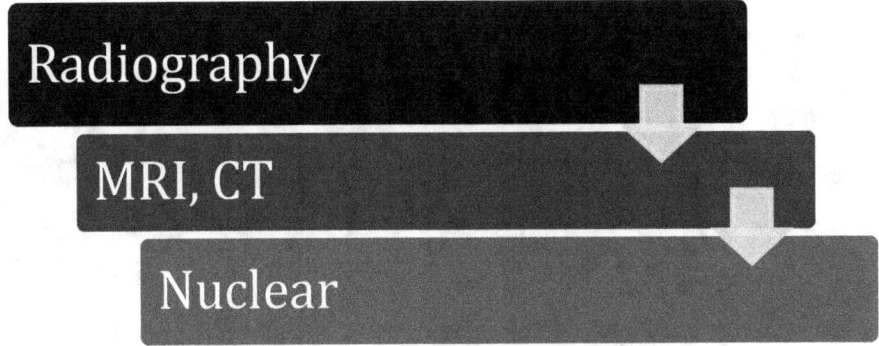

# Case 22-1

55-year-old man with 5-6 years of chronic episodic low back pain, history of severe iritis, and positive HLA-B27. On physical exam, the patient has mild pain with palpation of the sacroiliac joints. What is the best initial imaging study to evaluate his low back pain?

This scenario concerns the best initial imaging study for a patient with inflammatory sacroiliac or back symptoms and suspected spondyloarthropathy.

Sensible recommendation: XR SACROILIAC JOINTS

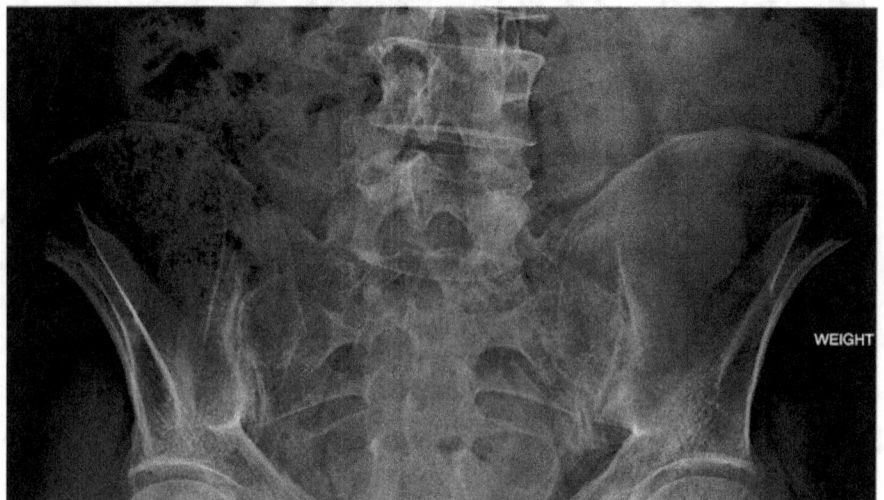

PA weightbearing radiograph of the sacroiliac joints demonstrates sacroiliac joint sclerosis and erosions consistent with bilateral asymmetric sacroiliitis.

Imaging of the patient with suspected spondyloarthropathy and low back pain should begin with radiographic examination. Radiographs are an efficient and cost-effective means to confirm the presence of sacroiliitis in the setting of inflammatory spondyloarthropathy or diagnose other common causes of chronic low back pain such as osteoarthritis.

# Case 22-2

44-year-old woman with progressive chronic low back pain for 5-6 years. The patient had and negative HLA-B27 and CRP and was treated for presumed osteoarthritis with anti-inflammatory medication and sacroiliac joint injections with minimal pain relief. Routine radiographic series of the sacroiliac joints demonstrated some sclerosis interpreted as either osteoarthritis or sacroiliitis. What is the next most appropriate study to further evaluate the sacroiliac joints?

This scenario concerns the next imaging study for a patient with chronic low back pain in whom sacroiliitis/spondyloarthropathy is suspected but radiographs are not definitive.

Sensible recommendation: MRI SACROILIAC JOINTS WO/W CONTRAST

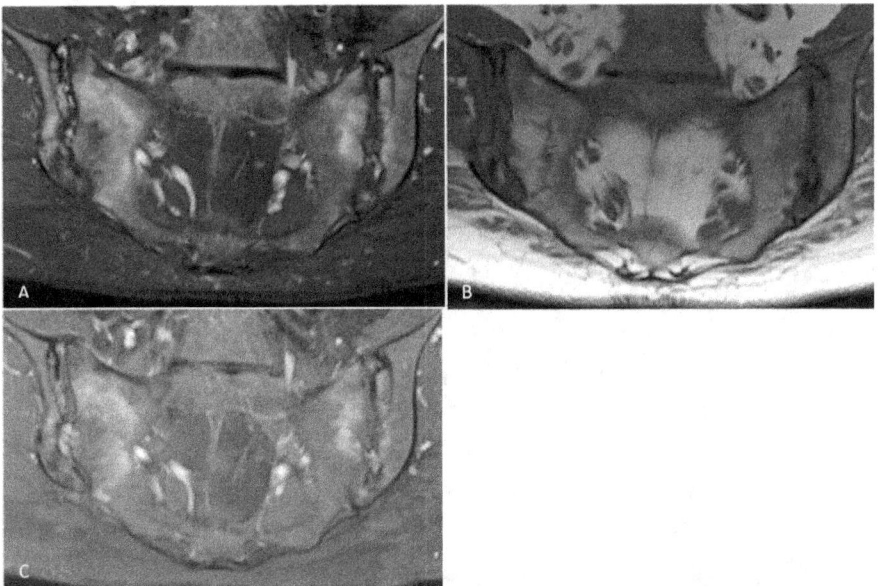

Coronal oblique T2FS (A), Coronal oblique T1 (B), and Coronal oblique T1 FS (C) with contrast shows findings of both acute and chronic sacroiliitis including acute osteitis/bone marrow edema, capsulitis, and synovitis, as well as chronic erosions and periarticular fat deposition. This patient was ultimately diagnosed with seronegative spondyloarthropathy.

MRI is the preferred examination in patients with chronic low back pain in the setting of suspected sacroiliitis/spondyloarthropathy and negative or equivocal radiographs. MRI allows for detection of both acute and chronic findings of sacroiliitis. Acute osteitis/bone marrow edema, enthesitis, capsulitis, and synovitis can be detected on MRI without contrast, but intravenous contrast administration may improve detection of these abnormalities. Findings of chronic sacroiliitis, such as subchondral sclerosis, erosions, periarticular fat deposition, and ankylosis can also be seen on MRI without contrast or CT without contrast.

# Case 22-3

A 26-year-old man presents to the rheumatology clinic with chronic low back pain and iridocyclitis. Initial lumbar spine and sacral radiographs are negative. What is the best next imaging study to further evaluate his symptoms?

This scenario involves low back pain in a patient with suspected axial spondyloarthropathy with initial negative lumbar spine and sacral radiographs.

Sensible recommendation: MRI SACROILIAC JOINTS WO CONTRAST

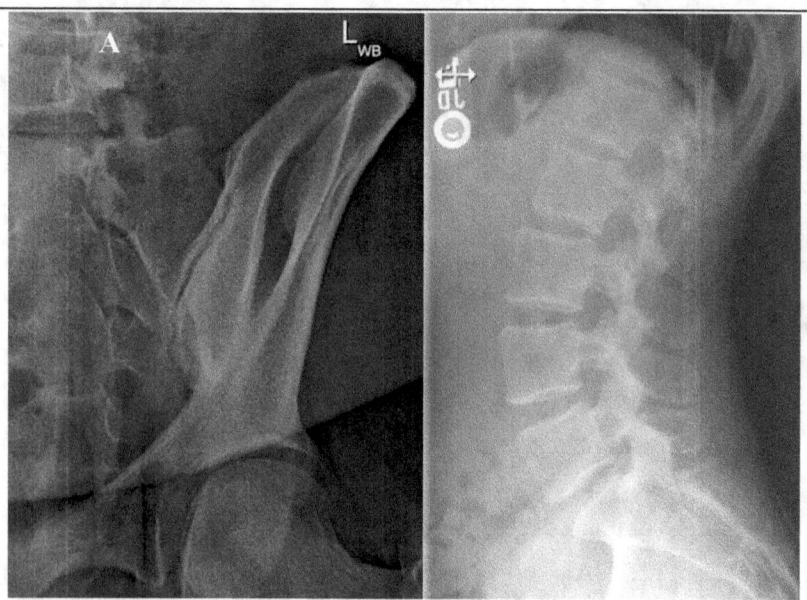

AP oblique view of the left sacroiliac joint (A) and lateral lumbar spine (B) radiographs are unremarkable.

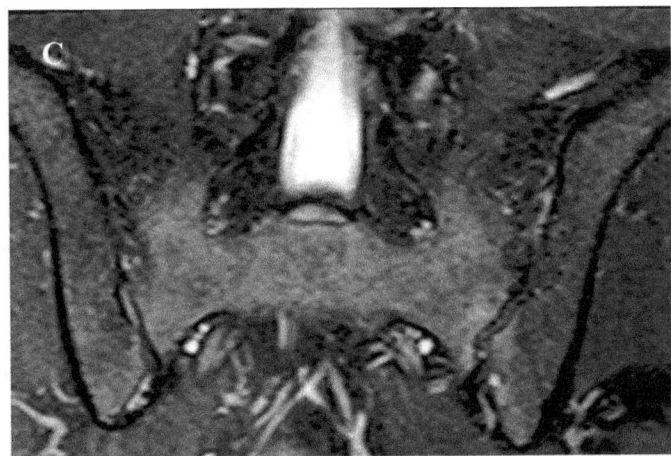

Coronal oblique T2 fat-saturated MR image (C) of the sacroiliac joints demonstrates asymmetric subchondral marrow edema of the left sacroiliac joint (white arrows).

Although lumbar and sacroiliac radiographs are the first study of choice in the initial evaluation of patients with suspected spondyloarthropathy, non-contrast enhanced MR study of the sacroiliac joints may aid in the diagnosis of sacroiliitis in a suspected patient with chronic low back pain as features of active and chronic sacroiliitis such as subchondral marrow edema and erosions are often more conspicuous on MRI. CT of the spine without intravenous contrast and MR spine with and without intravenous contrast may also be considered as complimentary studies to assess for syndesmophytes and vertebral body changes characteristic of SpA such as squaring of the vertebrae and Romanus lesions.

## Case 22-4

A 61-year-old man was referred for evaluation of chronic low back pain and positive HLA-B27 with concern for ankylosing spondylitis. His back pain has worsened over the last 2 to 3 years. Radiographs and MRI of his sacrum are negative. What is the most appropriate next imaging exam to evaluate his low back pain?

This scenario concerns the next imaging study for patients with suspected axial spondyloarthropathy, but negative radiographs and MRI of the sacroiliac joints.

Sensible recommendation: XR LUMBAR SPINE, MRI LUMBAR SPINE WO CONTRAST

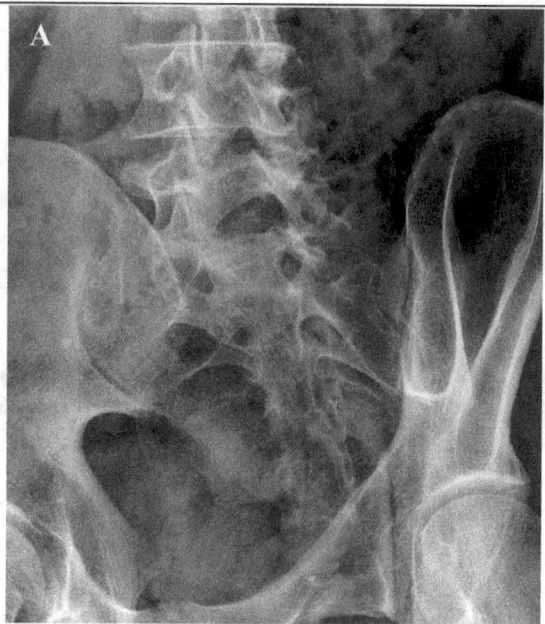

AP oblique radiograph of the right sacroiliac joint (A) is negative for sclerosis, sub-chondral demineralization, or erosions and demonstrates maintained joint space.

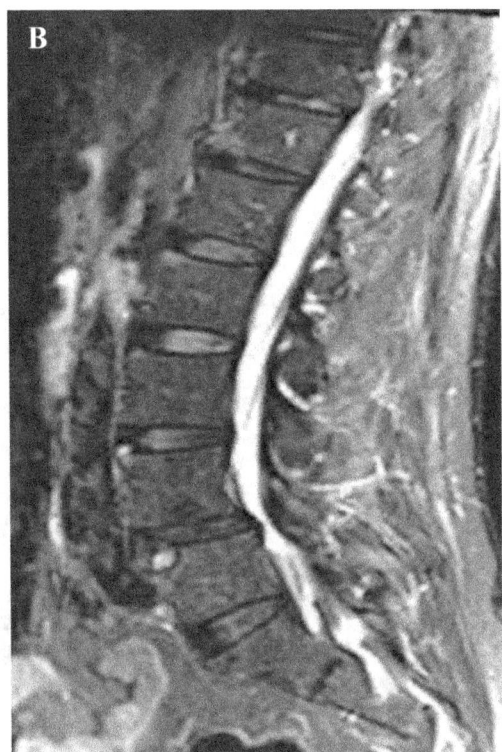

MRI of the lumbar spine (B); however, demonstrates increased STIR signal intensity of the anterior-superior aspects of multiple vertebral bodies consistent with Romanus lesions.

Although lumbar and sacroiliac radiographs are the first study of choice in the initial evaluation of patients with suspected spondyloarthropathy, noncontrast enhanced MR of the lumbar spine may aid in understanding the etiology of back pain in this patient population as features of SpA may be subtle on radiographs. MR is very sensitive in detection of bone marrow pathology as can be seen with Romanus lesions.

## Case 22-5

A 61-year-old man with past medical history of ankylosing spondylitis diagnosed in his 20s presents following a ground level fall. He is neurologically intact but is endorsing mild paraspinal lower neck pain.

This scenario concerns the imaging evaluation of an adult with history of spine ankylosis and suspected fracture.

Sensible recommendation: CT SPINE (area of interest), MRI SPINE WO CONTRAST

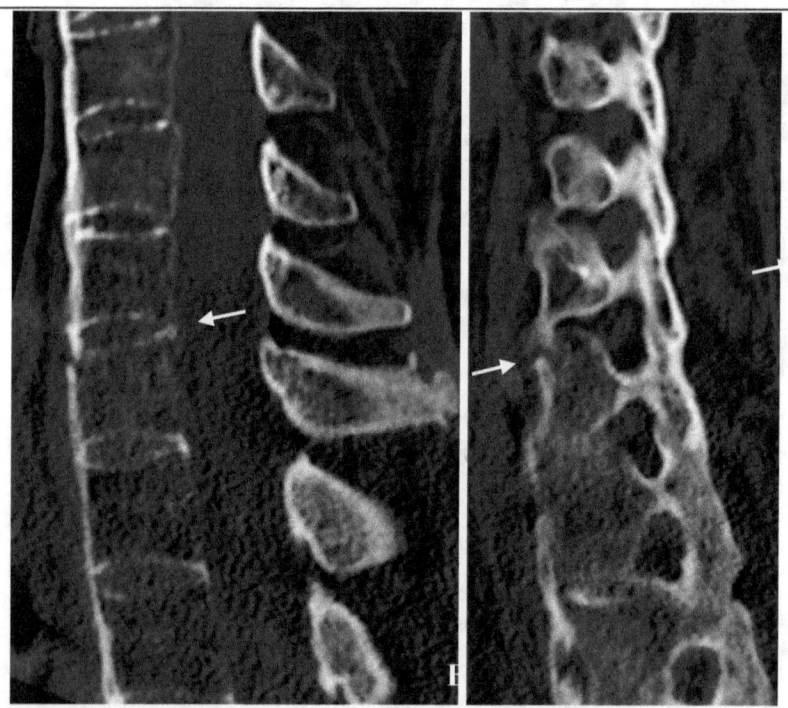

Sagittal midline (A) and paramidline (B) CT of the cervical spine demonstrates C7 three-column fracture (white arrows).

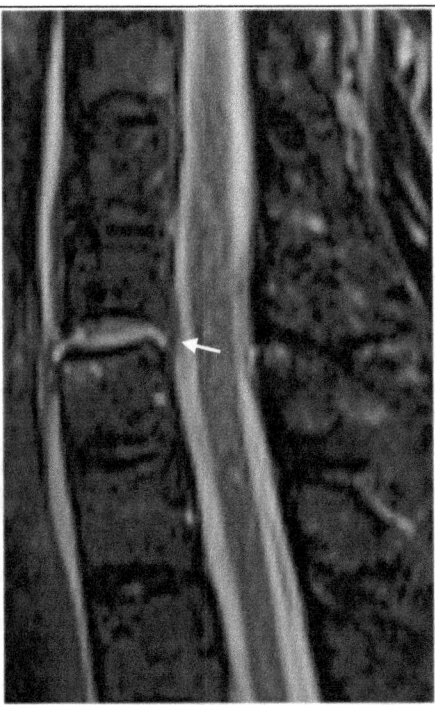

Sagittal STIR MRI of the cervical spine (C) shows fracturing of the anterior syn-desmophyte at this level with increased signal within the C6-C7 disc.

Patients with rigid spines such as this patient with spondyloarthropathy, are more susceptible to spinal fractures even after minor trauma. Ossification of the spinal ligaments alter the biomechanics of the spine and create long lever arms, limiting the ability of the spine to even absorb minimal impacts. Moreover, these patients often suffer diffuse demineralization of the osseous structures, further increasing susceptibility to fractures. These fractures are often nondisplaced and not perceptible on radiographs. As such, CT is very sensitive in detection of fractures in this patient population.

## Case 22-6

A 34-year-old man with a past medical history of ankylosing spondylitis, manifested with inflammatory low back pain for the last 10 years. Patient had previously been placed on 4 months of NSAID therapy without relief from symptoms. Subsequently, he was treated with Enbrel 50 mg SC/week and Celebrex 200 mg PRN. What imaging study is appropriate in evaluation of response to therapy in this patient?

This scenario concerns the imaging evaluation of an adult with known history of spondyloarthropathy with concerns for disease progression and/or evaluation of treatment response.

Sensible recommendation: MRI SPINE and/or SACROILIAC JOINTS WO CONTRAST

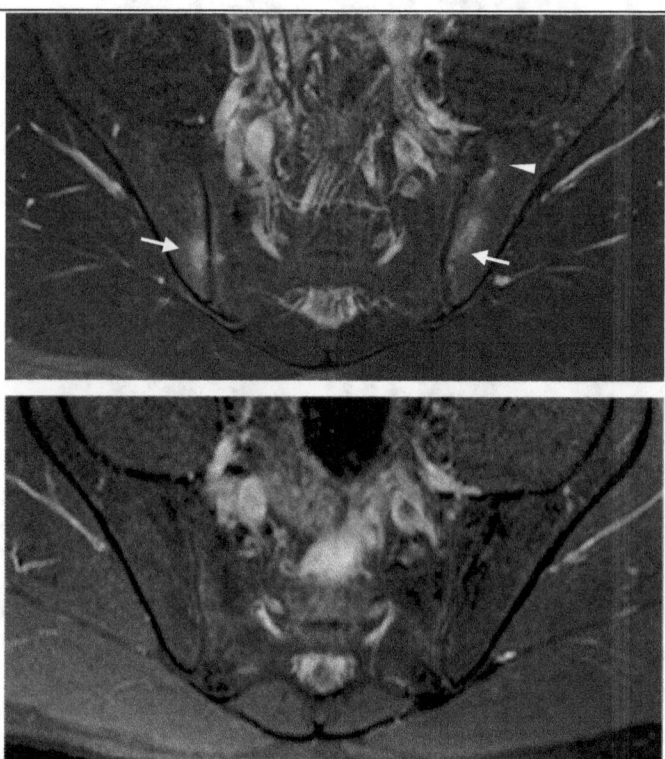

Coronal oblique T2 fat saturated MR (A) of the sacroiliac joints prior to therapy demonstrate subchondral marrow edema involving both sacroiliac joints (white arrows) with erosion of the left sacroiliac joint (white arrowhead). Post-treatment coronal oblique T2 fat saturated image (B) demonstrates resolution of active features of sacroiliitis.

Active features of sacroiliitis such as subchondral marrow edema, erosions, capsulitis/synovitis, enthesitis, and joint effusion can often be accurately depicted on MRI; hence, this modality is preferential in evaluating response to therapy or disease progression.

# References

1. Bernard SA, et al. American College of Radiology ACR Appropriateness Criteria in Chronic Back Pain. 2016. https://acsearch.acr.org/docs/3094107/Narrative. (accessed April 24, 2021)
2. Navallas, M., et al., Sacroiliitis associated with axial spondyloarthropathy: new concepts and latest trends. Radiographics, 2013. 33(4): p. 933-56.
3. Sepriano, A., et al., Is active sacroiliitis on MRI associated with radiographic damage in axial spondyloarthritis? Real-life data from the ASAS and DESIR cohorts. Rheumatology (Oxford), 2019. 58(5): p. 798-802.
4. Panwar, J., et al., Utility of CT imaging in differentiating sacroiliitis associated with spondyloarthritis from gouty sacroiliitis: a retrospective study. Clin Rheumatol, 2018. 37(3): p. 779-788.

# Chapter 23. Chronic or Nontraumatic Pelvis Pain

Hyojeong Lee, MD

Radiography is the initial exam for chronic or nontraumatic hip pain. MRI, US, or CT may be helpful for further evaluation, and the bone scan may have a problem-solving role.

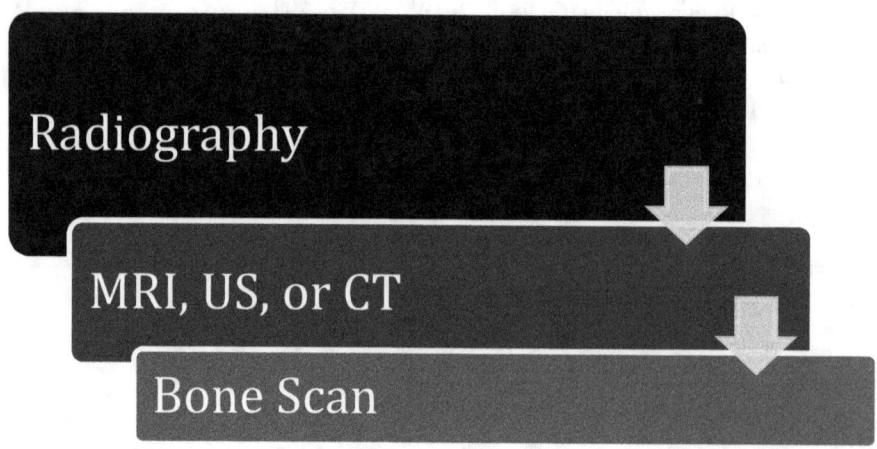

# Case 23-1

A 49-year-old woman presents with a 2-year history of progressing left pelvis pain radiating to left hip. She doesn't recall any injury. She thinks she has changed her gait related to right knee surgery 2 years ago. Pain is worse at night and occasionally wakes her from sleep. What is the most appropriate first imaging test?

This scenario concerns about a patient with chronic pelvic pain. First imaging study.

Sensible recommendation: XR PELVIS

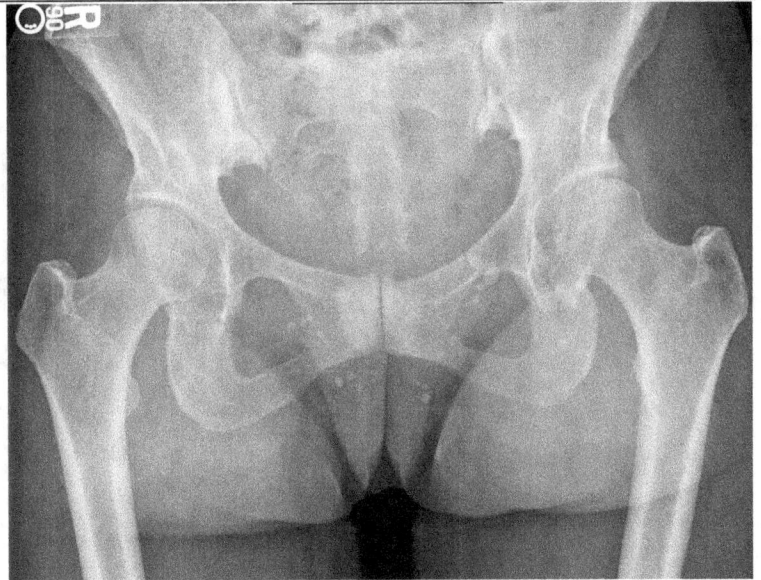

AP radiograph of the pelvis demonstrates subchondral sclerosis along both sacroiliac joints and the pubic symphysis (osteitis condensans ilii and pubis). There is also a unilateral transitional vertebra at left lumbosacral junction.

Chronic pelvic pain is a perplexing clinical problem. Symptoms may be related to numerous etiologies, including trauma, neoplasms, and arthropathies. Pain may be due to osseous, intra-articular, periarticular, or soft tissue pathology. Obtaining radiographs is a good first step to screen chronic pelvic pain. They may provide specific information for common disorders such as arthritis or less common disorders such as bone tumors. In many instances, such as osteoarthritis, they may be the only imaging necessary. The progression through the imaging armamentarium is not sequential and depends on the appearance of the radiographs and the suspected diagnosis.

# Case 23-2

A 53-year-old woman presents with a 2-year history of progressing left pelvis pain. Her pain is exacerbated with sitting and she is able to ambulate with reasonable comfort. AP radiograph of pelvis demonstrates a sclerotic lesion in the left ilium. What imaging test should be ordered next?

In this scenario, radiographs are nonspecific and an osseous or surrounding soft tissue abnormality is suspected, but not osteoid osteoma.

Sensible recommendation: MRI PELVIS WO/W CONTRAST

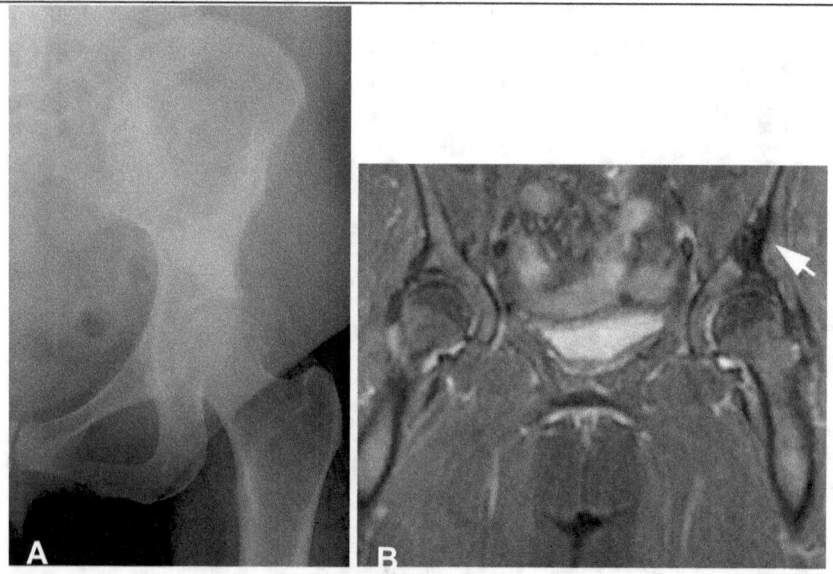

Primary bone tumor. AP radiograph of the left hip (A) shows a sclerotic focal bony lesion in the left acetabulum. Coronal T2 FS MRI of pelvis (B) shows a low signal intensity lesion in the left ilium with surrounding edema (arrow). Biopsy revealed a low-grade sclerosing osteosarcoma.

MRI is frequently performed after initial radiographs to detect osseous, articular, or soft tissue abnormalities. It is both highly sensitive and specific for detecting many abnormalities involving the hip or surrounding soft tissues and should in general be the next imaging technique used following radiographs. Other causes of a chronic pelvic pain for which MRI has been used with considerable success include radiographically occult fractures, acute and chronic soft tissue injuries, infection and inflammation, and tumors. In general, MR imaging is occasionally helpful in the diagnosis of tumor type. Radiographs remain superior for enabling prediction of the histologic diagnosis, with CT and MR imaging helpful in rare instances. MR is better than CT in showing the extent of tumor in marrow and soft tissues. Marrow lesions are often not visible on radiographs and may be subtle on CT scans. CT is better than MR imaging in showing pathologic fractures and mineralization.

## Case 23-3

A 45-year-old woman presents with chronic left hip pain. She is status post Roux-en-Y gastric bypass performed for treatment of morbid obesity complicated by diabetes mellitus, sleep apnea, hip and knee arthritis. Patient has had intermittent hip pain since the surgery. She has no risk factors for osteonecrosis, specifically, no alcohol use, or no prednisone use. She has no history of hip trauma. She reports no tingling, numbness, or weakness in the affected extremity. On physical exam, she has no pain with active straight-leg raise or with resisted straight-leg raise, but she has familiar groin pain with passive internal rotation. Radiograph of left hip shows mild osteoarthritis. She had an injection of left hip with anesthetic and corticosteroid, but it didn't improve her pain. What imaging exam should be ordered next?

This scenario concerns a patient with acute hip pain that is thought to be referred, but the clinician wishes to exclude an etiology in the hip. Initial radiographs were negative or equivocal.

Sensible recommendation: MRI PELVIS WO CONTRAST

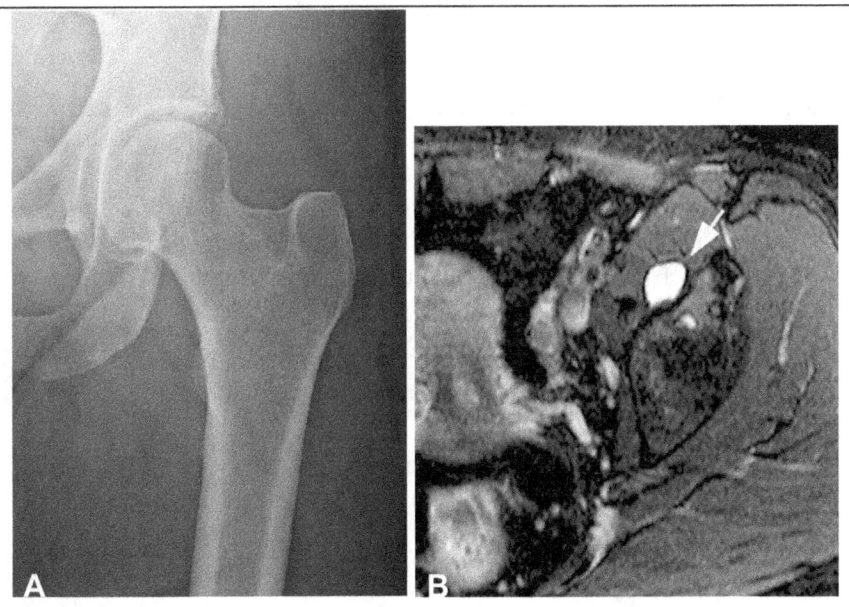

Iliopsoas bursitis. AP radiograph of the left hip (A) shows mild osteoarthritis of left hip. Axial T2 FS MRI (B) shows a fluid collection in the iliopsoas bursa (arrow). There is a small subchondral cyst at the acetabulum.

---

Diagnostic and therapeutic joint injections are useful tools for confirming the location of pain and in some cases helping in its control for a short period. Arthrocentesis is also critical in diagnosing the presence of infection or crystal disease. Local articular and extra-articular injections can define the symptomatic site and exclude referred symptoms. Intra-articular injection of a small amount of iodinated contrast medium under fluoroscopic guidance is used to confirm needle position.

The iliopsoas bursa is the single largest bursa in the human body, lying deep to the distal iliopsoas muscle complex and anterior to the superior hip joint. This bursa communicates with the hip joint in 15% of the population; thus, pathology in the iliopsoas bursa can also affect the hip joint. Iliopsoas bursitis is an inflammatory condition that causes groin pain. Rarely, patients present with a groin mass secondary to gross bursal distention. MRI is the investigation of choice for this condition as it more accurately defines the size and extent of the distended bursa and also allows evaluation of associated hip pathology. Fat-suppressed fluid-sensitive sequences typically show a rounded high-signal fluid collection posteromedial to the iliopsoas muscle. Management is most often nonoperative, consisting of rest, and rehabilitation therapy.

# Case 23-4

A 43-year-old man presents with chronic right groin pain. He has had 7 months of conservative therapy without relief and has been unable to resume playing soccer. Radiographs of the right hip and pelvis were normal. Pain is localized to the pubic and right groin region and is much worse with activity. There are no neurologic findings, and the patient is in otherwise good health The clinician suspects athletic pubalgia (sports hernia). What imaging exam should be ordered next?

This scenario concerns a patient with chronic groin pain that is not thought to be referred. Initial radiographs were negative or equivocal.

Sensible recommendation: MRI PELVIS WO CONTRAST

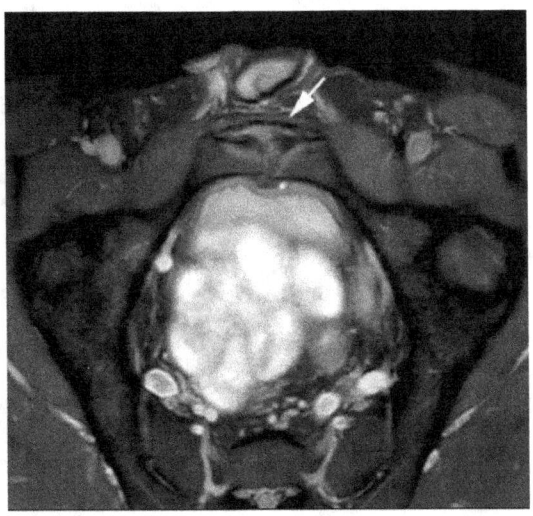

Oblique axial PD FS MRI at the level of the pubis shows separation of the common aponeurosis of the rectus abdominus and adductor muscles (arrow) from the surface of the pubis with abnormal high signal and adjacent marrow edema. These findings are diagnostic of "sports hernia.".

Chronic groin pain is a perplexing clinical problem. Symptoms may be related to numerous etiologies, including trauma, neoplasms, and arthropathies. Pain may be due to osseous, intra-articular, periarticular, or soft tissue pathology. MRI is frequently performed after initial radiographs to detect osseous and soft tissue abnormalities. It is both highly sensitive and specific for detecting many abnormalities involving the surrounding soft tissues and should, in general, be the first imaging technique used following radiographs. MRI is useful for examining surrounding soft tissue entities such as iliopsoas or subiliacus bursitis, athletic pubalgia, trochanteric bursitis, abductor tendinosis/tears, calcific tendonitis, and hamstring injuries and referred pain from spine or knee.

## Case 23-5

A 53-year-old woman presents several days after a rock-climbing injury with chronic left buttock pain that is much worse with sitting. Radiograph of left hip was read as normal. What imaging exam should be ordered next?

This scenario concerns a patient possible hamstring avulsion injury. Initial radiographs were negative or equivocal.

Sensible recommendation: MRI FEMUR WO CONTRAST

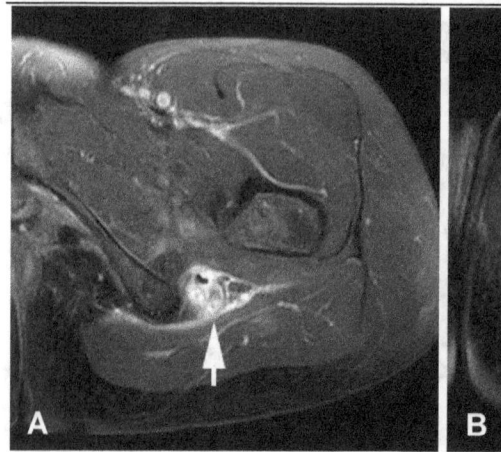 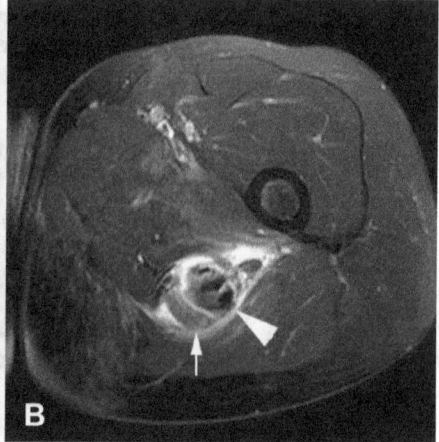

(A) Axial PD FS MRI left proximal thigh at the level of the ischium shows collection of fluid at the expected origin of the conjoint tendon of the biceps femoris and semitendinosus muscles (arrow). (B) At the level of the proximal femoral shaft, the avulsed conjoint tendon is seen (arrowhead) surrounded by fluid. The intact semimembranosus muscle is also seen (small arrow).

MRI is frequently performed after initial radiographs to detect osseous and soft tissue abnormalities. It is both highly sensitive and specific for detecting many abnormalities involving the surrounding soft tissues and should, in general, be the first imaging technique used following radiographs. MRI is useful for examining surrounding soft tissue entities such as iliopsoas or subiliacus bursitis, athletic pubalgia, trochanteric bursitis, abductor tendinosis/tears, calcific tendonitis, and hamstring injuries and referred pain from spine or knee. Contrast is not needed for MRI. For deep structures such as the hamstrings, US has poorer resolution than MRI and surgeons and patients may have more difficulty understanding the images.

## Case 23-6

89-year-old woman with a ground level fall several weeks ago. She was evaluated in the Emergency Department and radiographs were negative. She was sent home but had persistent pain. Pain is worse with long periods of sitting. Pain is worse on the right but centered over the lower sacrum/coccyx. Radiographs were normal, but follow-up whole body bone scan positive, with a typical linear pattern of abnormal uptake within the sacrum characteristic of insufficiency fracture. What is the next most appropriate step?

This scenario concerns further imaging to confirm a suspected sacral insufficiency fracture in an elderly patient. Initial radiographs normal, but bone scan hot in linear pattern typical for fracture.

Sensible recommendation: NO IMAGING

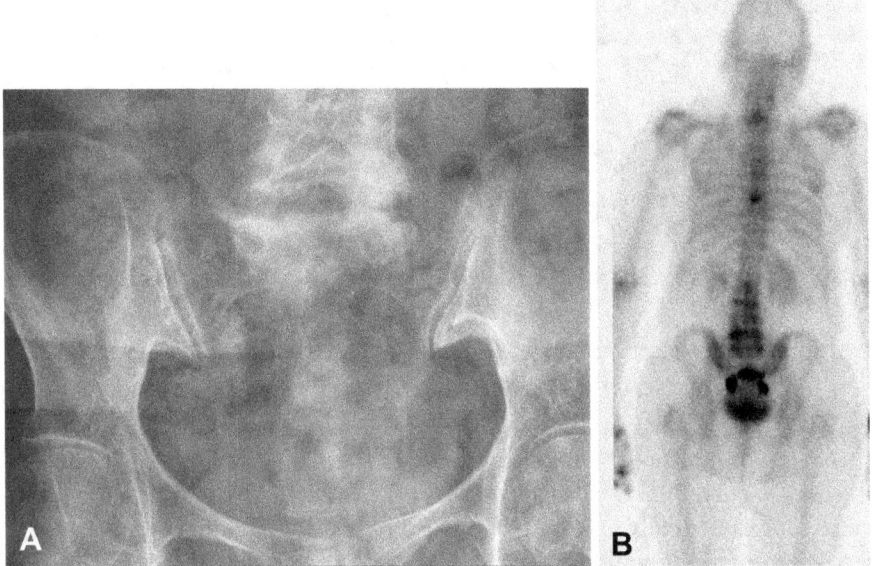

Frontal radiograph of the pelvis (A) demonstrates osteopenia, but no fracture. Follow-up whole body bone scan (B) demonstrates linear abnormal uptake within the sacrum in the characteristic H-pattern of bilateral insufficiency fractures.

When a sacral or pelvic insufficiency fracture is suspected, radiographs are normal, and the bone scan has a hot, linear pattern typical for the diagnosis, CT or MRI of the pelvis are not required, but may be used to confirm the diagnosis or find associated injuries. CT is particularly well suited for the diagnosis of stress fracture when it involves the sacrum. MRI is both sensitive and specific for the diagnosis of stress fracture.

## Case 23-7

70-year-old woman with osteoporosis and several weeks of severe right gluteal pain which radiates to her right hip and upper thigh after starting Tai Chi classes. She can walk relatively comfortably for short distances, though she could hardly walk without assistance several days prior. A pelvic radiographic series was interpreted as normal. Sacral insufficiency fracture is suspected in this osteoporotic patient; what is the next most appropriate modality to obtain to confirm the diagnosis?

This scenario concerns further imaging for a suspected insufficiency fracture (pelvis or hip). Initial radiographs normal.

Sensible recommendation: MRI PELVIS WO CONTRAST

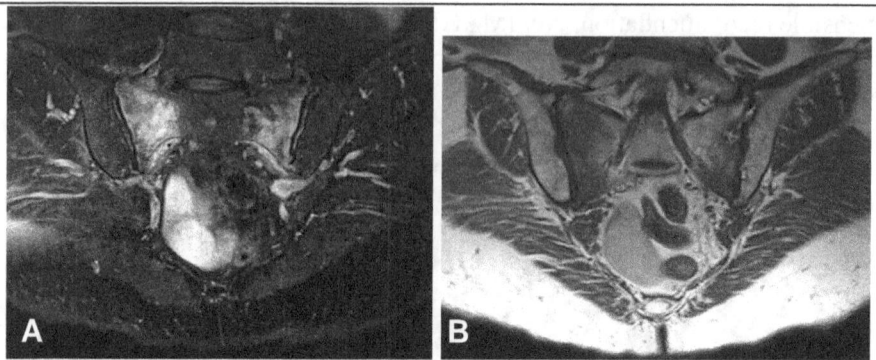

Axial T2 FS (A) and T1 MRI (B) demonstrate insufficiency fracture involving both the right and left hemisacrum.

When an insufficiency fracture is suspected in an osteoporotic patient or patient on long-term corticosteroid therapy, but with normal radiographs, repeat radiographs of the area of interest in 10-14 days, MRI of the area or interest, and Tc-99m bone scan with SPECT of the area of interest are all considered an equally appropriate next step. If the diagnosis is non-urgent, repeat radiographs could be obtained. If there is greater urgency, either MRI or bone scan can be obtained, with MRI considered superior due to potential false negative bone scan results in this cohort.

# Case 23-8

22-year-old female runner presents with 3 weeks of left groin pain. Three weeks ago, she went for a 15-mile run without any difficulty. When she got back to her car, she felt that her anterior left groin was quite tight and painful. The pain is somewhat dull and somewhat sharp and localized deep to the mid inguinal fold. She has been unable to get back to running the last 3 weeks as this reproduces her pain. She does not have any pain at rest or with walking but continues to feel like her anterior hip is tight, making it somewhat cumbersome to put her pants on. Which imaging test should be ordered first?

This scenario concerns the initial imaging exam for chronic groin pain. Suspected stress (fatigue) fracture, excluding vertebrae. First imaging study.

Sensible recommendation: XR PELVIS

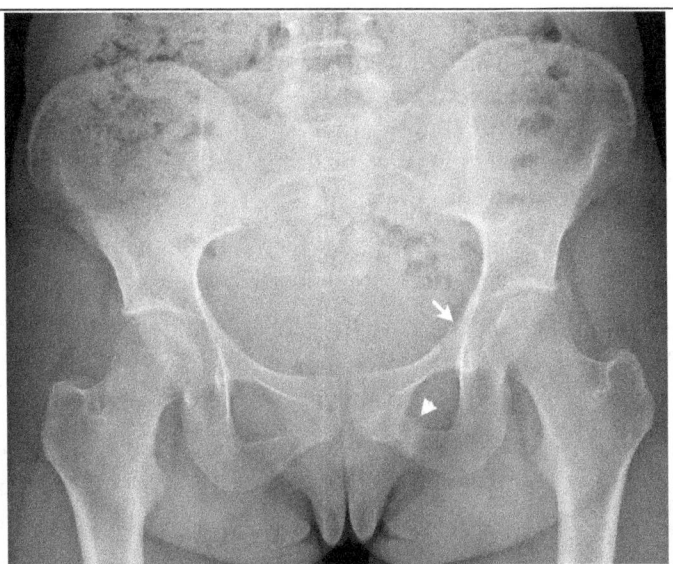

AP radiograph of pelvis demonstrates healing stress fractures at left pubic root (white arrow) and inferior obturator ring (white arrowhead).

In the setting of new or repetitive athletic activity, fatigue fractures can develop in patients with normal bone. Furthermore, certain athletic activities often result in specific sites of fatigue fracture, such as proximal femur and tibial stress fractures in runners, and tarsal navicular stress fractures in basketball players. Correlation of clinical history, pattern, and site recognition with radiographic findings is usually specific. Nevertheless, stress fractures are frequently occult on initial radiographs. Early radiographic findings are often nonspecific (subtle periosteal reaction, gray cortex sign) or even nonexistent. Late radiographic findings are often suggestive in appearance and include linear sclerosis (often perpendicular to the major trabecular lines), periosteal reaction, patchy endosteal sclerosis, and soft tissue swelling. Additionally, radiographs may remain negative depending on the timing of reimaging, the patient's metabolic bone status, and the type and location of the fracture. Thus, radiographs are specific but significantly insensitive. Despite this limitation, all authorities agree that radiographs should be the initial imaging modality; if the findings are conclusive, no further imaging need be performed.

# Case 23-9

29-year-old man presents with pain mainly in the joints in his hips, buttock, and lower back. He reports the onset of symptoms approximately 5-6 years ago. He describes increasing morning stiffness lasting 1-2 hours, especially in his lower back and hips. He gradually developed difficulty taking full, deep breath, as it caused sternal pain. He was not seen by a provider for the stiffness, instead used naproxen or other NSAIDs to help alleviate the pain. He notes it has been difficult to bend forward, to tie his shoes, and notes decreasing range of motion in his upper extremities. What is the most appropriate first imaging study?

This scenario concerns a patient presents with inflammatory sacroiliac or back symptoms. Suspected axial spondyloarthropathy. Initial evaluation.

Sensible recommendation: XR SACROILIAC JOINT, XR SPINE 2 VIEW, region of interest

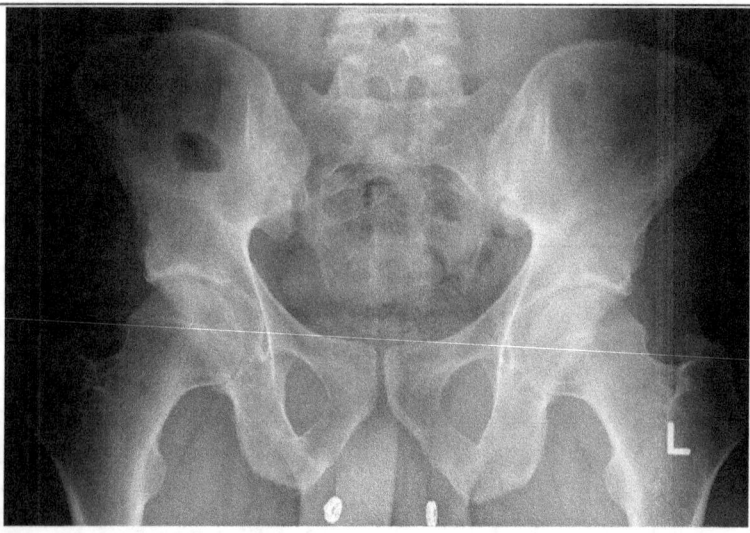

Ankylosing spondylitis. AP radiograph of pelvis demonstrates bony erosions associated with sclerosis involving both sacroiliac joints consistent with sacroiliitis. There is also diffuse joint space narrowing and erosions in both hips.

The axial spondyloarthropathies (axSpAs) are a group of inflammatory arthritides that include ankylosing spondylitis, psoriatic arthritis, reactive arthritis, and inflammatory bowel disease related spondyloarthropathies. These axSpAs involve the sacroiliac (SI) joints and/or the spine. It is estimated that as much as 5% of chronic back pain is caused by an underlying axSpA. Symptoms may begin in childhood or early adulthood and can lead to loss of mobility and function. As there is no one pathognomonic test, the diagnosis of axSpAs is often challenging and is based on a combination of physical exam, biological data (HLA-B27, C-reactive protein), and imaging findings. An axSpA typically presents prior to 45 years of age. The pain is chronic (3 months or more duration) and insidious in onset, with "inflamma-tory symptoms" that, depending of the criteria used, can include morning stiffness, pain that improves with exercise but not rest, pain that awakens in the second half of the night, and alternating buttock pain. There has been an evolution of the diagnostic criteria for the axSpAs. Assessment of Spondy-loArthritis International Society (ASAS) classification system includes combinations of clinical findings with or without imaging evidence of sacro-iliitis. The most pronounced change in the classification has been the inclusion of SI inflammatory lesions on magnetic resonance imaging (MRI) as an imaging means of early identification of patients with "pre-radio-graphic" spondyloarthropathy. Effective new biological therapies, such as the tumor necrosis factor-α antagonists, which have the potential to arrest disease progression and prevent the development of disability, make early diagnosis and treatment prior to radiographic joint damage essential. The in-itial imaging should begin with radiographic evaluation of the SI joints. For imaging of the SI joints, a standard anteroposterior (AP) radiograph of the pelvis may be sufficient. The ASAS recommends the whole pelvis with the hip joints be included as part of the initial screening AP imaging. Cervical, thoracic and lumbar spine radiographs with a minimum of an initial lateral projection should be obtained based on the regions of the patient's clinical symptoms. Decisions for advanced imaging should be made based on the re-sults of radiography and the clinical need for additional assessment.

## Case 23-10

33-year-old man presents with pain and discomfort in the posterior gluteal area for the last six years. It does not limit him or concern him except for several weeks out of the year during which he will have a "flare" of his symptoms. He denies any history of low back pain or stiffness. He cannot run because of his buttock pain. He denies any history of uveitis, rashes, fo-cal weakness, numbness, or tingling, and no history of oral or nasal ulcers. He has had completely normal GI symptoms that is normal bowel move-ments. Radiographs of his sacroiliac joints were non-diagnostic. What is the most appropriate next imaging study?

This scenario concerns a patient presents with inflammatory sacroiliac symptoms. Suspected axial spondyloarthropathy. Radiographs negative or equivocal.

Sensible recommendation: MRI PELVIS WO CONTRAST or MRI PELVIS WO/W CONTRAST

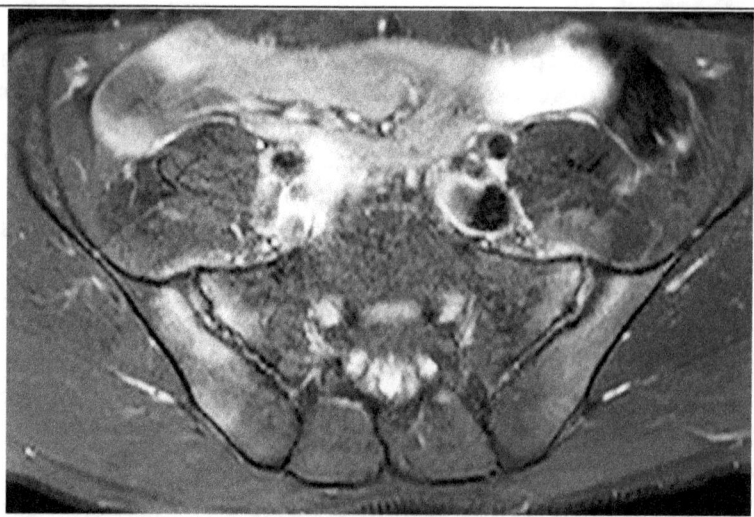

Ankylosing spondylitis. Axial T2 FS image of sacroiliac joints demonstrates sub-chondral edema and bony erosions involving bilateral sacroiliac joints.

CT of the SI joints without contrast may be helpful in cases when equivocal radiographic abnormalities exist, allowing identification of subtle erosions and soft tissue ossification. In the absence of radiographic findings, MRI of the SI joints is the best examination for the assessment of acute inflammatory changes. Intravenous gadolinium contrast-enhanced, T1-weighted, fat-saturated sequences may improve detection of subtle inflammatory lesions and differentiation of synovitis from joint fluid during the initial evaluation for axSpA. However, contrast-enhanced imaging has not been shown to significantly increase the diagnostic accuracy of MRI for sacroiliitis.

## Case 23-11

33-year-old man presents with chronic back pain for approximately the last 20 years. His back pain started when he was approximately 13 years old (20 years ago) as a teenager. He reports that his back pain is worst int he mid and low back. He reports daily constant pain of 5-6/10 that has progressively worsened over the past 20 years. He reports that pain is worse in the morning when he wakes up or if he rests for a prolonged period of time. He reports significant stiffness associated with the back pain. He recently started to have buttock pain and for that he has been taking naproxen 1-2 tablets daily. He reports it helps his pain but does not completely resolve it. Of note, the patient reports no loss of bowel or bladder control or symptoms of the urinary retention. The patient also reports no history of eye burning or abdominal pain, or bloody diarrhea in his past. Radiographs and MRI of his sacroiliac joints were negative. What is the most appropriate next imaging study?

This scenario concerns a patient presents with inflammatory sacroiliac symptoms. Suspected axial spondyloarthropathy. Negative radiographs and MRI of the sacroiliac joints.

Sensible recommendation: XR SPINE 2 VIEW, region of interest

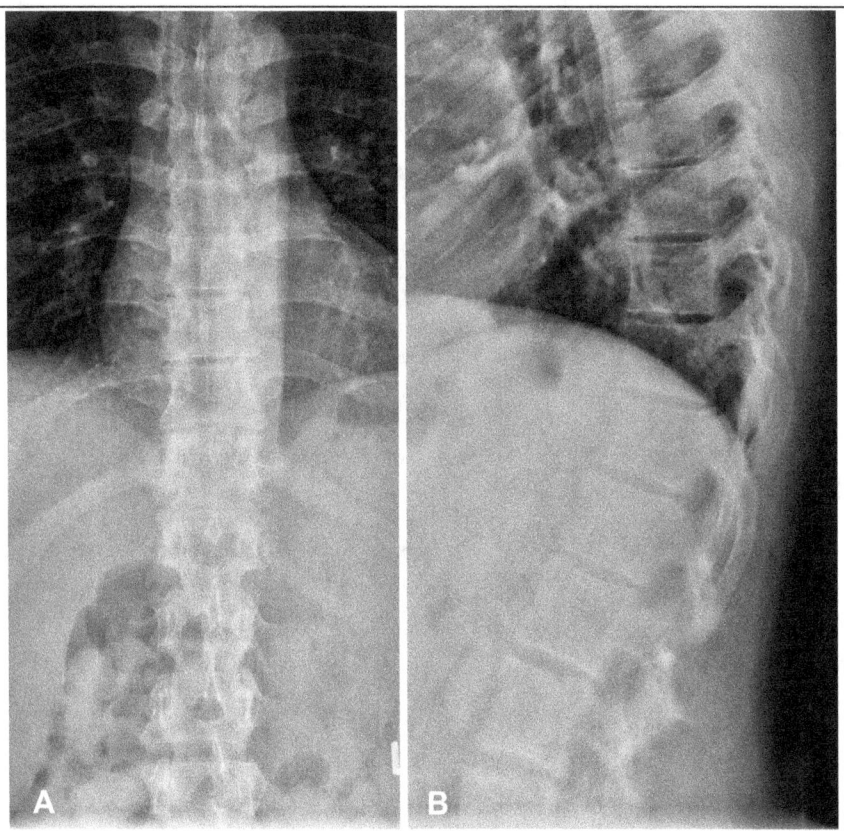

Ankylosing spondylitis. AP (A) and lateral (B) radiographs of thoracolumbar spine demonstrate squaring of vertebral bodies and scattered ankylosis of facet joints.

Isolated spine inflammatory involvement in the setting of normal SI joints has in the past been considered a rare occurrence but has since been recognized more frequently (6%–23%) on MR examinations. Lateral radiographs at minimum of the cervical and lumbar spine, if not already performed, may allow identification of findings that can help establish a diagnosis. CT may allow better visualization of subtle erosive changes or enthesopathic bone formation in the posterior elements or for evaluation of thoracic spine disease. If radiographs are normal and disease is unable to be confirmed by MRI of the sacroiliac joints, spine MRI may be helpful to support diagnosis.

## Case 23-12

85-year-old man presents with acute back pain after fall. He was on a ladder trying to pin something from a tree limb when he fell 5 feet. Patient is unsure if he had loss of consciousness at that time. Patient denies abdominal pain, nausea vomiting. Patient denies weakness or numbness in his arms or legs. He has history of ankylosing spondylolysis, and congestive heart failure with a pacemaker placed. Radiographs of thoracolumbar spine demonstrate ankylosis of thoracolumbar spines with widened intervertebral disc space at T11-12. What is the most appropriate next imaging study?

This scenario concerns a patient presents with spine ankyloses. Suspected fracture.

Sensible recommendation: CT SPINE WO CONTRAST, region of interest

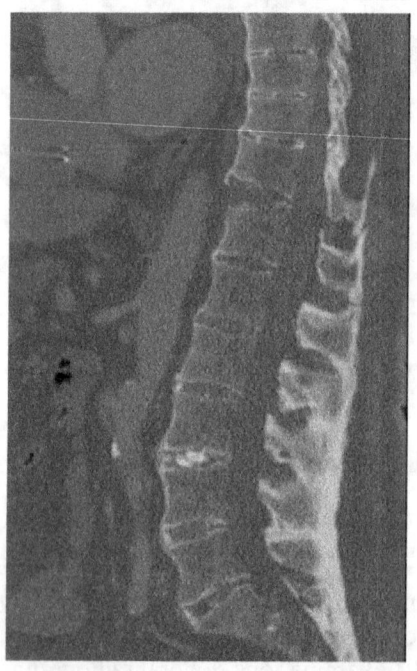

Sagittal CT image of thoracolumbar spine shows T11-T12 disc space hyperextension injury with over 1.5 cm of distraction anteriorly and compression of the posterior elements, as evidence by fracture of the calcified supraspinous ligament on image. There is a minimally displaced fracture of the right T12 superior facet.

AxSpA is associated with the development of both osteoporosis and ankylosis of the spine. Spinal fractures in the setting of ankylosis are frequently from low-energy mechanisms, such as a fall from standing or even in the absence of recognizable trauma as presumed insufficiency fractures. Many of these fractures involve all 3 columns of the spine and are unstable, with a high associated rate of neurologic injury. Radiographs are an inexpensive initial imaging method of evaluation but have a poor sensitivity for the presence or extent of fracture. CT with multiplanar reformatted images is necessary for exclusion of fracture of the spine in a patient with ankylosis and pain following any report of trauma. If neurological symptoms are present, MRI without contrast would be recommended for the evaluation for spinal cord, nerve root and ligamentous injuries.

# Case 23-13

30-year-old man presents with chronic low back pain secondary to Ankylosing spondylitis diagnosed 12 years ago. He was previously on infliximab with good response. He has also been on adalimumab. Over the last month, he feels like his arthritis symptoms are improving, but he has back pain that is sharp, located in left lateral thoracolumbar, and lower lumbosacral region. His thoracolumbar pain is most bothersome, rated 10/10 when it flairs. What is the most appropriate imaging for follow-up?

This scenario concerns a patient with known axial spondyloarthropathy. Follow-up for treatment response or disease progression.

Sensible recommendation: XR SACROILIAC JOINT, XR SPINE 2 VIEW, region of interest

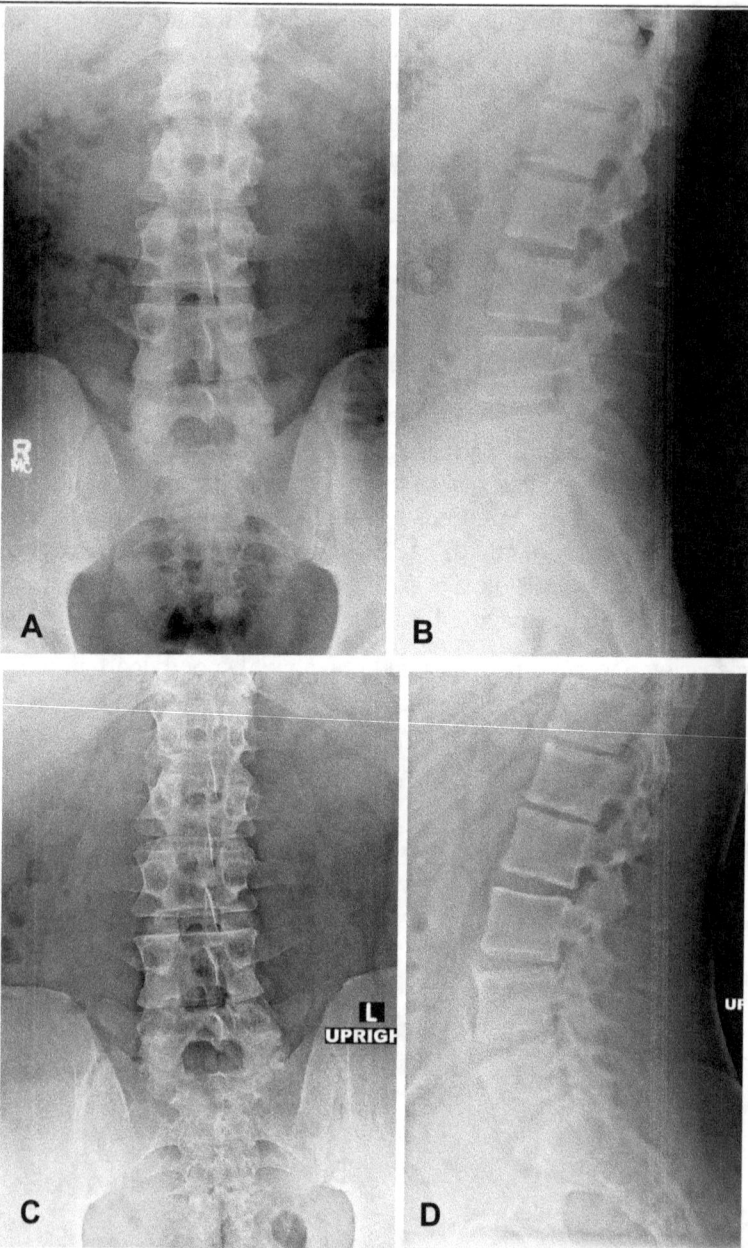

Ankylosing spondylitis. AP (A) and lateral (B) radiographs of lumbar spine, obtained 12 years ago demonstrate mild sacroiliitis and squaring of vertebral bodies. Follow-up AP (C) and lateral (D) radiographs of lumbar spine demonstrate sclerosis of corners of vertebral bodies (shiny corner sign) and endplates. Inflammatory sacroiliits has progressed.

In conjunction with clinical examination and laboratory biomarkers, conventional radiographs of the SI joints and symptomatic regions of the spine are the primary method of following structural progression of disease. The frequency of radiographic monitoring should be based on the patient's individual symptoms, with a general recommendation of no more frequently than every 2 years. MRI may be helpful for evaluation of persistent inflammation as a determination of treatment response. Gadolinium-enhanced imaging is not needed to identify active inflammatory lesions, which are equally well identified on fluid-sensitive fat-suppressed imaging (T2-weighted fat-saturated or STIR imaging).

# References

1.  Mintz DN, Roberts CC, Bencardino JT, Baccei SJ, Caird MS, Cassidy RC, Chang EY, Fox MG, Gyftopoulos S, Kransdorf MJ, Metter DF, Morrison WB, Rosenberg ZS, Shah NA, Small KM, Subhas N, Tambar S, Towers JD, Yu JS, Weissman BN. ACR Appropriateness Criteria(®) Chronic Hip Pain. J Am Coll Radiol. 2017 May;14(5S):S90-S102. doi: 10.1016/j.jacr.2017.01.035. Review. PMID: 28473098.
2.  American College of Radiology. ACR Appropriateness Criteria: Chronic hip pain, revised 2016. https://acsearch.acr.org/docs/69425/Narrative/ (accessed April 24, 2021).
3.  Bencardino JT, Stone TJ, Roberts CC, Appel M, Baccei SJ, Cassidy RC, Chang EY, Fox MG, Greenspan BS, Gyftopoulos S, Hochman MG, Jacobson JA, Mintz DN, Mlady GW, Newman JS, Rosenberg ZS, Shah NA, Small KM, Weissman BN. ACR Appropriateness Criteria(®) Stress (Fatigue/Insufficiency) Fracture, Including Sacrum, Excluding Other Vertebrae. J Am Coll Radiol. 2017 May;14(5S):S293-S306. doi: 10.1016/j.jacr.2017.02.035. Review. PMID: 28473086.
4.  American College of Radiology. ACR Appropriateness Criteria: Stress (Fatigue/Insufficiency) Fracture, Including Sacrum, Excluding Other Vertebrae, revised 2016. https://acsearch.acr.org/docs/69435/Narrative/ (accessed April 24, 2021).
5.  American College of Radiology. ACR Appropriateness Criteria: Chronic Back Pain: Suspected Sacroiliitis/Spondyloarthropathy, 2016. https://acsearch.acr.org/docs/3094107/Narrative/ (accessed April 24, 2021).

# Chapter 24. Chronic or Nontraumatic Hip Pain

Hyojeong Lee, MD

Radiography is the initial exam for chronic or nontraumatic hip pain. MRI, US, or CT may be helpful for further evaluation, and the bone scan may have a problem-solving role.

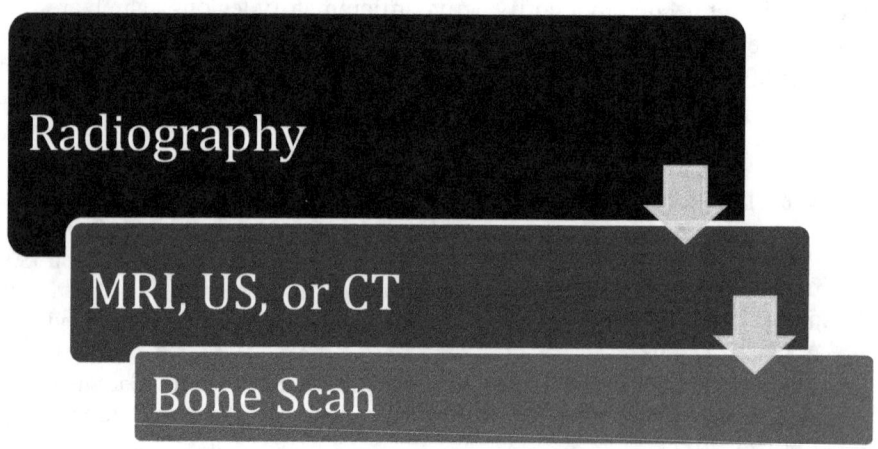

# Case 24-1

28-year-old man presents with a several year history of right hip pain. His hip pain began gradually; there was no history of trauma or discrete injury. The pain is located diffusely about the hip, thigh, knee and low-back. It is worse with weight bearing, and relieved by NSAIDs. What is the most appropriate first imaging study?

This scenario concerns a patient with chronic hip pain. First imaging study.

Sensible recommendation: XR PELVIS AND HIP

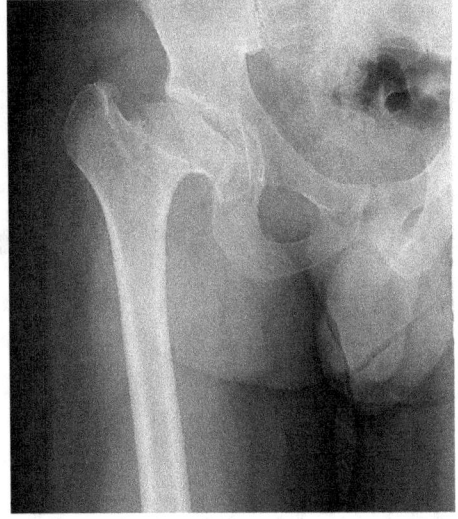

Frontal radiograph of right hip demonstrates dysplastic appearance of right hip; coxa magna, coxa plana and coxa vara. Findings are consistent with a sequela of prior LCP (Legg- Calve- Perthes) disease.

Depending on history and physical examination, imaging may not be necessary to evaluate all hip pain. Radiographs should be obtained first in most, if not all, cases and may provide specific information for common disorders such as arthritis or less common disorders such as primary bone tumors. For certain disorders, such as dysplasia or femoroacetabular impingement (FAI), specialized views such as the false profile or a Dunn view can provide more detailed evaluation of the anatomy. Radiography is an excellent screening tool. Whether the radiographs are normal or not, they are often of considerable value for the selection of additional imaging. For OA, a common entity, physical examination and radiography may be better than MRI and have reasonable sensitivity and specificity.

# Case 24-2

81-year-old woman with a five-month history of right hip pain. She doesn't have history of injury. On physical exam, her right greater trochanter is point tender to palpation and she has myofascial para-articular trigger points. AP radiograph of her right hip shows minimal arthritic changes and osteopenia. What imaging exam should be ordered next?

This scenario concerns a patient with chronic hip pain. Radiographs negative, equivocal, or nondiagnostic. Suspect extra- articular noninfectious soft tissue abnormality, such as tendonitis. Next imaging study.

Sensible recommendation: MRI HIP WO CONTRAST

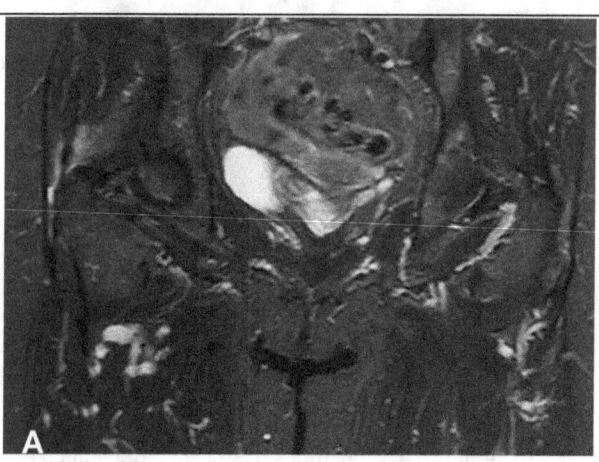

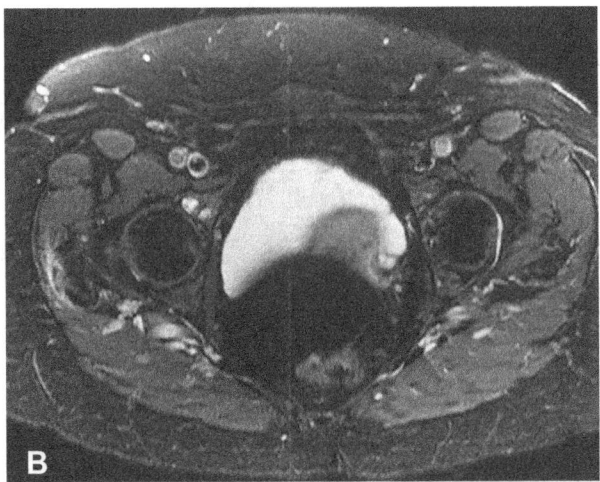

Coronal (A) and axial (B) T2 FS MRI of hip demonstrate edema around right gluteus medius tendon, in keeping with tendinitis.

MRI is frequently performed after initial radiographs to detect osseous and soft tissue abnormalities of hip. It is both highly sensitive and specific for detecting many abnormalities involving the surrounding soft tissues and should, in general, be the first imaging technique used following radiographs. MRI is useful for examining surrounding soft tissue entities such as iliopsoas or subiliacus bursitis, athletic pubalgia, trochanteric bursitis, abductor tendinosis/tears, calcific tendonitis, and hamstring injuries. Other causes of a chronically painful hip for which MRI has been used with considerable success include acute and chronic soft tissue injuries, inflammation, and tumors. IV gadolinium chelate agents or US can be used to differentiate between joint fluid and synovitis. IV contrast is rarely needed for MRI.

## Case 24-3

53-year-old woman who is a marathon runner presents with chronic left hip pain. Her pain started about a year ago. She tore her adductor muscle about two years ago while she was training for marathon. She feels like she never fully recovered from her injury. The pain is more in her ischial region now. AP radiograph of her left hip shows minimal arthritic changes. What imaging exam should be ordered next?

This scenario concerns a patient with chronic hip pain. Radiographs negative, equivocal, or nondiagnostic. Suspect impingement. Next imaging study.

Sensible recommendation: MRI HIP WO CONTRAST or MRI HIP AR-

THROGRAPHY

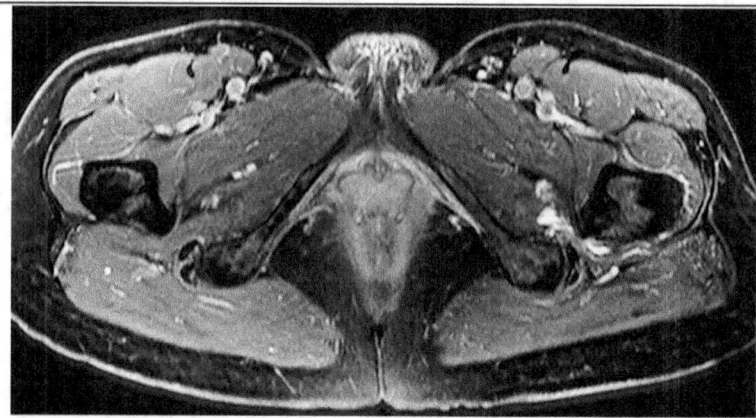

Ischiofemoral impingement. Axial T2 FS MR image of the hip shows asymmetric narrowing of left ischiofemoral space associated with partial thickness tear of left quadratus femoris.

Osseous abnormalities are often evident on radiographs (incidence unverified), but cross-sectional imaging is more sensitive for many abnormalities.

Intrinsic bony abnormalities include fracture, osteonecrosis, and tumor. Extrinsic bony pathology includes dysplasia and the impingement syndromes, both intra-articular (FAI) and extra-articular (ischiopelvic, ischiotrochanteric, subspinous, and femoropelvic). MRI is sensitive and specific diagnosing those abnormalities. MRI and CT arthrography are useful for evaluating articular cartilage and labrum of the hip.

## Case 24-4

A 33-year-old man presents with right groin pain for 6 months. He is an avid hockey player who has been playing ice hockey for about two years. He started physical therapy, took about a month off from hockey, and began to feel better and then got back to hockey. He went back into a tournament where he played for three days in a row and it increased his pain significantly. He discontinued hockey for the last month and a half, except for about two to three weeks ago he played hockey and thought he was going to do it to a lesser degree, but it seemed to flare things up again unfortunately. He still has a chronic soreness in his right groin and he describes it sometimes as deep. It does not really radiate, and there is no low back pain nor any numbness or tingling paresthesia, nor left-sided symptoms. Radiograph right hip is obtained and reported as normal (not shown). What imaging exam should be ordered next?

This scenario concerns a patient with chronic hip pain and suspected acetabular labral tear or femoroacetabular impingement. Initial radiographs were negative or equivocal.

Sensible recommendation: MRI HIP ARTHROGRAPHY

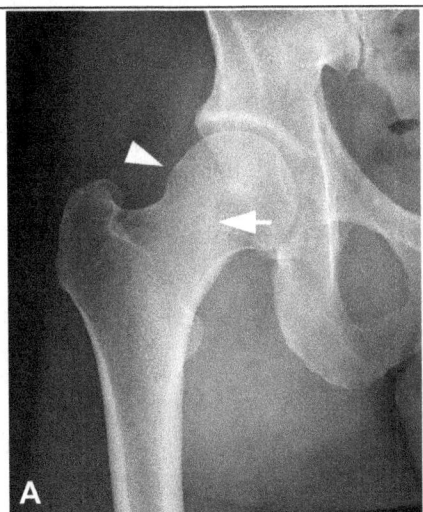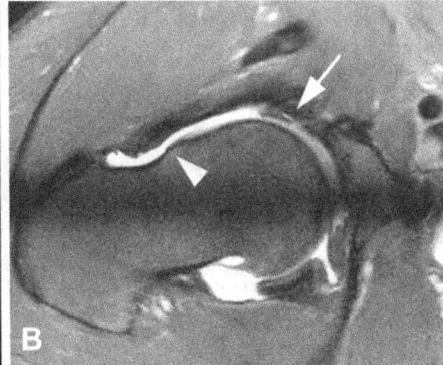

Femoroacetabular impingement. AP radiograph of the right hip (A) shows aspherical femoral head, and a bump at the head-neck junction (arrowhead. There is a synovial herniation pit (arrow). Radial T2 FS MR arthrogram image of the right hip (B) shows superior labral tear (arrow) and a femoral bump (arrowhead).

For evaluating labral tears, MR arthrography should probably be used. Direct MR arthrography with the intra-articular injection of a dilute (1:200) solution of Gd-chelate in saline has been established as a reliable technique for diagnosing acetabular labral tears that are frequently associated with femoroacetabular impingement (FAI) syndrome and may be an effective tool in assessing acetabular cartilage delamination.

High-resolution MRI with 3T may improve the visualization of the acetabular labrum and the hyaline articular cartilage. Indirect MR arthrography, in which Gd-chelate contrast is administered by IV injection and diffuses into the joint space through the synovium, has been proposed as an alternative to direct MR arthrography for detecting intra-articular disorders. It is faster and easier to perform than direct arthrography and does not require fluoroscopy. It suffers from less consistent enhancement of the joint space as well as inability to distend the joint capsule. Its value in assessing the hyaline articular cartilage and the acetabular labrum of the hip is uncertain. Hip cartilage abnormalities also can be successfully evaluated by high-resolution CT arthrography. Three-dimensional CT is an accurate tool for quantifying the femoral head-neck concavity, for providing a noninvasive assessment of hips at risk of FAI, and for assessing the femoral offset in osteoarthritis hip. CT is also useful in evaluating hip dysplasia, including the medial acetabular bone stock, in preoperative planning for hip replacement.

# Case 24-5

23-year-old man presents with chronic bilateral, left greater than the right hip pain. His hip pain started back to injury in basketball practice two years ago, worsening over time, limiting activities such as running or jumping. Pelvic radiographs demonstrate bilateral hip osteoarthritis. The clinician wants to evaluate articular cartilage status of hips. What is the most appropriate next imaging study?

This scenario concerns a patient with chronic hip pain. Evaluate articular cartilage. Next test after radiographs.

Sensible recommendation: MRI HIP WO CONTRAST or MRI HIP ARTHROGRAPHY

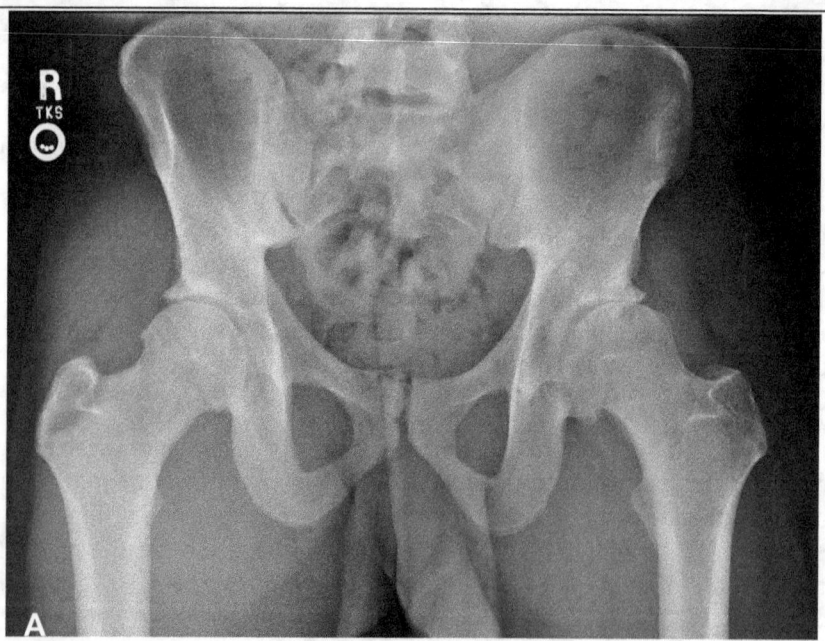

Osteoarthritis. AP radiograph of the pelvis (A) shows osteoarthritis in both hips. The left hip shows obliterated superior joint space narrowing associated with a subchondral cyst in the left femoral head.

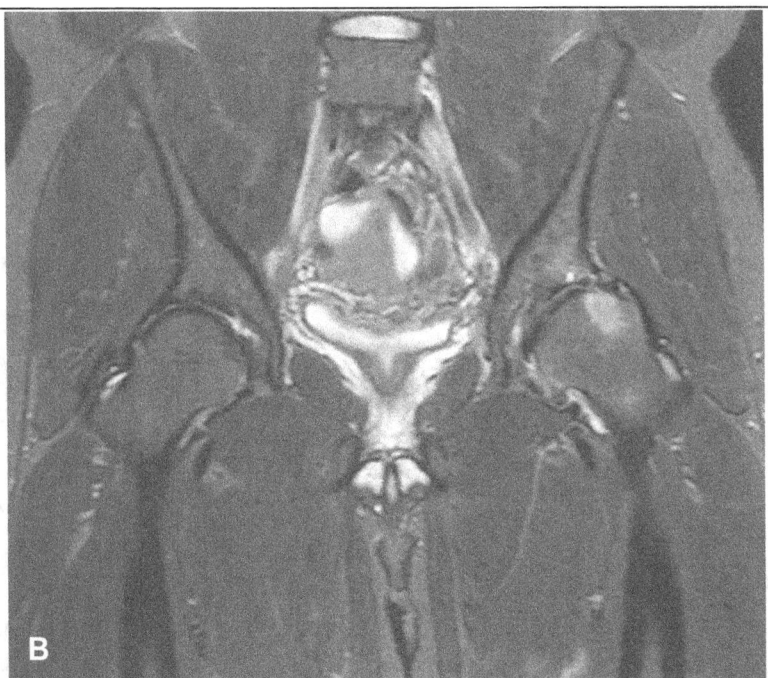

Coronal T2 FS MR image of both hips (B) shows articular cartilage thinning with osteophytosis in the right hip, and loss of articular cartilage of left hip associated with subchondral cysts, subchondral edema and osteophytosis.

Direct visualization of articular cartilage is possible using those imaging techniques that provide either intrinsic contrast (MRI and US) or extrinsic contrast (any type of arthrography). Different methods of chondral imaging are possible on routine MRI and there are ultrastructural techniques (T2 mapping, T1rho, dGEMRIC, sodium imaging) that are mostly used for research. MRI, MR arthrography, and CT arthrography can all give excellent delineation of articular cartilage. Grading systems for cartilage are primarily used for research.

# Case 24-6

39-year-old woman presents with a chronic left hip pain, worsening during the last two weeks. She has history of IVDU (in remission), endometrial cancer status post radical hysterectomy, radiation and chemotherapy. She fell on her left hip about two weeks ago, and since that time, she has had significant pain with ambulating, and actually cannot ambulate without a walker. When she moves her hip - especially with extension - she feels a popping and clicking noise. She has not noted any numbness, or tingling. She had a fever to 102 degrees during the last 2 weeks associated with night sweats. Plain radiographs of pelvis were reported as septic arthritis of left hip. What is the most appropriate next imaging study?

This scenario concerns a patient with chronic hip pain. Arthritis of uncertain type. Radiographs positive. Infection is a consideration.

Sensible recommendation: MRI HIP WO/W CONTRAST, XR JOINT ASPIRATION HIP

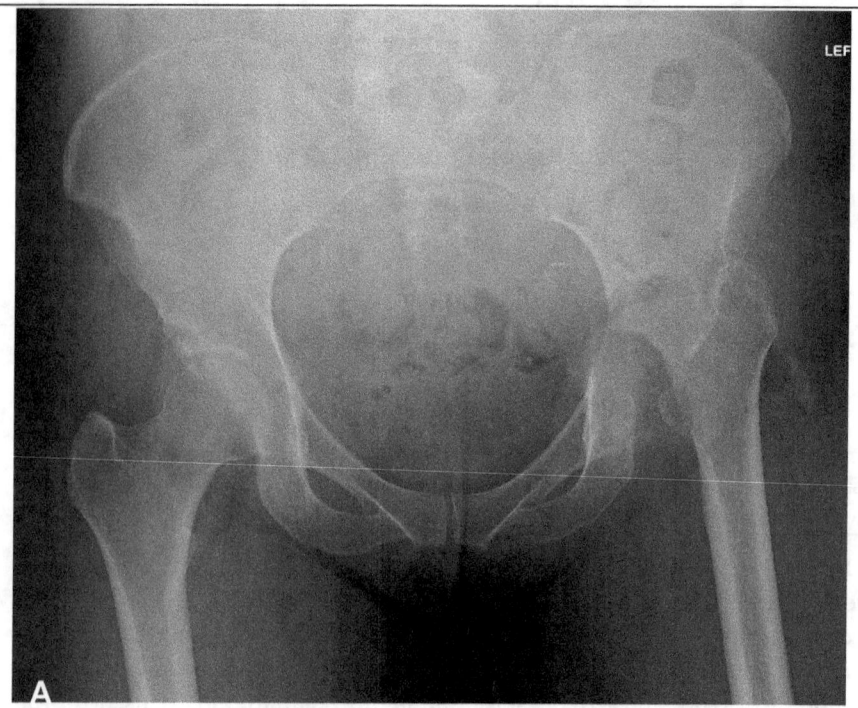

Septic arthritis. AP radiograph of the pelvis (A) shows destruction of left hip. The femoral head and acetabulum are resorbed associated with superior migration of femoral shaft supero-laterally.

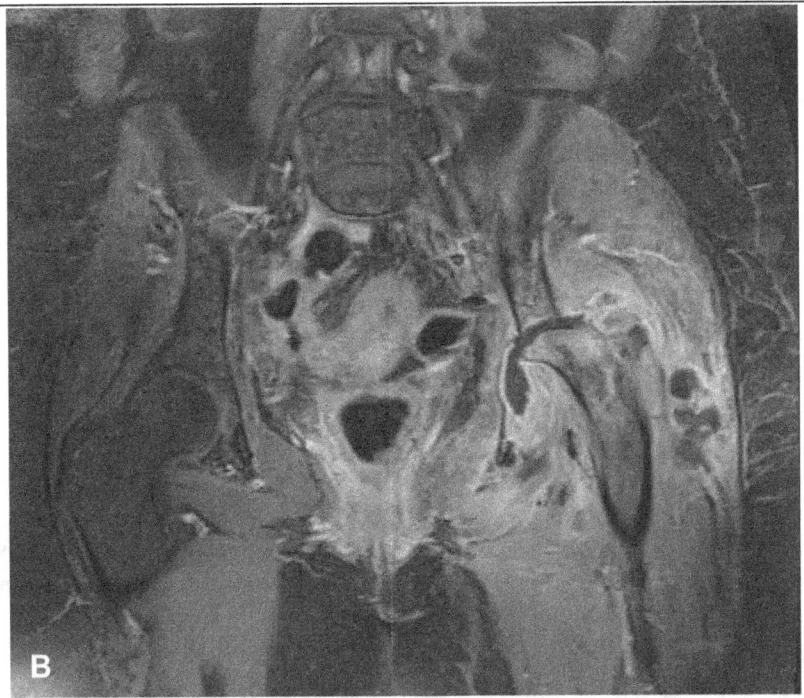

Coronal post-contrast T1 FS MR image of both hips (B) shows bony erosions of left hip, synovitis and joint effusion. Multiple lobulated intra-muscular abscesses are present in the left thigh muscles.

A rheumatologic evaluation may be appropriate, including bloodwork and evaluation for other areas of abnormality, perhaps with bone scan or 18F-fluoride PET. The best way to exclude septic arthritis is by joint aspiration. MRI is a noninvasive option. In the pediatric population, where debridement will be performed, US may be used to identify the effusion before joint aspiration or surgery. If an infectious etiology leads to chronic pain, less aggressive organisms must be considered. Although CT scan can demonstrate erosions and enthesophytes before radiography, it has not been shown to specifically evaluate infection.

## Case 24-7

A 25-year-old woman presents with chronic right hip pain for the past year. She had no traumatic event to her right hip. She denies any problems with her hips as a child. At the time she was working as a bank teller and she felt that maybe standing all day contributed to her hip pain. Her pain is mostly in her groin, although she does get some pain over her greater trochanteric area. She also gets a painful popping sensation. The pain can last anywhere from hours even to weeks depending on how much pain she has. Her pain is brought on by activity such as walking, especially stair climbing and coaching soccer. There is nothing particular that makes the pain better. She denies any other medical problems. She has had blood work in the past, apparently for inflammatory disorders and she reports that this is normal. AP radiograph of the hip shows subchondral cysts in the acetabulum associated with mild joint space narrowing and osteophytosis. What imaging exam should be ordered next?

This scenario concerns a patient with chronic hip pain whose initial radiographs were suggestive of synovial osteochondromatosis or pigmented villonodular synovitis (PVNS). Next imaging study.

Sensible recommendation: MRI HIP WO CONTRAST

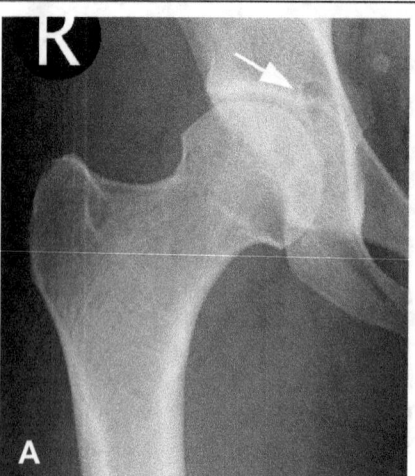

PVNS. AP radiograph of the right hip (A) shows subchondral cysts in the acetabulum (arrow) associated with mild joint space narrowing and osteophytosis. Coronal T2 FS MRI (B) shows diffuse synovitis in the right hip. Axial GRE MRI (C) shows magnetic susceptibility (arrowhead) throughout the synovitis with significant blooming (signal dropout). There are erosions associated with this involving the superior aspect of the acetabulum (arrow).

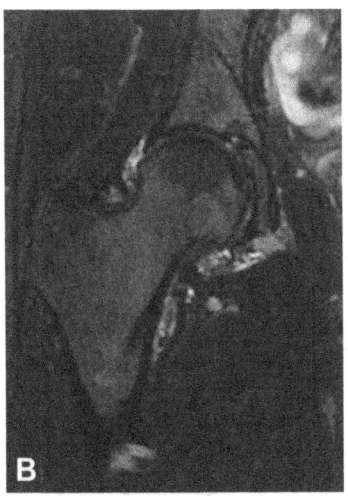
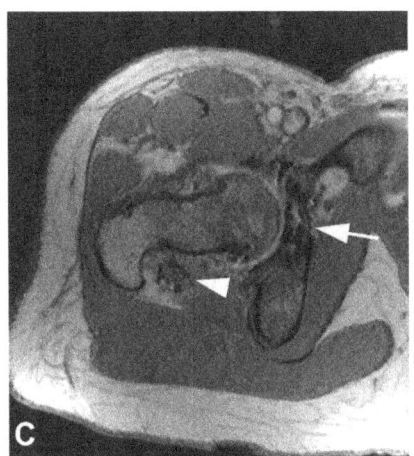

MRI is frequently performed after initial radiographs to detect osseous, articular, or soft tissue abnormalities. It is both highly sensitive and specific for detecting many abnormalities involving the hip or surrounding soft tissues and should in general be the first imaging technique used following radiographs. Generally, if the arthritis has an atypical appearance on radiographs, MRI may be helpful for further characterization and the intravenous contrast is rarely needed.

PVNS is an uncommon benign neoplastic process that may involve the synovium of the joint diffusely or focally (called PVNS) or that may occur extra-articularly in a bursa or tendon sheath (called giant cell tumor of tendon sheath). The knee, followed by the hip, is the most common location for PVNS. Radiographs reveal nonspecific features of a joint effusion. Extrinsic erosion of bone (on both sides of the joint) may also be seen and is most frequent with intra-articular involvement of the hip (>90% of cases). Cross-sectional imaging reveals diffuse involvement of the synovium. The MR imaging findings of prominent low signal intensity (seen with T2-weighting) and blooming artifact from the hemosiderin (seen with gradient-echo sequences) are nearly pathognomonic of this diagnosis. In addition, MR imaging is optimal for evaluating lesion extent.

## Case 24-8

47-year-old man presents with a three-month history of right hip pain with gradual onset. He states that he notices some clicking and popping in his right hip joint occasionally when he makes sudden rotational movements. He reports the pain is a deep pain, occasionally sharp, located over his right lateral hip. He has surgical history of prior lumbar discectomy. Radiographs of right hip shows mild osteoarthritis. What is the most appropriate next imaging study?

This scenario concerns a patient with chronic hip pain and low back, pelvic, or knee pathology. Want to exclude hip as the source. Radiographs negative, equivocal, or showing mild osteoarthritis.

Sensible recommendation: MRI HIP WO CONTRAST

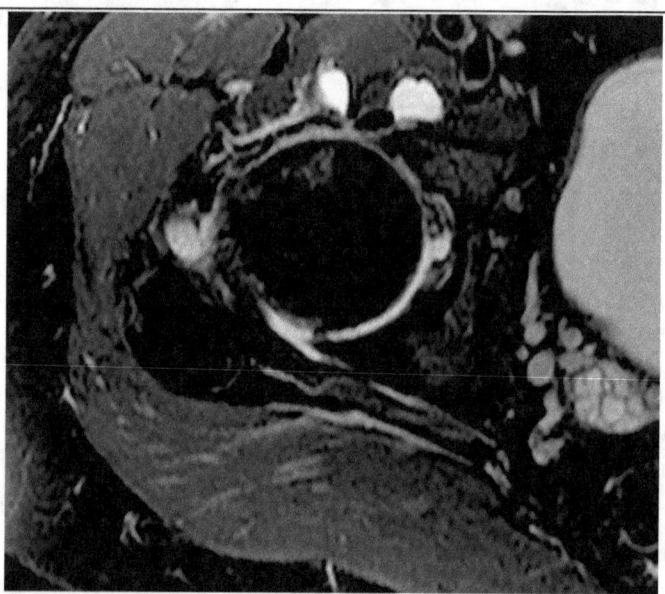

Axial T2 FS MR image of right hip shows mild osteoarthritis of right hip with small joint effusion and a communicating iliopsoas bursitis.

MRI is frequently performed after initial radiographs to detect osseous and soft tissue abnormalities of hip. It is both highly sensitive and specific for detecting many abnormalities involving the surrounding soft tissues and should, in general, be the first imaging technique used following radiographs. MRI is useful for examining surrounding soft tissue entities such as iliopsoas or subiliacus bursitis, athletic pubalgia, trochanteric bursitis, abductor tendinosis/tears, calcific tendonitis, and hamstring injuries.

## Case 24-9

A 15-year-old girl presents with right hip pain for a month. She is a sophomore who joined the cross-country team 2 months ago. She had never been a runner before, and she had been running about 10-15 miles per week. A month ago, she noted severe right anterior hip pain and she was unable to continue running. She used crutches for a week and gradually got off them but has still been limping with a significantly antalgic gait (but without crutches). She feels her pain has improved but she is not able to normalize her gait pattern. Her hip radiographs were normal. Which imaging test should be ordered first?

This scenario concerns the next imaging exam for chronic hip pain. Suspected stress (fatigue) fracture. Negative radiographs. Next imaging study.

Sensible recommendation: MRI HIP WO CONTRAST

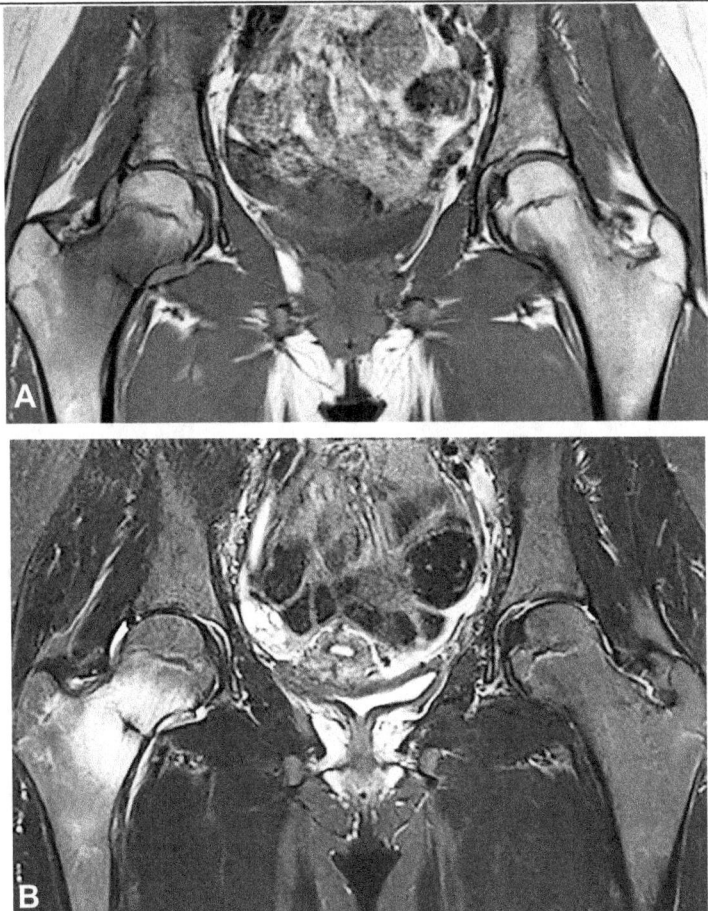

MRI of right hip coronal T1 (A) and T2 FS (B) images demonstrate a medial compression type stress fracture of the right femoral neck.

Stress fractures in the femur most often occur in the femoral neck and represent up to 7% of all stress fractures. Lateral "tension-type" femoral neck stress fractures are inherently unstable and prone to displacement and are high-risk fractures, often necessitating percutaneous screw fixation. Medial "compression-type" femoral neck stress fractures are low risk and can be treated with a non–weight-bearing regimen. Finally, stress fractures of the femoral head are high risk in healthy patients and, if not recognized promptly, have increased rates of delayed union, nonunion, displacement, and avascular necrosis. Given the importance of recognizing these high-risk fractures in the femoral head and neck, MRI is the preferred second-line study after initial negative radiographs to prevent delayed diagnosis.

# Case 24-10

An 88-year-old Asian female presents with weakness in her left thigh while weightbearing. This is clearly worse with standing and walking. Walking is worse than standing. Over the period of several weeks, this weakness evolved into what she clearly describes as pain. When asked to point out the location, she points to the posterolateral aspect of her subtrochanteric thigh. She denies any numbness or tingling in her lower extremities. She denies any constitutional symptoms. She is taking bisphosphonate to prevent osteoporosis. The clinician is concerned about possible insufficiency fracture. What is the most appropriate first imaging exam?

This scenario concerns the initial imaging exam for suspected stress (insufficiency) fracture, pelvis or hip. First imaging study.

Sensible recommendation: XR PELVIS AND HIP

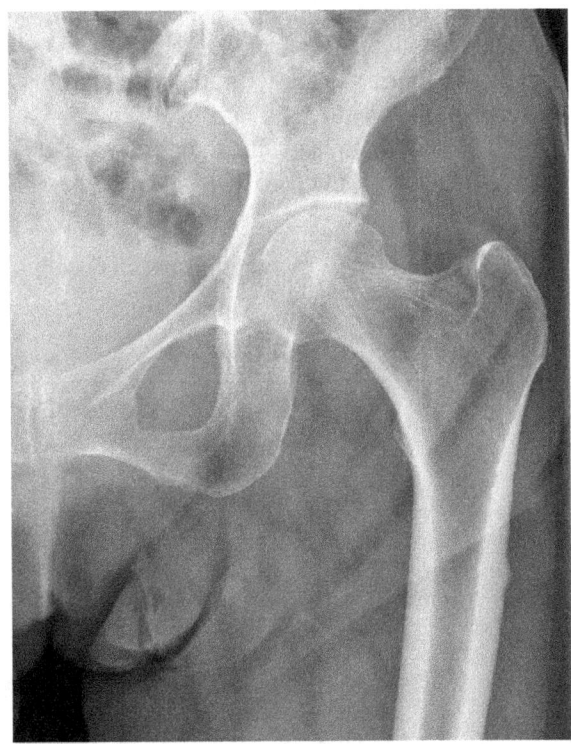

AP radiograph of the left hip shows a focal beaking of the proximal lateral cortex of left femur consistent with a bisphosphonate-related insufficiency fracture.

Pelvic and hip insufficiency fractures have varied presentations and often insidious onset. Patients frequently present with intractable lower back or pelvic pain, with loss of mobility and independence and symptom exacerbation with weight bearing. Insufficiency fractures occur in patients with abnormal bone, be it from osteoporosis, irradiated bone, or resumption of activity post-arthroplasty as typical examples. Radiographs should be the initial imaging modality. Radiographs may be more likely to be negative initially in older or osteoporotic patients with insufficiency fractures, particularly when they occur in the pelvis or sacrum where there is more overlapping soft tissue. However, if the findings are conclusive for insufficiency fracture, no further imaging is needed.

## Case 24-11

A 28-year-old man presents with left hip pain for four months. His pain has gradually increased in severity and became a shooting constant pain in the left hip. He reports that the pain is most pronounced when he is supine and attempting to sleep at night. He also reports that the pain is exacerbated when he walks and when he performs twisting motions at the hips. He denies any history of steroid use, or any trauma to the left hip. He has history of a motorcycle collision years ago but does not recall any specific trauma to the hip itself. He drinks 2-3 beers per day with heavier use on the weekends. He also has a remote history of IV drug use and cocaine use. What imaging exam should be ordered?

This scenario concerns the initial imaging study for an adult or child with clinically suspected osteonecrosis of the hip.

Sensible recommendation: XR PELVIS AND XR HIP

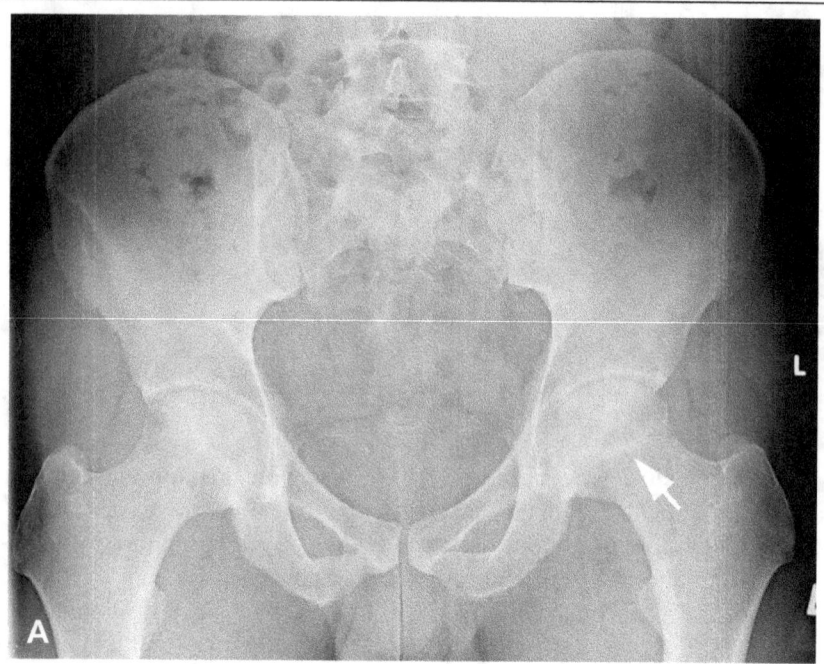

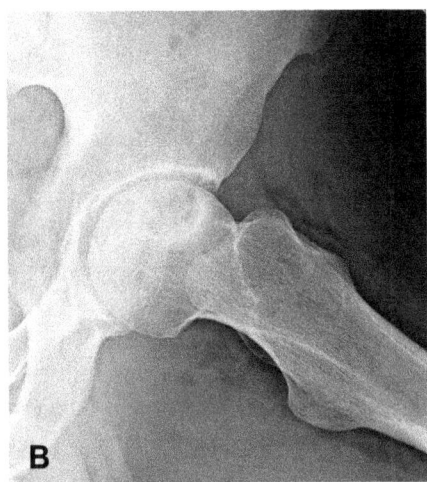

Osteonecrosis. AP radiograph of pelvis (A) demonstrates subtle subchondral sclerosis at the left femoral head (arrow in A). Frog-leg lateral radiograph of left hip (B) shows round subchondral lucency at the left femoral head with a well-defined serpentine sclerosis.

Osteonecrosis (often termed avascular necrosis with involvement of the epiphyseal regions) is a relatively common disease in which there is ischemic death of the cellular elements of bone and marrow. The femoral heads are the most commonly affected sites, with estimates of symptomatic femoral head osteonecrosis of 2 to 4.5 per patient year, resulting in 10,000 to 20,000 new cases annually in the United States. Because the majority of patients are asymptomatic, this incidence likely significantly underestimates the true prevalence of osteonecrosis. Osteonecrosis affects both children and adults and there are numerous predisposing causes, including dislocation of the hip, femoral neck fracture, corticosteroid usage, alcoholism, collagen vascular disease, hemoglobinopathies, Gaucher disease, caisson disease, and some skeletal dysplasias. There are no specific physical findings or laboratory examinations that can reliably establish the diagnosis of osteonecrosis. Clinically suspected osteonecrosis can be confirmed only by diagnostic imaging or biopsy. Imaging methods that can assist in establishing the diagnosis include radiography, computed tomography (CT), radionuclide bone scintigraphy, and MRI wo/w contrast. These methods vary considerably in their cost, diagnostic accuracy, and the information provided.

Radiographs should be obtained as the initial study in every patient suspected to have osteonecrosis. Radiographs are the least expensive and most widely available imaging technology. In the presence of osteonecrosis, the radiographic findings may be normal, abnormal, or equivocal. Both anteroposterior of the pelvis and frog-leg lateral views of the hip should be obtained because articular collapse or cortical depression may be seen on only 1 of the 2 projections.

## Case 24-12

A 24-year-old man presents with left hip pain. The patient's history dates back to four years ago when he was diagnosed with ALL. He underwent a stem cell transplant and has been maintained on a tapering dose of prednisone. He first noted hip pain about two months ago. He says some days it is fairly bad and other days it is fairly mild. He feels that the pain is getting worse gradually and accompanied by instability and a sharp, dull ache. He says that avoiding rotation or weight-bearing improves his symptoms. Stretching or bearing weight worsens his symptoms. Initial radiographs of both hips showed normal right hip, and a questionable subchondral lucency at his left femoral head. What imaging exam should be ordered next?

This scenario concerns the next appropriate imaging study for an adult with clinically suspected osteonecrosis of the hip. Initial radiographs may have been negative or suspicious for osteonecrosis.

Sensible recommendation: MRI HIP WO CONTRAST

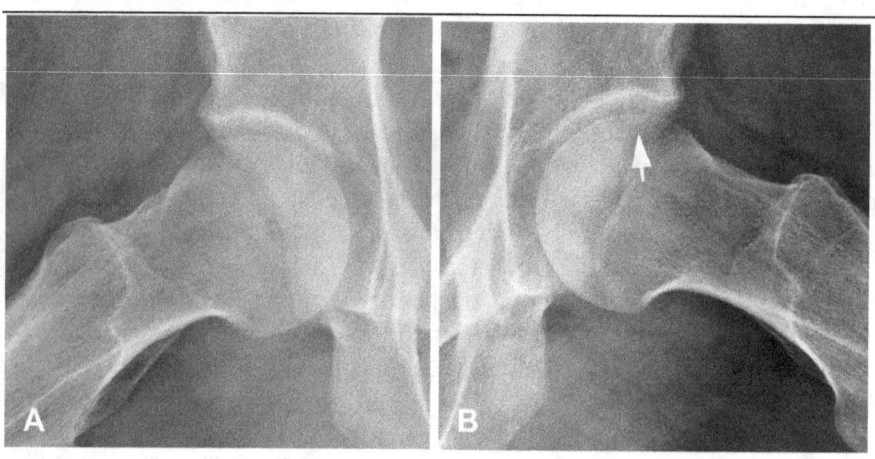

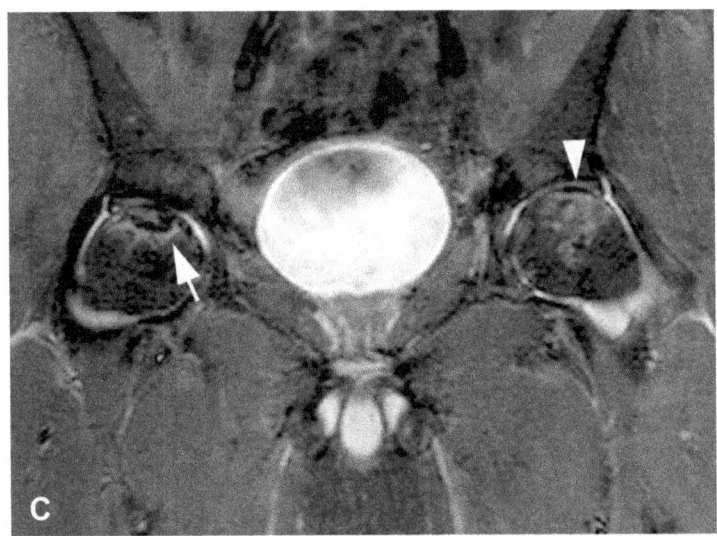

Frog-leg lateral right hip radiograph (A) is normal. Frog-leg lateral left hip radio-graph (B) shows a questionable subchondral lucency at left femoral head (arrow). Coronal STIR MRI (C) shows osteonecrosis in both femoral heads. The right femoral head contour is normal with subchondral double lines (arrow in C). The left femoral head shows osteonecrosis and flattened lateral femoral head (arrowhead in C), associated with prominent surrounding edema.

In the adult patient with suspected osteonecrosis of the hip and normal or suspicious radiographs but clinically requiring further radiologic assessment, MRI is the modality of choice. MRI is generally considered the most sensitive and specific radiologic method of assessment for identification of osteonecrosis, with accuracy of 97 to 100% in several series. In adult patients with radiographically proven, occult, or equivocal osteonecrosis, MRI may be indicated for diagnosis, evaluation of extent or volume of disease, and evidence of articular collapse, if clinically important to guide optimal treatment. Nontraumatic osteonecrosis is bilateral in 70 to 80% of cases, which further increases the extent of disability in the setting of femoral head collapse. The high incidence of bilateral involvement of osteonecrosis in systemic disease with the use of corticosteroids often requires imaging of the contralateral hip.

Intravenous contrast is typically not used or necessary for the diagnosis or evaluation of femoral head osteonecrosis. This technique may be useful to suggest foci of osteonecrosis subsequent to femoral neck fracture, which has been reported in up to 75% of cases. CT (MDCT) can be useful for preoperative assessment if not adequately evaluated by MRI. In adults, CT with multiplanar reconstruction has been reported to be less sensitive than bone scintigraphy and MRI. If bone scintigraphy is to be undertaken, it is suggested that the study be done using pinhole collimation and SPECT with scatter correction and iterative reconstruction algorithms. The addition of single-photon emission CT (SPECT) may improve the accuracy of radionuclide imaging for diagnosing osteonecrosis.

# Case 24-13

A 27-year-old woman presents with left hip pain. The patient reports that about 4 months ago she started having left lateral hip pain that was intermittent and actually improved with walking and was worse with sitting. The symptoms are worse with flexing her left hip and improved with resting. She denies any loss of sensation or loss of bowel and bladder control. She denies any previous hip, knee, or back injuries. Of note, she is status post resection of a fourth ventricle epidermoid tumor. Post-operatively, she was treated with a couple weeks of steroids. Frog-leg left hip radiograph shows femoral avascular necrosis with subchondral lucency and articular surface step off. Surgery is contemplated. What imaging test should be ordered next?

This scenario concerns an adult with a painful hip and radiographs that show osteonecrosis with femoral head collapse. What imaging is most appropriate for surgical planning?

Sensible recommendation: MRI HIP WO CONTRAST

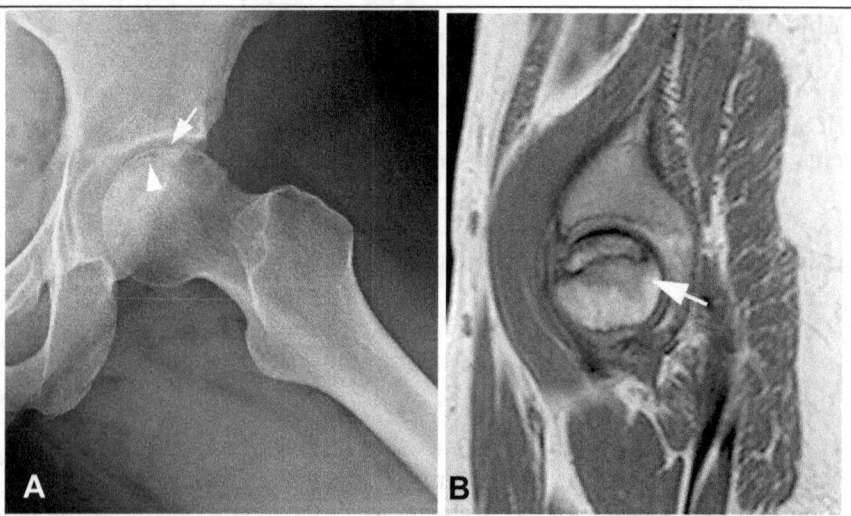

Osteonecrosis. Frog-leg lateral left hip radiograph (A) shows femoral osteonecrosis. There is subchondral curvilinear lucency (arrowhead), and subtle articular surface step off (arrow). Sagittal T1 MRI (B) shows osteonecrosis of left femoral head with articular surface collapse and surrounding hypointense marrow edema (arrow in B).

In the adult or child patient with pain and radiographic evidence of articular collapse resulting from femoral head osteonecrosis and with surgical intervention contemplated for treatment, further imaging assessment is typically required. MRI is useful to determine the degree and location of articular collapse, which is optimally evaluated in the sagittal imaging plane, and the status of the contralateral hip. The sagittal plane has been emphasized as optimal in evaluating articular collapse on MRI. Various staging systems have in common progression from radiologically occult disease to positive imaging manifestations of osteonecrosis, followed by femoral head collapse and subsequent development of secondary osteoarthritis. The volume of joint effusion, presence of prominent edema about the focus of osteonecrosis, patient age (over 40 years), and body mass index (greater than 24kg/m) have been associated with increased stage and likelihood of femoral head collapse.

# Case 24-14

A 51-year-old man presents with acute on chronic left hip pain. He rates his hip pain as 10/10 and equally worse with mobility or rest. His pain started after he fell on his left hip several months ago. He is able to ambulate with aid of a walking cane. He has history of chronic alcohol abuse and a gunshot injury with a possible retained bullet fragment in his chest. Radiograph of left hip shows left femoral head osteonecrosis with articular surface collapse. The clinician is still suspicious for an occult fracture. What imaging exam should be ordered next?

This scenario concerns an adult or child with clinically suspected osteonecrosis. Initial radiographs were positive but MRI is contraindicated and imaging for surgical planning is needed.

Sensible recommendation: CT HIP WO CONTRAST

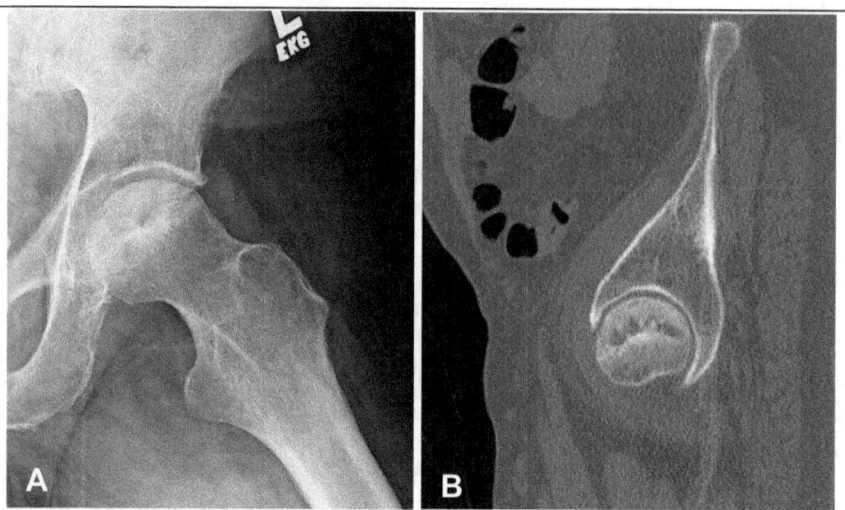

Frog-leg lateral left hip radiograph (A) shows femoral head osteonecrosis. There is subchondral curvilinear lucency and sclerosis at left femoral head. Sagittal refor-matted CT image (B) shows femoral head avascular necrosis involving about 50% of the femoral head.

The imaging assessment of a patient who cannot undergo MRI but requires further radiologic evaluation can be performed with either bone scintigraphy or CT. CT, although less sensitive than MRI and bone scintigraphy for de-tection of early femoral head osteonecrosis, is more specific and has the advantage of allowing anatomic assessment (particularly in patients with ab-normal radiographs). Osteonecrosis of the femoral head that is more chronic is well seen on CT evaluation. In addition, similar to MRI, sagittal and coro-nal MDCT allows assessment of the volume of femoral head involvement, the presence of articular collapse, and early secondary degenerative disease. The use of intravenous contrast is not needed for CT evaluation of femoral head osteonecrosis. The CT assessment of femoral head osteonecrosis in this clinical scenario is important to guide the need and types of further treat-ment that may be required.

Bone scintigraphy should be performed with high-resolution pinhole colli-mation and is particularly useful in patients with normal radiographs. More recently, SPECT has been shown to improve the diagnostic accuracy of this technique. The disadvantage of bone scintigraphy in assessment of osteone-crosis is the lack of anatomic evaluation and specificity.

# References

1. Mintz DN, Roberts CC, Bencardino JT, Baccei SJ, Caird MS, Cassidy RC, Chang EY, Fox MG, Gyftopoulos S, Kransdorf MJ, Metter DF, Morrison WB, Rosenberg ZS, Shah NA, Small KM, Subhas N, Tambar S, Towers JD, Yu JS, Weissman BN. ACR Appropriateness Criteria(®) Chronic Hip Pain. J Am Coll Radiol. 2017 May;14(5S):S90-S102. doi: 10.1016/j.jacr.2017.01.035. Review. PMID: 28473098.

2. American College of Radiology. ACR Appropriateness Criteria: Chronic hip pain. American College of Radiology, 2013, revised 2016. https://acsearch.acr.org/docs/69425/Narrative/ (accessed April 24, 2021).

3. Yoon LS, Palmer WE, Kassarjian A. Evaluation of radial-sequence imaging in detecting acetabular labral tears at hip MR arthrography. Skeletal Radiol. 2007;36(11):1029-1033.

4. Kavanagh EC, Koulouris G, Ford S, McMahon P, Johnson C, Eustace SJ. MR imaging of groin pain in the athlete. Semin Musculoskelet Radiol. 2006 Sep;10(3):197-207.

5. Murphey MD1, Rhee JH, Lewis RB, Fanburg-Smith JC, Flemming DJ, Walker EA. Pigmented villonodular synovitis: radiologic-pathologic correlation. Radiographics. 2008 Sep-Oct;28(5):1493-518.

6. Bencardino JT, Stone TJ, Roberts CC, Appel M, Baccei SJ, Cassidy RC, Chang EY,Fox MG, Greenspan BS, Gyftopoulos S, Hochman MG, Jacobson JA, Mintz DN, Mlady GW, Newman JS, Rosenberg ZS, Shah NA, Small KM, Weissman BN. ACR

7. Appropriateness Criteria(®) Stress (Fatigue/Insufficiency) Fracture, Including Sacrum, Excluding Other Vertebrae. J Am Coll Radiol. 2017 May;14(5S):S293-S306. doi: 10.1016/j.jacr.2017.02.035. Review. PMID: 28473086.

8. American College of Radiology. ACR Appropriateness Criteria: Stress (Fatigue/Insufficiency) Fracture, Including Sacrum, Excluding Other Vertebrae. American College of Radiology, revised 2016. https://acsearch.acr.org/docs/69435/Narrative/ (accessed April 24, 2021).

9. American College of Radiology. ACR Appropriateness Criteria: Osteonecrosis of the Hip. American College of Radiology, revised 2015. https://acsearch.acr.org/docs/69420/Narrative/ (accessed April 24, 2021).

10. Murphey MD, Foreman KL, Klassen-Fischer MK, Fox MG, Chung EM, Kransdorf MJ. From the radiologic pathology archives imaging of osteonecrosis: radiologic-pathologic correlation. Radiographics. 2014;34(4):1003-1028. PMID:25019438.

11. Ikemura S, Yamamoto T, Motomura G, Nakashima Y, Mawatari T, Iwamoto Y. MRI evaluation of collapsed femoral heads in patients 60 years old or older: Differentiation of subchondral insufficiency fracture from osteonecrosis of the femoral head. AJR Am J Roentgenol. 2010;195(1):W63-68.

12. Shimizu K, Moriya H, Akita T, Sakamoto M, Suguro T. Prediction of collapse with magnetic resonance imaging of avascular necrosis of the femoral head. J Bone Joint Surg Am. 1994;76(2):215-223. PMID: 8113255.

13. Stevens K, Tao C, Lee SU, et al. Subchondral fractures in osteonecrosis of the femoral head: comparison of radiography, CT, and MR imaging. AJR Am J Roentgenol. 2003;180(2):363-368. PMID 12540435.

# Chapter 25. Chronic or Nontraumatic Knee Pain

Lindsay Stratchko, DO, Eric Walker, MD, Jonelle Petscavage-Thomas, MD

Radiography is the best initial exam for chronic or nontraumatic knee pain. MRI would typically be the next step for joint or soft tissue evaluation, and CT and bone scan may have a role in problem-solving.

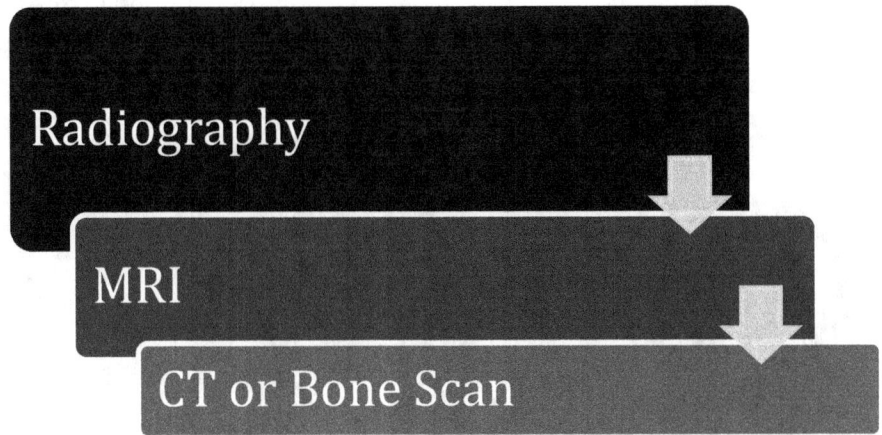

# Case 25-1

A 79-year-old woman presents with a several year history of left anterior knee pain. The woman denies any trauma or surgery to her left knee. Her past medical history is significant for hypertension, hyperlipidemia and hypothyroidism. She is status post hysterectomy and right shoulder rotator cuff repair. She has not undergone any diagnostic imaging thus far. What is the most appropriate initial imaging study?

This scenario concerns the initial imaging exam for a child or adult greater than or equal to 5 years of age with chronic anterior (patellofemoral) knee pain.

Sensible recommendation: XR KNEE 3 VIEW (AP, lateral, sunrise)

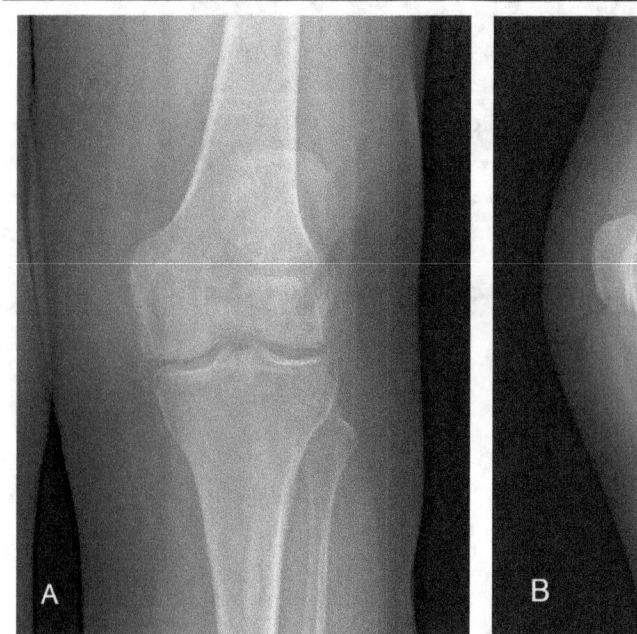
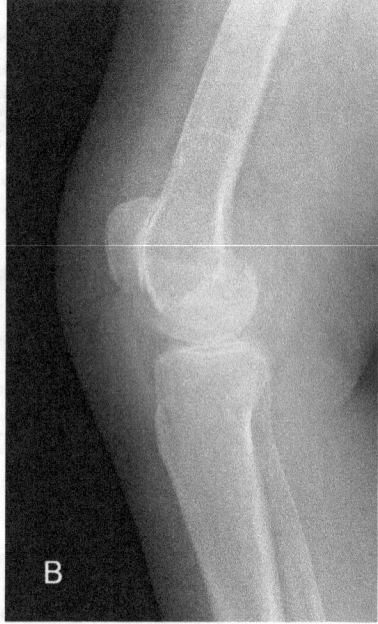

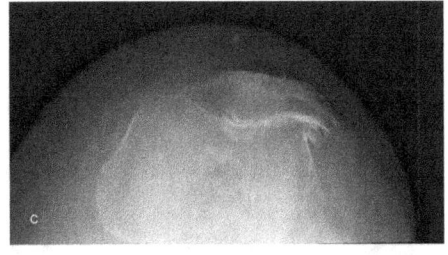

AP (A), Lateral (B) and Sunrise (C) left knee radiographs show lateral subluxation of the patella as well as patellofemoral bone-on-bone articulation, marginal osteophytes, subchondral cysts and sclerosis, findings of patellofemoral osteoarthritis (Kellgren-Lawrence Stage IV). Note is also made of chondrocalcinosis of the menisci.

Nontraumatic anterior knee pain suggests patellofemoral pathology, which should be initially investigated with radiography. Signs of patellofemoral osteoarthritis and findings to suggest maltracking can be identified with radiographs. In addition to the anteroposterior knee radiograph, lateral and sunrise knee radiographs should be included in evaluation of the patellofemoral compartment. Common findings of degenerative osteoarthritis include patellofemoral joint space narrowing, subchondral sclerosis (eburnation), subchondral cystic change and osteophytes. Findings of patellar maltracking include a shallow trochlear groove and lateral subluxation of the patella. If initial radiographs are nondiagnostic, MRI may be helpful in evaluating for additional etiologies of the patient's persistent pain.

## Case 25-2

A 58-year-old man presents for evaluation of his right knee pain. His pain has been progressively worsening over the past year and he currently requires daily NSAID's to manage his discomfort while working as an electrician. He has not had any recent falls or trauma to his right knee. He is otherwise healthy, stating he likes to walk at least two miles a day. His only surgery includes appendectomy at age 10. What is the best initial imaging test to evaluate this patient's right knee pain?

This scenario concerns the initial imaging exam for a child or adult greater than or equal to 5 years of age with chronic, nonlocalized knee pain.

Sensible recommendation: XR KNEE 4 VIEW

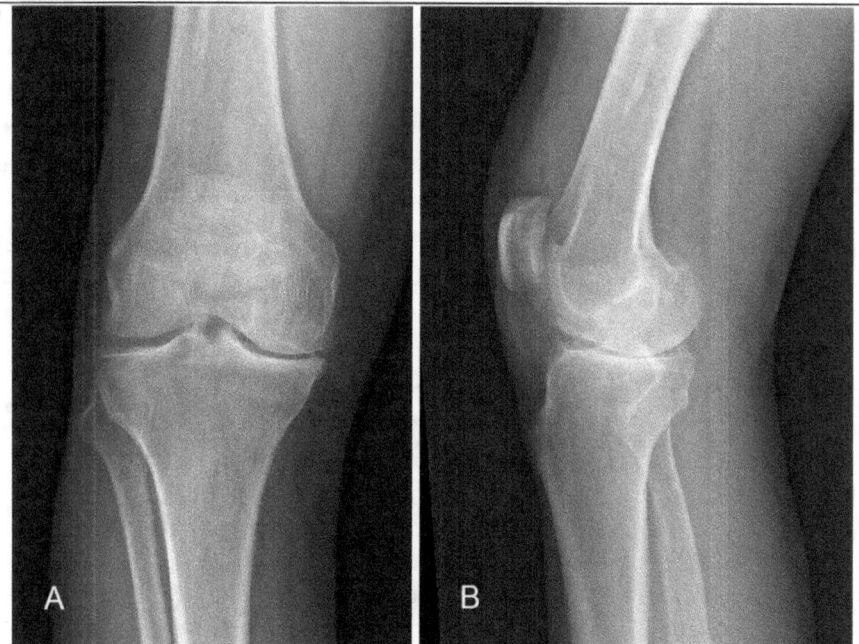

AP (A) and Lateral (B) right knee radiographs show tricompartmental marginal osteophytes, subchondral sclerosis and joint space narrowing, most notably in the medial femorotibial compartment. These are findings of moderate osteoarthritis (Kellgren-Lawrence Stage III).

Osteoarthritis is the most common cause of nontraumatic knee pain in the adult and should initially be evaluated with radiographs. Findings of osteoarthritis include joint space narrowing, osteophytes, subchondral cystic change and sclerosis (eburnation). Standing knee radiographs more accurately depict the degree of joint space narrowing than supine radiographs, which is helpful in grading the severity of degenerative joint disease. Further imaging with MRI may ultimately be necessary, particularly if there is concern for meniscal pathology or internal derangement.

## Case 25-3

A 16-year-old female presents with worsening medial right knee pain throughout her field hockey season. She has had several falls during practice, but no particular inciting injury that she can recall. The patient was initially evaluated at an urgent care center two weeks prior. Radiographs at that time demonstrated a moderate knee joint effusion. What is the most appropriate next imaging test to order to evaluate this patient's ongoing right knee pain?

This scenario concerns the next imaging exam for adult or child greater than or equal to 5 years of age with chronic knee pain. Initial knee radiograph negative or demonstrates joint effusion. Next imaging procedure.

Sensible recommendation: MRI KNEE WO CONTRAST

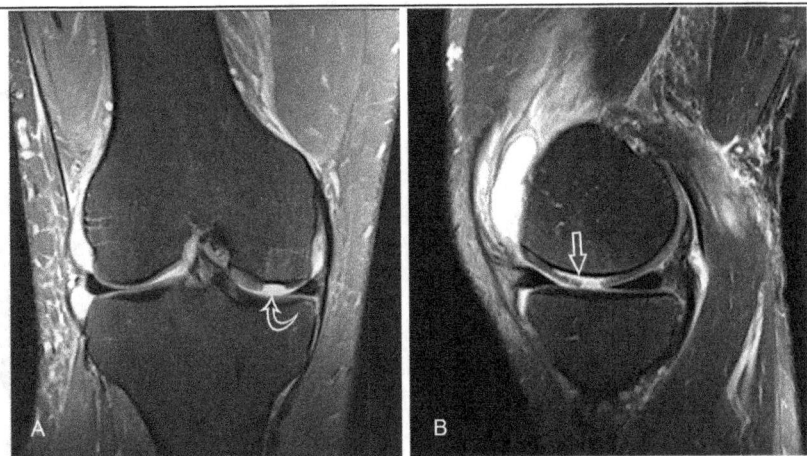

Coronal (A) and sagittal (B) PD FS MRI demonstrate a focal area of articular cartilage loss (curved arrow) of the medial femoral condyle with anterior and posterior delamination (arrow) of the cartilage noted on the sagittal image.

When initial knee radiographs are normal or show a nonspecific joint effusion, MRI without intravenous contrast is the most appropriate next imaging test. MRI is more sensitive in the evaluation of ligaments, tendons, menisci and cartilage when compared to radiography, providing additional diagnostic information in patients with persistent pain. Fluid-sensitive sequences can identify soft tissue and bone marrow edema, which can clue the reader into mechanism of injury (i.e. pivot shift) and reveal pathology to explain the patient's pain. Intravenous contrast is helpful in the evaluation for synovitis.

## Case 25-4

A 58-year-old man presents for evaluation of right knee pain after playing tennis for a few weeks. He states that the pain gets significantly better within a day or two after rest. He has not noticed any swelling or joint instability. He states that most of his pain is right under the kneecap. His initial knee radiographs were negative. What is the most appropriate next imaging study?

This scenario concerns the next imaging exam for adult or child greater than or equal to 5 years of age with chronic, anterior (patellofemoral) knee pain.

Knee radiographs were normal or demonstrated a joint effusion.

Sensible recommendation: MRI KNEE WO CONTRAST

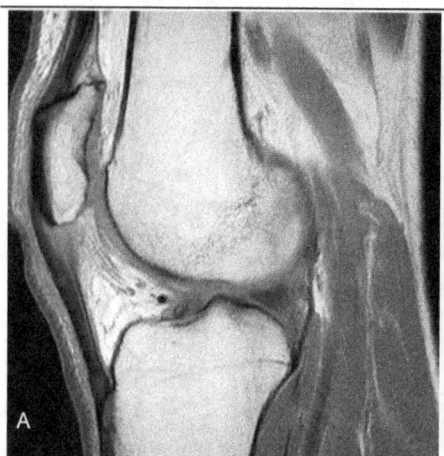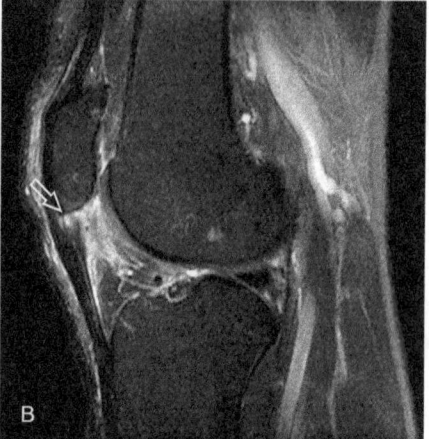

Sagittal PD MRI (A) and T2 FS MRI (B) reveal thickening and increased signal within the proximal patellar tendon. The T2 FS image demonstrates adjacent edema within the surrounding subcutaneous and infrapatellar fat and a small partial tear (arrow) within the patellar tendon proximally. He was treated with physical therapy and anti-inflammatory medications.

Nontraumatic anterior knee pain is attributed to several entities, some of which can be identified on knee radiographs. When pain is persistent and knee radiographs are normal or show nonspecific findings, MRI is the most appropriate next imaging test. MRI is more sensitive in detecting patello-femoral cartilage loss compared to radiography, particularly in early stages when the joint space is preserved. Additional causes of chronic anterior knee pain that can be evaluated with MRI include abnormal alignment of the patella in relation to the femur, either by lateral subluxation (patellofemoral maltracking, patellofemoral pain syndrome) or lateral tilt (excessive lateral pressure syndrome). Jumper's knee or patellar tendinosis is a common condition particularly prevalent in sports involving jumping and heavy landing, rapid acceleration or deceleration and kicking, such as basketball, volleyball, soccer, tennis, long jump and high jump. A few other causes of anterior knee pain include synovial plica syndrome, bursitis, quadriceps fat pad syndrome, and quadriceps tendinopathy.

## Case 25-5

An 18-year-old male is presenting for further evaluation of abnormal left knee radiographs. He initially presented to the Emergency Department with left knee pain after falling off a ladder. He is otherwise healthy and without a surgical history. Emergency Department radiographs showed a crescentic lucency at the lateral aspect of the medial femoral condyle concerning for osteochondritis dissecans. What is most appropriate next imaging study to evaluate stability of the osteochondral fragment?

This scenario concerns the next imaging exam for an adult or child greater than or equal to 5 years of age with chronic knee pain. Initial knee radiograph demonstrates osteochondritis dissecans (OCD), loose bodies, or history of cartilage or meniscal repair. Next imaging procedure.

Sensible recommendation: MRI KNEE WO CONTRAST

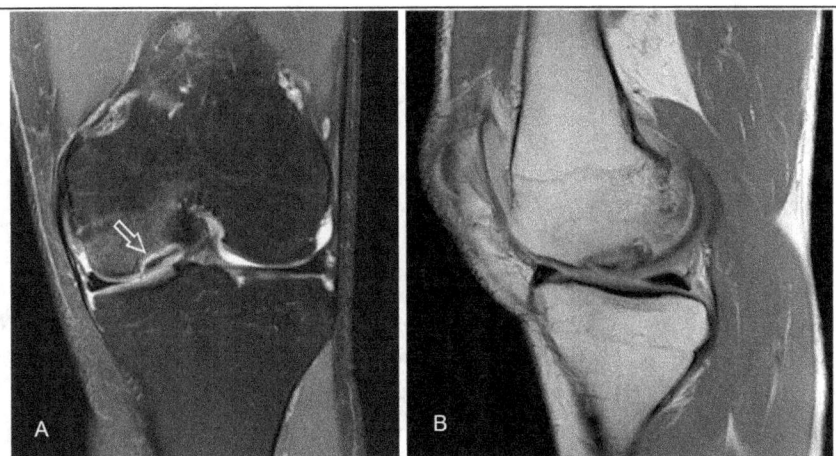

Coronal PD FS MRI (A) and sagittal PD MRI (B) of the left knee show a nondisplaced, osteochondral injury involving the lateral aspect of the medial femoral condyle. The high signal intensity (fluid) around the fragment on the coronal image, called the rim sign (arrow), suggests a detached, unstable lesion often requiring surgical intervention.

The most common location for osteochondral injuries in the pediatric population are the femoral condyles. High-grade, displaced osteochondral injuries with intra-articular loose bodies can be seen on knee radiographs, but lower grade injuries are difficult to distinguish without further imaging. Knee MRI without intravenous contrast is the most appropriate imaging study to evaluate the degree of detachment and displacement of the osteochondral fragment. Intra-articular contrast injection and MR arthrography may be helpful in delineating detachment; however, it is often not necessary. CT is a reasonable alternative if MRI is contraindicated.

# Case 25-6

A 64-year-old man presents with a two-day history of left lateral knee pain, redness and swelling. Past medical history includes hyperlipidemia and several episodes of pancreatitis secondary to alcohol consumption. The patient denies trauma, fever or chills. He presented to his primary care provider and left knee radiographs were obtained. The radiographs showed erosive changes of the lateral femoral condyle with overlying nodular soft tissue swelling consistent with gout. What is the most appropriate next imaging test?

This scenario concerns the next imaging exam for an adult with chronic knee pain. Initial knee radiograph demonstrates degenerative changes or chondrocalcinosis. Next imaging procedure.

Sensible recommendation: NO IMAGING, if diagnosis is clinically concordant.

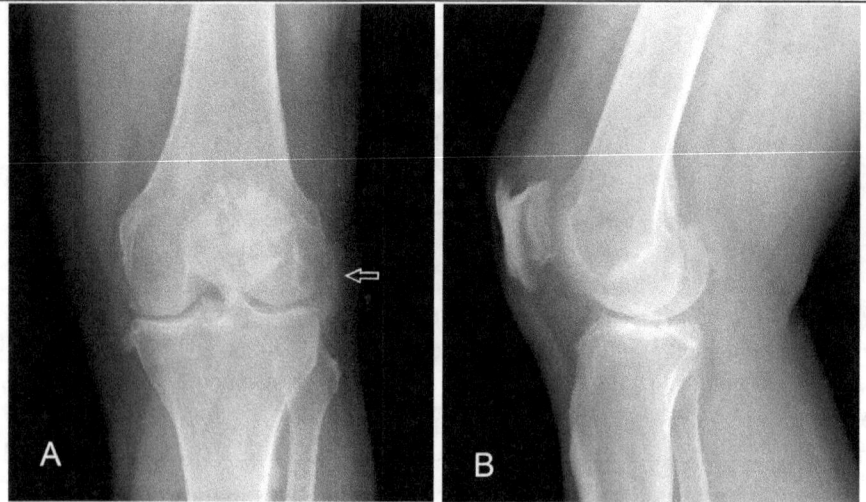

AP (A) and Lateral (B) left knee radiographs show large erosions of the lateral femoral condyle, seen in the setting of gout. There is nodular soft tissue swelling of the lateral knee adjacent to the erosions consistent with tophi (arrow).

Additional imaging is typically not appropriate if initial knee radiographs identify a reasonable source of the patient's pain. As previously described, osteoarthritis has classic radiographic findings and is one of the most common causes of nontraumatic knee pain in the adult. Findings to suggest specific crystalline arthropathies can also be identified without cross sectional imaging. Dual-energy CT without contrast may be indicated if gout or mixed crystal disease is a consideration. Otherwise, CT is not commonly used as a diagnostic test to evaluate patients with osteoarthritis or chondro-calcinosis. MRI without contrast is not usually indicated in patients for whom radiographs are diagnostic of osteoarthritis unless symptoms are not explained by the radiographic findings (eg, stress fractures) or the appropriate treatment option requires additional imaging. If an effusion is present, US- or fluoroscopically guided joint aspiration can be performed for synovial fluid analysis if there is concern for crystal disease or infection.

## Case 25-7

A 28-year-old presents with right knee pain. The pain has been present for the past several months and is not relieved with over-the-counter analgesics. There was no history of trauma. The patient's past medical history is significant for acute myeloid leukemia in remission after treatment with chemotherapy and high dose steroids. Initial radiographs show mixed sclerosis and lucency of bilateral femoral condyles with articular surface irregularity of the medial femoral condyle consistent with avascular necrosis and subchondral collapse. What is the most appropriate next imaging study to evaluate the patient's avascular necrosis?

This scenario concerns the next imaging exam for an adult with chronic knee pain. Previous radiographs demonstrated avascular necrosis.

Sensible recommendation: MRI KNEE WO CONTRAST

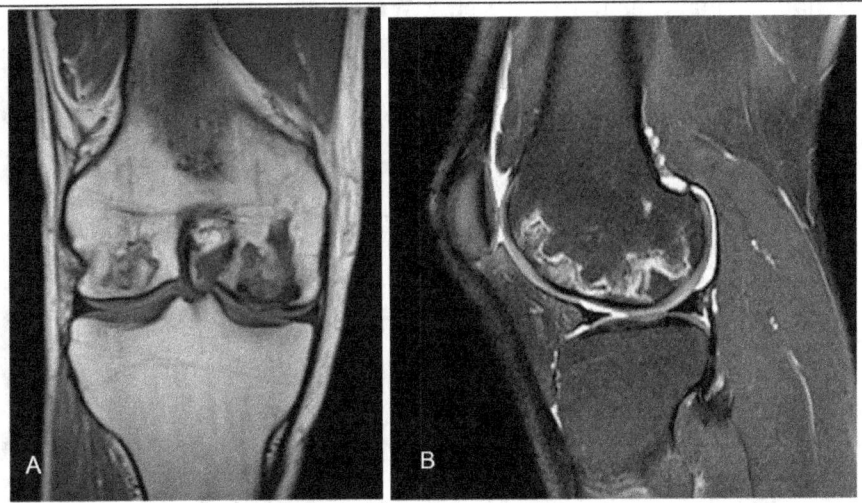

Coronal T1 MRI (A) and sagittal T2 FS MRI (B) show serpiginous mixed T2 signal within bilateral femoral condyles with linear parallel low and high T2 signal (double line sign). There is subchondral collapse and articular surface irregularity of the medial femoral condyle on the coronal image.

Avascular necrosis (AVN) can be secondary to many entities including, but not limited to, steroid use, alcohol, trauma, sickle cell disease, and pancreatitis. Radiographic appearance ranges from normal to collapse of the affected articular surface with secondary degenerative changes. MRI is indicated when pain persists with normal radiographs or if further imaging is needed for treatment planning. AVN of the knee is often managed conservatively; however, arthroscopic intervention may be indicated to remove small unstable fragments. If a large percentage of the articular surface area is involved, the patient often will require total knee arthroplasty.

# Case 25-8

A 37-year-old presents to the Emergency Department with diffuse right knee pain, swelling and inability to bear weight after a fall while skiing. The patient had significant pain during physical examination, limiting evaluation of stability. Initial radiographs showed a subtle depression of the lateral femoral condyle (deep lateral femoral notch sign) and a large joint effusion. What is the most appropriate next imaging study to perform?

This scenario concerns the next imaging exam for an adult or child greater than or equal to 5 years of age with chronic knee pain. Initial knee radiograph demonstrates signs of prior osseous injury (ie, Segond fracture, tibial spine avulsion, etc.). Next imaging procedure.

Sensible recommendation: MRI KNEE WO CONTRAST

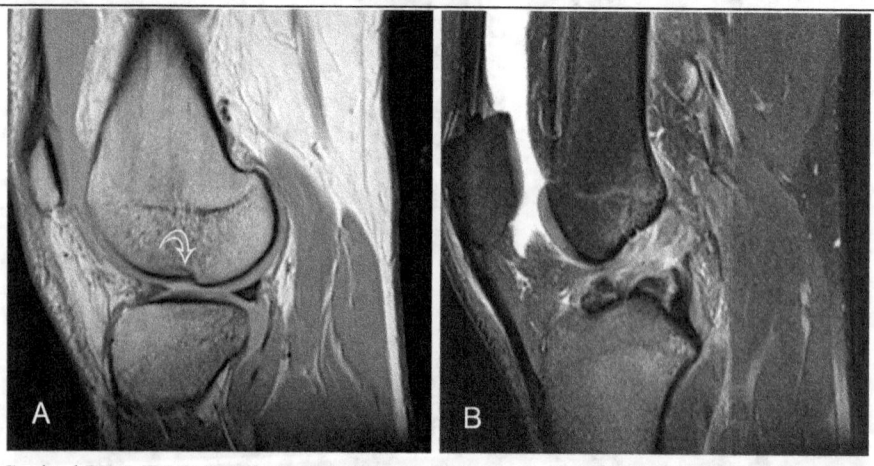

Sagittal PD MRI (A) at the level of the lateral femoral condyle. There is a depression of the lateral femoral condyle articular surface correlating with the deep lateral femoral notch in the patient's history (curved arrow). Sagittal T2 FS MRI (B) at the intercondylar notch reveals high T2 signal intensity within the intercondylar notch in the expected region of the ACL consistent with complete tear. There is a moderate sized joint effusion and bone marrow edema in the posterior tibial plateau.

Secondary signs of internal derangement can be identified on knee radiographs. Findings such as a Segond fracture of the lateral tibial plateau or a deep lateral femoral condylar notch are highly associated with anterior cruciate ligament tears. If these subtle findings are encountered on radiography, MRI should be performed to evaluate for associated ligamentous, capsular, and meniscal pathology. In the case of pivot shift mechanism of injury, anterior cruciate ligament and medial collateral ligament tears are often seen along with meniscal tears. If MRI is contraindicated, CT arthrography can be used to further assess for internal derangement.

# References

1. American College of Radiology. ACR Appropriateness Criteria: Nontraumatic Knee Pain. American College of Radiology, revised 2018. https://acsearch.acr.org/docs/69432/Narrative/ (accessed April 24, 2021).
2. Jacobson JA, Girish G, Jiang Y, Sabb BJ. Radiographic evaluation of arthritis: degenerative joint disease and variations. Radiology. 2008 Sep;248(3):737-47. doi: 10.1148/radiol.2483062112. Review.
3. Kellgren JH, Lawrence JS. Radiological assessment of osteo-arthrosis. Ann Rheum Dis. 1957 Dec; 16 (4):494-502.
4. Yu JS, Petersilge C, Sartoris DJ, Pathria MN, Resnick D. MR imaging of injuries of the extensor mechanism of the knee. Radiographics. 1994 May;14(3):541-51.
5. Sanders TG, Paruchuri NB, Zlatkin MB. MRI of osteochondral defects of the lateral femoral condyle: incidence and pattern of injury after transient lateral dislocation of the patella. AJR Am J Roentgenol. 2006;187 (5): 1332-7. doi:10.2214/AJR.05.1471
6. Resnick D, Niwayama G, Goergen TG et-al. Clinical, radiographic and pathologic abnormalities in calcium pyrophosphate dihydrate deposition disease (CPPD): pseudogout. Radiology. 1977;122 (1): 1-15. doi:10.1148/122.1.1
7. Steinberg ME, Hayken GD, Steinberg DR. A quantitative system for staging avascular necrosis. J Bone Joint Surg Br. 1995;77 (1): 34-41.
8. Pao DG. The lateral femoral notch sign. Radiology. 2001;219 (3): 800-1.

# Chapter 26. Chronic and Nontraumatic Ankle Pain

Kimia Kani, MD

Radiography is the initial exam for chronic and nontraumatic ankle pain. One of MRI, CT, or US may be the next step, but sometimes more than one is indicated. The bone scan has a limited role.

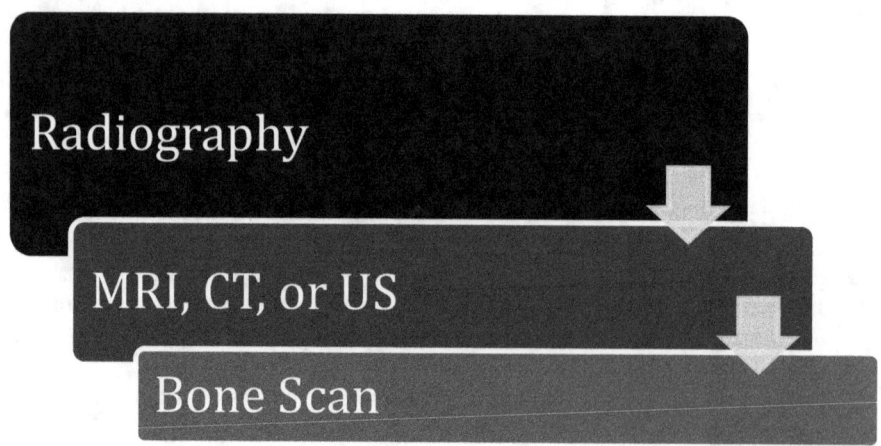

# Case 26-1

A 32-year-old man presents with chronic left ankle pain. He has a known history of multifocal hemangioendotheliomas of the left lower extremity, lungs and liver. What imaging test should be ordered initially?

This scenario is concerned with the most appropriate initial imaging study for chronic ankle pain.

Sensible recommendation: XR ANKLE 3 VIEW

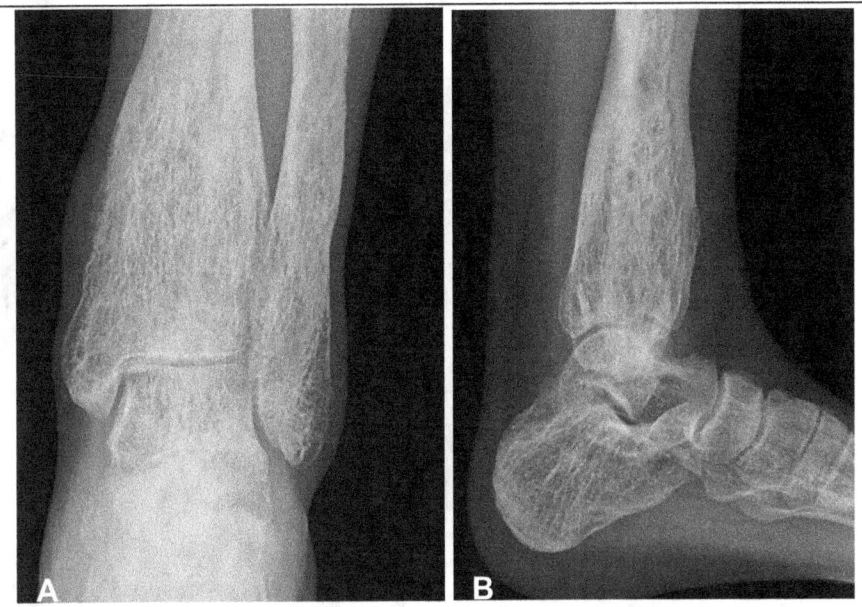

AP (A) and lateral (B) radiographs of the left ankle demonstrate lucent, expansile lesions of the distal tibia, distal fibula, talus and calcaneus, with coarse trabeculations and thinning of the cortex. The calcaneus is dysplastic. Findings have been stable from ankle radiographs obtained 10 years ago (not shown) and are compatible with known hemangioendotheliomas.

Ankle pain is considered chronic when symptoms persist more than 6 weeks. Radiographs are the most appropriate initial imaging study for evaluation of chronic ankle pain. Ankle radiographs may be obtained without or with weight-bearing, and typically include anteroposterior (AP), lateral and mortise views.

# Case 26-2

A 58-year-old man presents with several-month history of left hindfoot pain which is mainly occurring during weight-bearing and ambulatory activities.

On physical examination, hindfoot is in significant valgus and is not reducible. He has some tenderness to palpation over the peroneal tendons distal and posterior to the fibula and over the sinus tarsi. Ankle radiographs demonstrate multiple sites of osteoarthritis. What is the best imaging study to order next?

This scenario is concerned with the next appropriate imaging study for chronic ankle pain where initial radiographs show multiple sites of degenerative joint disease in the hindfoot.

Sensible recommendation: MRI ANKLE WO CONTRAST, CT ANKLE WO CONTRAST, or XR JOINT INJECTION, region of interest

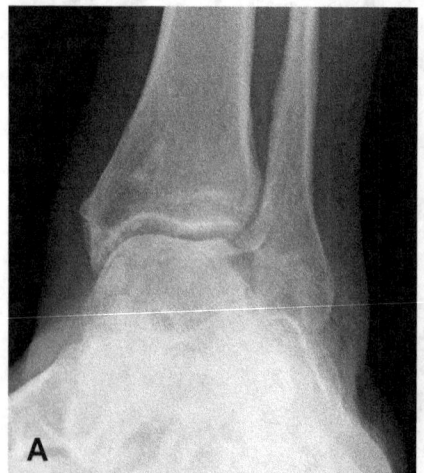
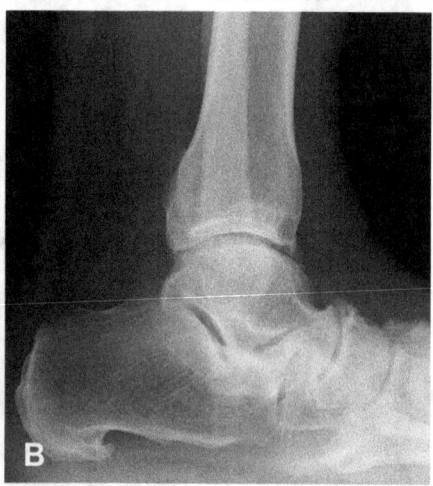

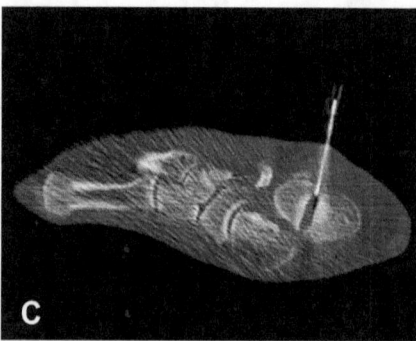

Mortise (A) and lateral (B) weight-bearing left ankle radiographs show pes planovalgus and moderate osteoarthritis of the ankle, posterior subtalar, talonavicular and calcaneocuboid joints. Using CT guidance (C) Kenalog and bupivacaine were injected into the posterior subtalar joint.

Precise treatment of chronic ankle and foot pain depends on accurate assessment of the site of origin and cause of pain. Most often a diagnosis is based upon medical history, physical examination and one or more imaging studies. However, this assessment can be difficult especially in the presence of multilevel osteoarthritis, where the localization and degree of clinical symptoms do not necessarily correlate with the sites and severity of imaging findings. In such cases, image-guided anesthetic (with or without corticosteroid) injection of joints and/or tendon sheaths to identify the source of pain, may be valuable in clinical decision making and patient treatment. MRI ANKLE WO CONTRAST may also be an appropriate next best examination, especially when ligament, muscle-tendon, or stress injuries are suspected clinically as well as for evaluation of cartilage integrity. CT ANKLE WO CONTRAST may be helpful for preoperative planning when osteoarthritis is evident.

## Case 26-3

30-year-old woman presents with right anterolateral ankle pain after inverting her ankle twice in a row seven months ago. Right ankle radiographs are negative but an osteochondral injury is suspected. What imaging studies should be ordered?

This scenario is concerned with the next study for a patient with suspected osteochondral injury with negative initial ankle radiographs.

Sensible recommendation: MRI ANKLE WO CONTRAST

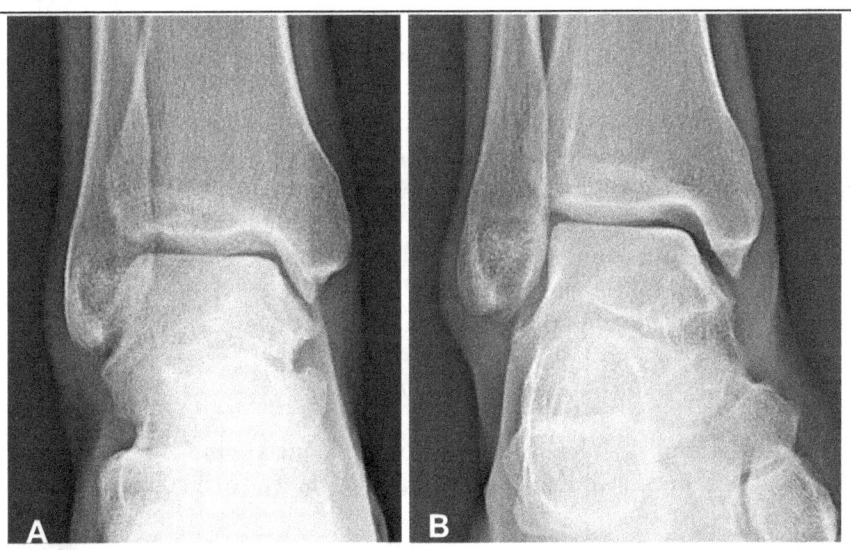

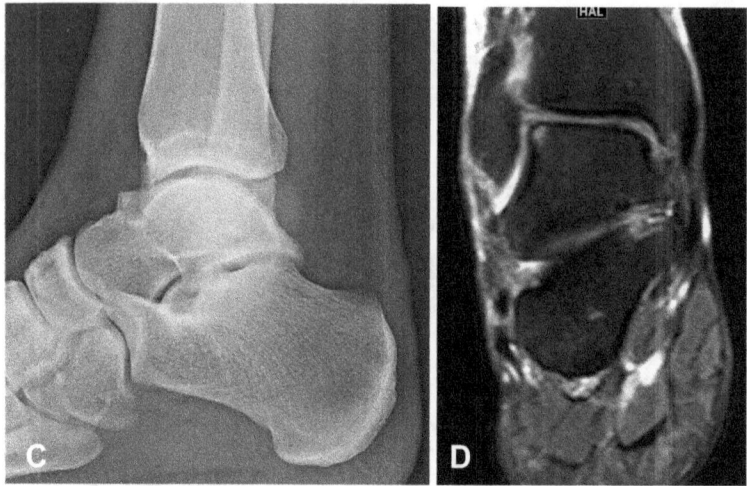

AP (A), mortise (B) and lateral (C) right ankle radiographs are normal. Coronal T2 FS MRI (D) of the right ankle shows an osteochondral lesion (seen as focal sub-chondral edema) of the lateral shoulder of the talar dome.

Osteochondral lesions (OCLS) may involve the talar dome, and less commonly the tibal plafond and tarsal navicular bone. Usually OCLS can be attributed to a traumatic event, although non-traumatic OCLS can also occur. Radiographs may fail to detect OCLS in up to 50% of cases. In patients with negative ankle radiographs and suspected osteochondral injury, MRI ankle is the most appropriate next study. MRI can accurately evaluate and determine the stability of an OCL. In addition to morphologic assessment, a variety of MRI techniques have the potential to provide biochemical and physiological information about the cartilage. A potential pitfall is that due to bone marrow edema, the true extent of the bony component of an OCL may be overestimated on MRI, which may affect treatment planning. MR arthrography (or CT arthrography) may be an appropriate next imaging study, as the instilled intra-articular contrast will outline the cartilage defect. CT ankle is less appropriate at the next imaging study, since cartilage cannot be directly evaluated with this modality.

## Case 26-4

An 85-year-old man with a history of gout presented to the foot and ankle clinic with pain and swelling of the left ankle. He was treated with colchicine and his dose of prophylactic allopurinol was increased, but his pain failed to respond adequately to therapy. Radiographs of the ankle were obtained and showed soft tissue swelling. A tendon abnormality was suspected clinically. What imaging test should be ordered at this point?

This scenario is concerned with the next study for a patient with suspected tendon abnormality with negative initial ankle radiographs.

Sensible recommendation: MRI ANKLE WO CONTRAST or US ANKLE, region of interest

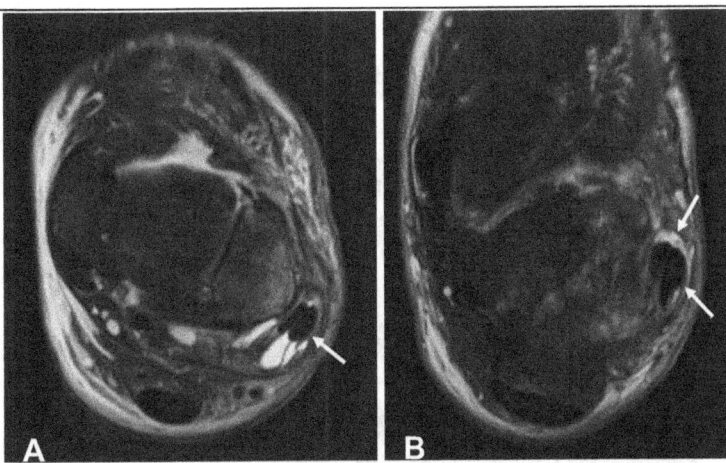

Axial T2 FS MRI at (A) and distal (B) to the lateral malleolus. The peroneal tendons are anteriorly subluxated from the retromalleolar groove (A). There is thickening of the peroneal tendons and distention of the common peroneal tendon sheath (arrows) with associated linear low-signal-intensity bands. Findings are suggestive of stenosing tenosynovitis. Reactive bone marrow edema is seen in the lateral malleolus.

Tendon abnormalities include tendinopathy, tenosynovitis, tendon tear (partial or complete) and tendon subluxation or dislocation. MRI and US can both effectively demonstrate ankle tendon abnormalities, although US results are more dependent on operator expertise and do not screen for alternative diagnoses. An exception is the significant advantage of US over MRI in the dynamic assessment of tendon subluxation or dislocation. In addition, US guided injections (including anesthetics and/or steroids) into the ankle tendon sheath or the Achilles paratenon may be useful for both diagnostic and therapeutic purposes.

## Case 26-5

44-year-old woman presents with left ankle pain which has been present since a ski injury 7 weeks ago. The pain is localized around the lateral malleolus and is made worse by activity. Physical examination of the left ankle demonstrates microinstability with a positive anterior drawer sign. Radiographs of the left ankle are negative for fracture. What imaging test should be ordered next?

This scenario is concerned with the next study for a patient with suspected ankle instability with negative initial ankle radiographs.

Sensible recommendation: MRI ANKLE WO CONTRAST

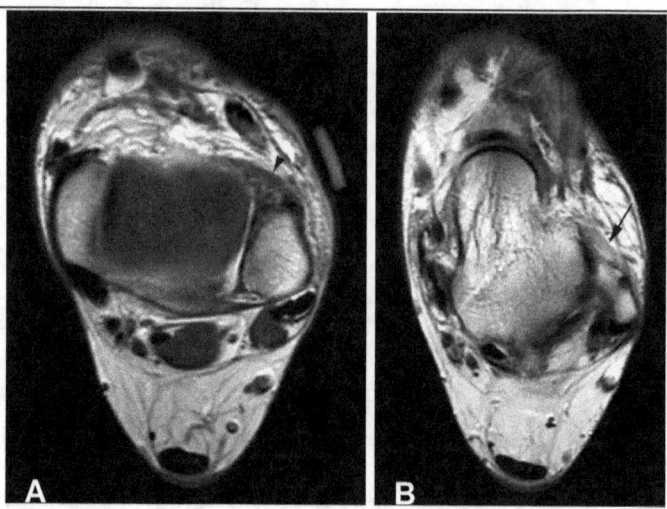

Axial PD MRI through the syndesmosis (A) and distal aspect of the lateral malleolus (B). Thickening and intermediate signal intensity of the anterior tibiofibular (arrowhead) and anterior talofibular (arrow) ligaments are indicative of partial thickness ligamentous tears.

Ankle sprains are the most common sports-related injury, and usually result from inversion forces to the lateral collateral ligament (LCL) complex. The LCL complex is usually torn in a predictable manner: anterior talofibular ligament is torn first, followed by the calcaneofibular ligament, and only with extreme inversion the posterior talofibular ligament is torn. Most ankle sprains respond to non-surgical treatment, but 20-30% develop chronic ankle instability. Chronic ankle instability (CAI) is defined as recurrent giving away of ankle for at least 6 months despite adequate nonsurgical treatment. CAI is usually a combination of mechanical (secondary to ligament tears) and functional (due to proprioceptive and muscular deficits) instability. Radiographic assessment of ankle instability includes standing anteroposterior, lateral and mortise views. Hindfoot alignment may be assessed on comparative hindfoot alignment or long axial view radiographs. In the absence of definite findings on standard radiographs, MRI ANKLE WO CONTRAST is the most appropriate imaging study. MRI has been proven to provide excellent evaluation of the ankle ligaments, with the additional advantage of demonstrating associated injuries, such as tendon abnormalities and osteochondral lesions.

# Case 26-6

A 30-year-old man presents for follow up of left ankle pain. He sustained a dorsiflexion/inversion type injury to his left ankle 10 months ago. The patient states that his ankle pain is unchanged and continues to be located in the posteromedial portion of the ankle, in spite of conservative therapy. His symptoms are only present occasionally during or after activity (such as soccer, running). He denies any pain with regular ambulation. Radiographs of the left ankle demonstrate a prominent os trigonum but are otherwise unremarkable. Ankle impingement syndrome is suspected clinically. What imaging study should be ordered next?

This scenario is concerned with the next study for a patient with suspected ankle impingement syndrome. Initial radiographs are negative or suggestive of impingement.

Sensible recommendation: MRI ANKLE WO CONTRAST

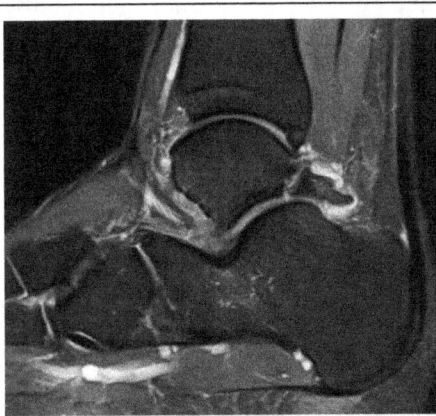

Sagittal T2 FS MRI shows a prominent os trigonum with bone marrow edema that in conjunction with the clinical findings is suggestive of posterior ankle impingement syndrome.

Ankle impingement is an important cause of chronic ankle pain particularly in the professional athlete. Ankle impingement results from an initial ankle sprain and/or repeated microtrauma, that over time results in abnormal osseous and soft tissue thickening. Impingement syndromes can occur in the anterolateral, anterior, anteromedial, posteromedial and posterior aspects of the ankle joint. Anterior and posterior impingement syndromes usually have important osseous abnormalities, while soft tissue abnormalities predominate in the other types of impingement syndromes. Impingement syndromes are usually a clinical diagnosis and imaging beyond conventional radiographs is not always necessary. MRI ANKLE WO CONTRAST may be especially useful for evaluating patients with an uncertain clinical diagnosis, excluding pathologies that may mimic or coexist with impingement syndromes, and for surgical planning. Nevertheless, the reported sensitivities and specificities of MRI for evaluation of soft tissue abnormalities in anterolateral impingement varies widely, and there are only limited reports on the use of MRI for other types of impingement syndromes. Capsular distention by intra-articular contrast injection on MR arthrography and CT arthrography, permits accurate evaluation of the capsular recesses especially in anterolateral and anteromedial impingement syndromes. Ultrasound may be used for diagnosis and for guiding injection of steroid and/or local anesthetics (for example at sites of focal capsular thickening) for symptom ablation and aiding clinical diagnosis.

## Case 26-7

A 20-year-old female pole vaulter presents to the sports clinic for evaluation of right midfoot pain. The pain started 8 months ago, without a specific injury She is unable to jump or hop without pain. On physical examination there is tenderness over the navicular and talar neck. Right ankle and foot radiographs are unremarkable. What imaging test is the most appropriate next study?

This scenario is concerned with the next study for a patient with chronic ankle pain of uncertain etiology. Initial radiographs are negative.

Sensible recommendation: MRI ANKLE WO CONTRAST

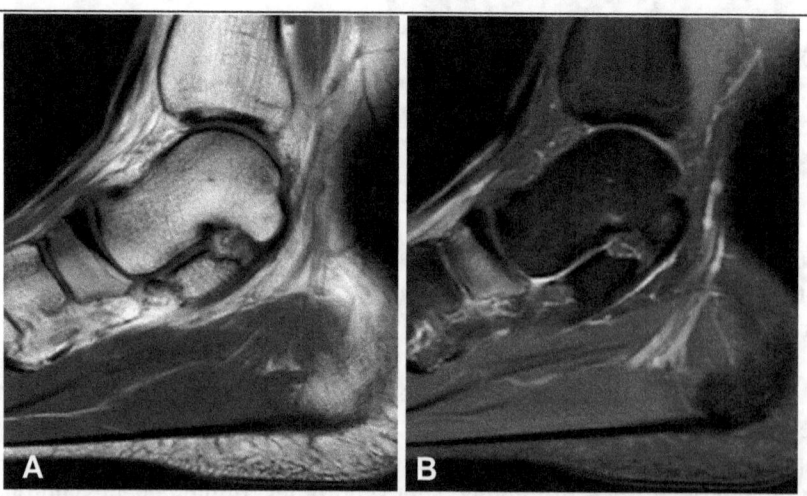

Sagittal T1 MRI (A) and T2 FS MRI (B) show relatively diffuse navicular bone marrow edema that is hyperintense on the T2-weighted and partially hypointense on the T1-weighted images. No fracture line is seen. Findings are suggestive of stress injury (grade III). There is also stress-adaptive sclerosis of the proximal aspect of the navicular.

In the presence of chronic ankle pain and normal radiographs further imaging is primarily directed by clinical findings. MRI ANKLE WO CONTRAST permits a global assessment of anatomic structures and is usually the most appropriate next study. US can be considered in the presence of focal symptoms, peripheral-nerve related symptoms, or especially due to its dynamic assessment capabilities, when symptoms are present during specific movements or positions. If there is a concern for fracture, both MRI and CT could be considered, although MRI is more sensitive for detecting osseous stress injuries and soft tissue injuries.

# Case 26-8

21-year-old woman presents with an aching right lateral ankle, which had swelling and a modest warmth. She reported no injury but admits that she runs about 3-4 times a week, 3 miles at a time. She was also given indomethacin, but she admits that she never went to get it filled. She has an upcoming race in a few weeks. Initial radiographs were negative. Stress fracture is suspected, and the diagnosis must be established; what is the most appropriate next imaging study?

This scenario concerns further evaluation for a suspected stress fracture in patient with a need-to-know diagnosis. Initial radiographs were normal.

Sensible recommendation: MRI ANKLE WO CONTRAST

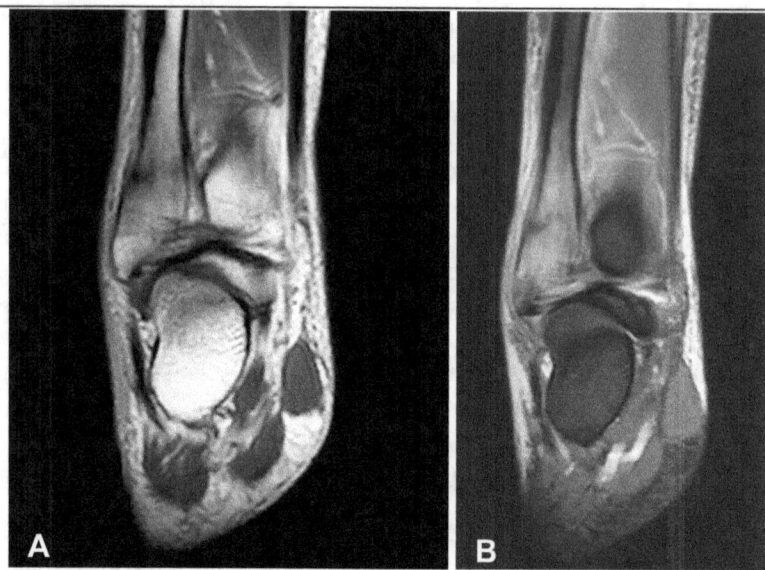

Coronal T1(A) and T2 FS (B) images of right ankle demonstrate a stress fracture involving the distal fibular metaphysis.

When establishing the diagnosis of stress fracture is considered necessary, repeat radiographs in 10-14 days are recommended. If the patient or clinician are anxious or can't wait to have the diagnosis made, or repeat radiographs remain negative, MRI is the favored next imaging modality. Notably, radiographs may remain negative depending on the timing of reimaging, the patient's metabolic bone status, and the type and location of the fracture. MRI is highly accurate and demonstrates stress reactions as early as bone scan, with similar sensitivity, and with improved specificity.

# Case 26-9

20-year-old male basketball player with right distal/medial shin pain. The patient had recently joined the men's college basketball team and had ramped up his activity, playing for 4 hours per day. He is tender to palpation along the medial border of the tibia. Radiographs obtained were interpreted as normal, and although the bone scan is hot, it is considered non-specific. What is the next appropriate imaging modality to obtain?

Suspect stress fracture, not hip or sacrum. Radiographs normal. Bone scan positive but nonspecific.

Sensible recommendation: XR ANKLE 3 VIEW after 10-14 days or MRI ANKLE WO CONTRAST

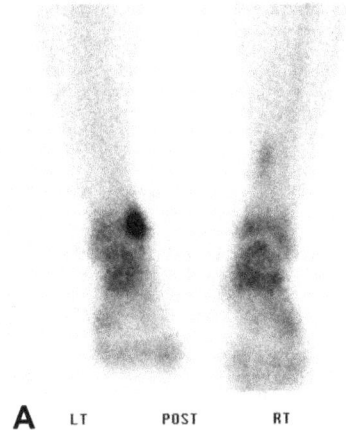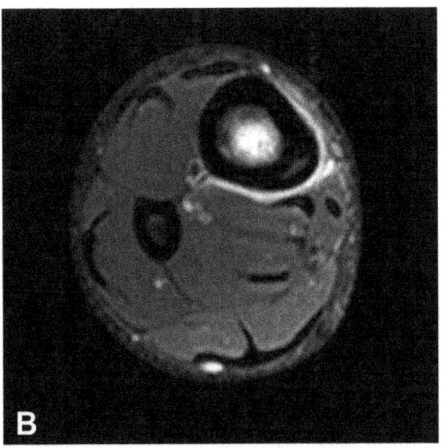

Bone scan (A) of the lower extremities demonstrates increased uptake at the right distal tibia, interpreted as non-specific. Axial T2 FS MRI (B) demonstrates periosteal and bone marrow edema compatible with stress reaction involving the right tibia.

When a stress fracture is suspected, radiographs prove to be normal, and a bone scan appears positive however non-specific, MRI WO CONTRAST of the area of interest is recommended. Because of a lack of sensitivity with bone scan (with synovitis, arthritis, degenerative joint disease, stress reactions, and tumors appearing similar), supplemental imaging with MRI may be necessary to formulate a conclusive diagnosis or to avoid false positive diagnoses. When the patient is an athlete and there is concern regarding appropriate return to play, MRI provides more information.

# References

1. Chang EY, Tadros AS, Amini B, Bell AM, Bernard SA, Fox MG, Gorbachova T, Ha AS, Lee KS, Metter DF, Mooar PA, Shah NA, Singer AD, Smith SE, Taljanovic MS, Thiele R, Kransdorf MJ. ACR Appropriateness Criteria(®) Chronic Ankle Pain. J Am Coll Radiol. 2018 May;15(5S):S26-S38. doi: 10.1016/j.jacr.2018.03.016. PMID: 29724425.
2. American College of Radiology. ACR Appropriateness Criteria: Chronic Ankle Pain. American College of Radiology, revised 2017. https://acsearch.acr.org/docs/69422/Narrative/ (accessed April 24, 2021).
3. Chronic ankle pain. American College of Radiology. ACR Appropriateness Criteria. DeSmet AA, Dalinka MK, Alazraki N, et al. Radiology. 2000 Jun;215 Suppl:321-32.
4. Bencardino JT, Stone TJ, Roberts CC, Appel M, Baccei SJ, Cassidy RC, Chang EY, Fox MG, Greenspan BS, Gyftopoulos S, Hochman MG, Jacobson JA,

Mintz DN, Mlady GW, Newman JS, Rosenberg ZS, Shah NA, Small KM, Weissman BN. ACR Appropriateness Criteria(®) Stress (Fa-tigue/Insufficiency) Fracture, Including Sacrum, Excluding Other Vertebrae. J Am Coll Radiol. 2017 May;14(5S):S293-S306. doi: 10.1016/j.jacr.2017.02.035. Review. PMID: 28473086.

5.  American College of Radiology. ACR Appropriateness Criteria: Stress (Fatigue/Insufficiency) Fracture, Including Sacrum, Excluding Other Vertebrae. American College of Radiology, revised 2016. https://acsearch.acr.org/docs/69435/Narrative/ (accessed April 24, 2021).

# Chapter 27. Chronic or Nontraumatic Foot Pain

Kimia Kani, MD

Radiography is the initial exam for chronic or nontraumatic foot pain. One of MRI, CT, or US may be the next step, but sometimes more than one is indicated. The bone scan has a limited role.

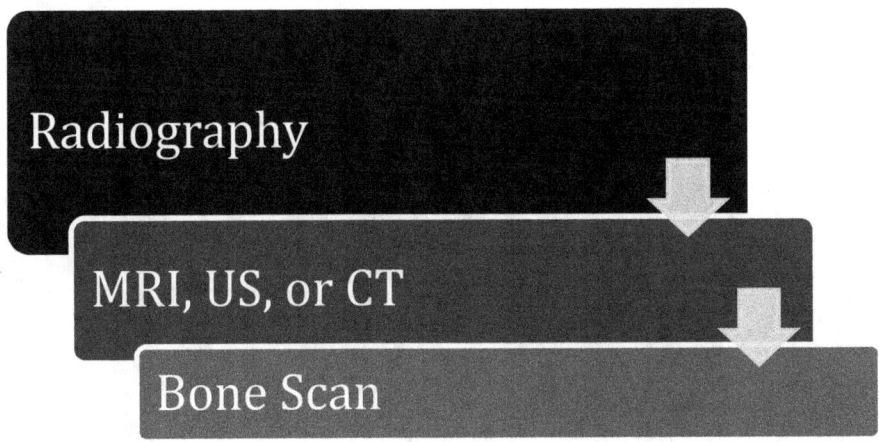

# Case 27-1

A 56-year-old woman presents with painful bunions of her feet. She reports bunions most of her adult life, but now the bunions are painful regardless of the width of her footwear. On physical examination, she had bilateral hallux valgus. What is the most appropriate initial imaging study?

This scenario is concerned with the initial imaging study for a patient with chronic foot pain of unknown etiology.

Sensible recommendation: XR FOOT 3 VIEW

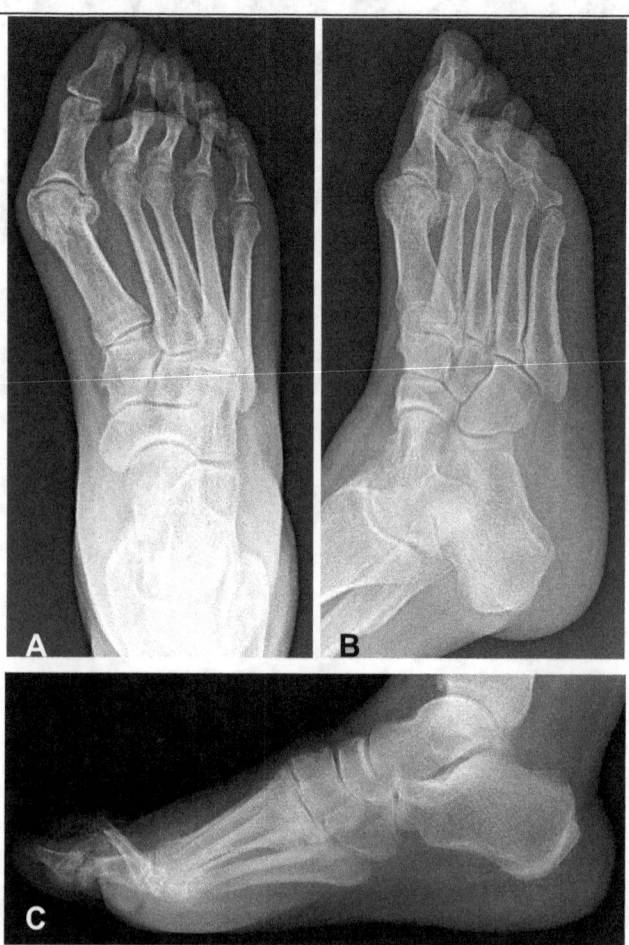

AP (A), oblique (B) and lateral (C) radiographs of the right foot show prominent bunion deformity with degenerative arthritis at the first metatarsophalangeal joint and overriding of the second toe. Radiographs of her left foot (not shown) demonstrated similar findings.

Foot pain is considered chronic when symptoms persist more than 6 weeks. Radiographs are the most appropriate initial imaging study for evaluation of chronic foot pain. Foot radiographs may be obtained without or with weight-bearing, and typically include anteroposterior, oblique and lateral views.

## Case 27-2

A 43-year-old man presents with many years of left foot pain. On physical examination there is left flatfoot deformity with hindfoot valgus. Left ankle and foot radiographs are equivocal for tarsal coalition. What imaging studies should be ordered next?

This scenario is concerned with the next imaging study for a patient, adult or child, with chronic painful rigid flat foot. Initial radiographs unremarkable or equivocal and clinical concern for tarsal coalition.

Sensible recommendation: CT FOOT WO CONTRAST or MRI FOOT WO CONTRAST

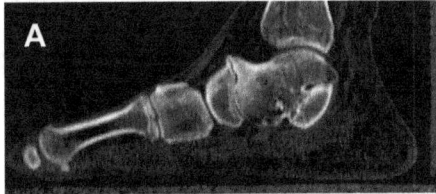 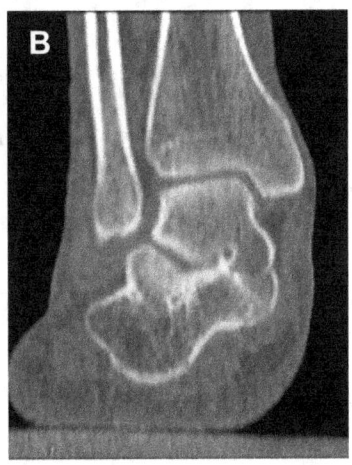

Sagittal (A) and coronal (B) reconstructed CT images of the left foot with simulated weight-bearing. There is osseous coalition of the middle subtalar joint, advanced talonavicular osteoarthritis and pes planovalgus.

Tarsal coalition is an osseous, cartilaginous or fibrous union between two or more tarsal bones. The condition is usually congenital, and most commonly affects the calcaneonavicular joint and the middle facet of the subtalar joint, sometimes bilaterally. Tarsal coalition may be asymptomatic. Symptomatic patients classically present in the second decade of life with chronic pain and a rigid flatfoot on clinical examination. Standard weight-bearing ankle and foot radiographs are the initial imaging evaluation and may be supplemented with a Harris-Beath view (for evaluation of the middle and posterior subtalar joints) and weight-bearing hindfoot alignment radiographs. Osseous tarsal coalition is seen as a bridging bony bar between the involved bones. Nonosseous coalition is seen as a narrowed and irregular cleft between the involved bones (the surrounding bones are hypertrophic and may show cyst formation and sclerosis). On radiographs the site of coalition may be seen directly or especially for subtalar coalitions, the associated secondary signs of tarsal coalition may be the only clues for the diagnosis of this condition. CT FOOT WO CONTRAST and MRI FOOT WO CONTRAST are alternative methods for evaluation of tarsal coalition. CT examination may include evaluation of the contralateral foot. MRI of the foot may permit distinction of cartilaginous from fibrous coalitions, assessment of bone marrow edema, and evaluation of adjacent soft tissues (e.g., associated tenosynovitis due to altered biomechanics).

# Case 27-3

A 39-year-old man presented with pain, stiffness, swelling and discoloration of his right foot. He reports a mild right ankle sprain 7 weeks ago. On physical examination of his right foot, the skin has a mottled appearance and the foot is swollen and sensitive to the slightest touch. Radiographs of the ankle and foot demonstrate mild diffuse osteopenia but are otherwise unremarkable. What imaging test should be ordered at this point?

This scenario is concerned with the next imaging study for a patient with negative radiographs and clinical concern for complex regional pain syndrome type I.

Sensible recommendation: Tc-99m BONE SCAN

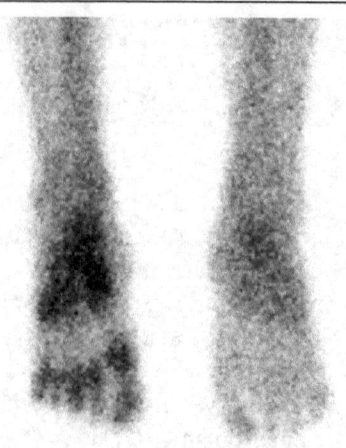

Delayed spot nuclear image after injection of 99m Tc-MDP shows increased uptake in the right foot and ankle with periarticular accentuation.

Complex regional pain syndrome (CRPS) is characterized by a triad of sensory, motor and autonomic dysfunction that usually involves one of the extremities after an initial event. CRPS is divided into two types that are mostly similar clinically, except for the presence of nerve injury in type II. The initial event in CRPS type I may or may not be traumatic, and may include minor injury, fracture or elective surgery of the affected extremity. The predominate features of CRPS are chronic pain and temperature differences between the affected and contralateral limb. This condition has the potential to result in long-term disability, especially with late diagnosis and treatment of the disease. CRPS type I is primarily a clinical diagnosis of exclusion. Imaging is used to primarily exclude other conditions. Radiographs may demonstrate nonspecific osteopenia of the affected region, that may be the result of disuse. Tc-99m bone scan is the most appropriate study for supporting the clinical diagnosis of CRPS type 1. On the delayed images, the classic finding of this condition is diffuse increased radiotracer uptake throughout the foot with periarticular accentuation. MRI is nonspecific and may demonstrate variable findings such as periarticular marrow edema, soft tissue swelling, joint effusions and in the later stages of disease muscle atrophy.

# Case 27-4

46-year-old woman presents with worsening pain over her right second metatarsophalangeal joint and there is a clinical concern for Freiberg infraction. What is the most appropriate initial imaging study?

This scenario concerns the initial study for a patient, adult or child, with chronic pain and tenderness over head of second metatarsal and clinical concern for Freiberg infraction.

Sensible recommendation: XR FOOT 3 VIEW

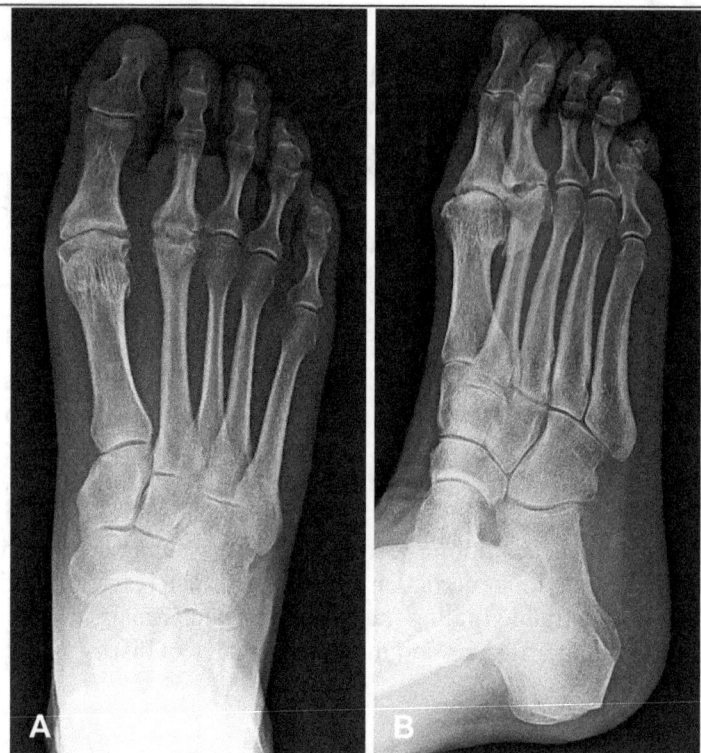

AP (A) and oblique (B) radiographs of the right foot show flattening, fragmentation and sclerosis of the second metatarsal head. There is secondary osteoarthritis of the second metatarsophalangeal joint. First metatarsophalangeal osteoarthritis is also noted.

Freiberg infraction is a disorder that usually affects the second or third metatarsal heads. The pathophysiology of this condition is likely multifactorial and includes trauma, vascular compromise, genetic predisposition and altered biomechanics. This condition most commonly affects adolescent females and patients may complain of pain and tenderness of the affected metatarsophalangeal joint. Diagnosis of this condition is typically made clinically and confirmed with radiography. Radiographic changes are characteristic and may include increased density, subchondral lucencies, flattening, collapse, and fragmentation of the metatarsal head. Widening in the later stages arthrosis of the involved metatarsophalangeal joint may ensue. Spontaneous healing with remodeling may occur especially in the early stages of the disease. Early in the disease process, radiographs will be normal and the diagnosis may be suggested with Tc-99m bone scans or MRI. On bone scans, early disease is seen as a photopenic center in the metatarsal head with a hyperactive collar. On MRI, early findings include nonspecific low signal intensity changes in the metatarsal head on T1-weighted images, with corresponding increased signal intensity on the fluid-sensitive sequences.

# Case 27-5

28-year-old mailman presents with persistent pain and swelling of his left foot. He has history of acute on chronic foot injury, with the most recent injury occurring 8 weeks ago. On physical examination there is swelling along the talonavicular aspect of the left foot with bony asymmetry and local tenderness. Radiographs demonstrate a prominent type 2 accessory navicular bone. What imaging test should be ordered next?

This scenario concerns the next study for a patient with chronic pain and tenderness over the hindfoot, unresponsive to conservative therapy. Radiographs showed an accessory ossicle at the site.

Sensible recommendation: MRI FOOT WO CONTRAST

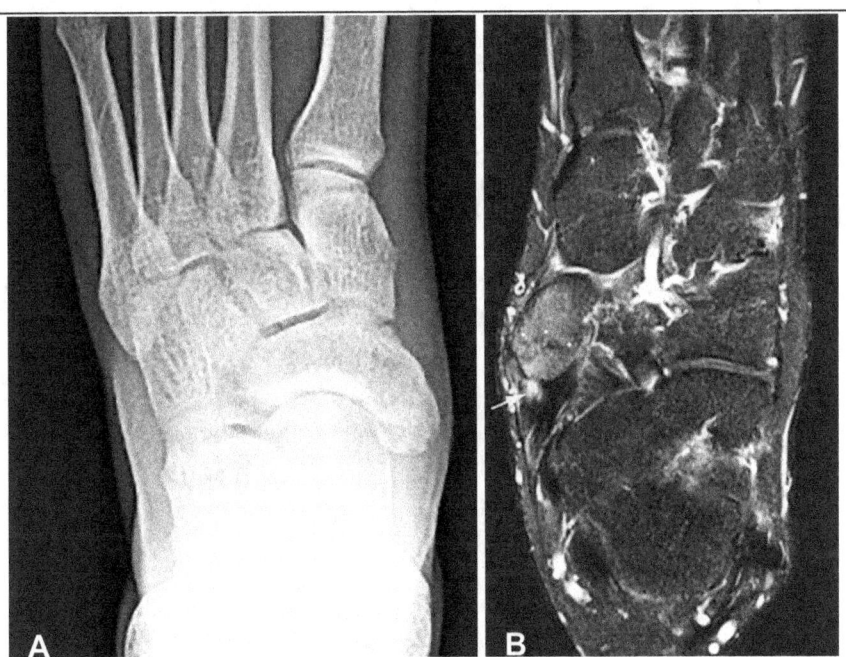

AP radiograph (A) of the left mid-foot shows a prominent type II accessory navicular bone. Axial T2 FS MRI (B) shows bone marrow edema of the accessory navicular and the adjacent posteromedial navicular tuberosity (the intervening synchondrosis is demarcated by white dots). There is a partial thickness tear (arrow) of the posterior tibial tendon at level of attachment to the accessory navicular.

A variety of accessory ossicles have been described in the foot and ankle. The most common accessory ossicles are the os trigonum, the accessory navicular and the os intermetatarseum. While usually asymptomatic, accessory ossicles can cause pain secondary to trauma (e.g., fracture of the accessory ossicle), degenerative changes at the synchondrosis, or repetitive impingement of the neighboring soft tissues. Some accessory navicular types may be associated with posterior tibial tendon dysfunction and/or flat-foot deformity. MRI is the most appropriate imaging study for evaluation of potentially symptomatic accessory ossicles. Various combinations of degenerative or traumatic changes, bone marrow edema, joint effusion, tenosynovitis, tendon tear, or adventitial bursa formation may be seen at or in the vicinity of the symptomatic accessory ossicle. Bone scintigraphy may be appropriate (especially if MRI is unavailable), and demonstrates increased uptake at level of the symptomatic accessory ossicle. Image-guided injection of the os trigonum synchondrosis with local anesthetics (possibly with corticosteroids) affords a direct method of confirming the site of pain and may assist in surgical planning.

# Case 27-6

A 49-year-old woman with a history of rheumatoid arthritis presents with progressive and chronic right foot pain. She attributes her pain to prominent rheumatoid nodules along the plantar surface of her right forefoot which give her discomfort while walking. She comes to the orthopedics clinic today to see whether there is any surgical management available for her nodules. Radiographs demonstrate well-corticated metatarsophalangeal erosions. What imaging test should be performed to more specifically characterize and localize the soft tissue nodules for preoperative planning?

This scenario concerns the next study for a patient where there is clinical concern for inflammatory arthropathy, including rheumatoid arthritis, and the initial radiograph is nonspecific.

Sensible recommendation: MRI FOOT WO/W CONTRAST

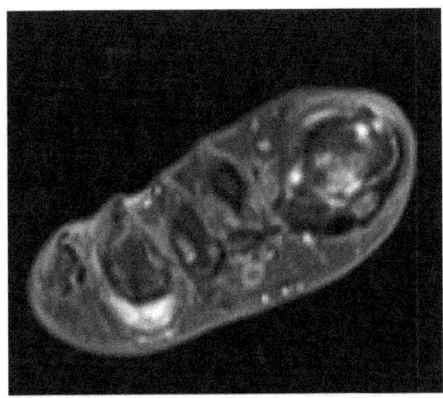

Short axis T1 FS Gd MRI of the right foot shows an enhancing nodule along the plantar aspect of the fourth metatarsal head and a rim enhancing nodule along the plantar aspect of the second metatarsal head. Additional enhancing nodules were seen along the plantar surface of the forefoot (not shown).

Radiographs are the initial and most important imaging test for evaluating arthritis. MRI (especially contrast-enhanced MRI) can be helpful for further evaluation of patients with inflammatory arthropathies. The addition of contrast improves visualization and differentiation of inflamed synovium and pannus from the neighboring joint, tendon sheath or bursal fluid, and is useful for assessing the response to therapy. MRI can detect the stigmata of inflammatory arthropathies at an earlier stage, before changes become evident on radiographs or patients becomes symptomatic in the ankle/foot. MRI can be used for exact assessment of the sites of involvement (which may be helpful for diagnosing a specific type of inflammatory arthropathy, especially in the early stages of disease), extent of disease, and disease complications. US (using both gray scale and power Doppler US) may be an appropriate next study, especially as a complement to clinical examination of the patient in daily clinical practice. Detection of inflammatory soft tissue and bone erosions is possible with US, although somewhat dependent on the skill of the US operator.

## Case 27-7

64-year-old woman presents for evaluation of chronic right medial heel pain. Her symptoms are exacerbated by walking. Radiographs of the right ankle and foot are unremarkable. What imaging study should be performed next?

This scenario concerns the next study for a patient with localized pain at the plantar aspect of the heel and clinical concern for plantar fasciitis. Initial radiographs are negative.

Sensible recommendation: MRI FOOT WO CONTRAST

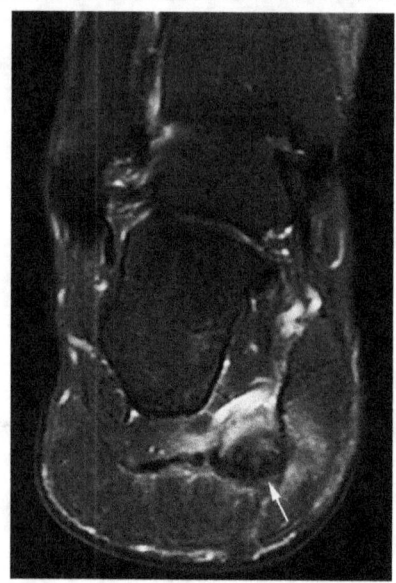

Coronal T2 FS MRI demonstrates non-homogeneous signal intensity and pronounced thickening of the central component of the plantar aponeurosis, with high T2 signal intensity in the surrounding soft tissues. Findings are diagnostic of plantar fasciopathy.

Plantar fasciopathy is the most common cause of plantar heel pain. It can arise from stress of repetitive trauma, or be secondary to systemic conditions (e.g., seronegative spondyloarthropathies, rheumatoid arthritis, or gout). When there is a clinical concern for plantar fasciopathy, radiographs may be performed initially. Although radiography is typically insensitive to plantar fasciopathy, it may be of value especially in delineating other causes of heel pain (e.g. stress fracture or tumor), predisposing foot deformities (on weight bearing radiographs), or erosions. In patients who have an atypical presentation, an unclear diagnosis, or who have failed conservative management, further imaging with ultrasound or preferably MRI may be of value.

## Case 27-8

49-year-old woman presents with complaints of right foot numbness and tingling. She has history of ganglion cyst excision from her right tarsal tunnel for similar symptoms, with resultant improvement of her numbness and tingling. However, over the last few months she reports recurrent numbness and tingling along the plantar aspect of her right foot. Radiographs of the ankle and foot are unremarkable. What imaging test should be ordered next?

This scenario concerns a patient with burning pain and paresthesia along the plantar surface of the foot and toes and clinical concern for tarsal tunnel syndrome. Initial radiographs were negative.

Sensible recommendation: MRI FOOT WO CONTRAST

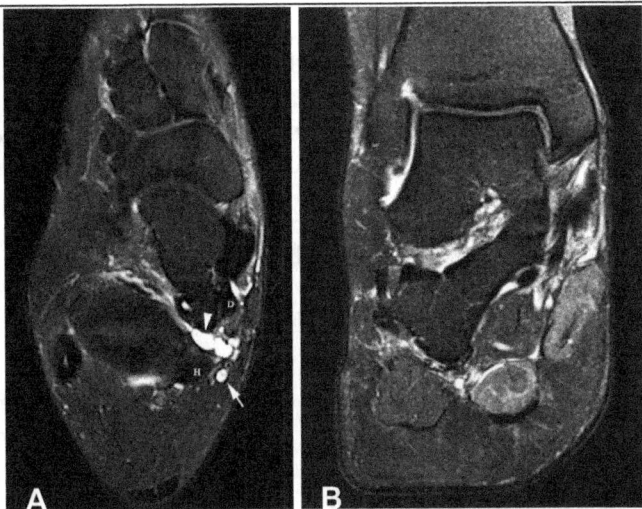

Axial (A) and coronal (B) T2 FS MRI of the right ankle. On the axial image observe the recurrent ganglion cyst (arrowhead) in the tarsal tunnel. The cyst is located between the flexor digitorum longus (D) and flexor hallucis longus (H) tendons and abuts the neurovascular bundle (arrow). Coronal image shows denervation signal changes in the abductor hallucis and flexor digitorum brevis muscles.

Tarsal tunnel syndrome results from entrapment of the posterior tibial nerve and/or its branches in the tarsal tunnel. This compressive neuropathy may result from trauma (fracture, surgery, and scarring), space-occupying lesions (ganglion cyst, tumor, anomalous muscle, and varicosities), foot deformities, or systemic diseases such as diabetes mellitus. Nevertheless, in up to 40% of cases an underlying cause for tarsal tunnel syndrome cannot be identified. Patients classically complain of burning pain and paresthesia along the plantar aspect of the foot and toes that worsen with activity. MRI is the most appropriate modality for evaluation of tarsal tunnel syndrome as it permits identification of potential causes of nerve entrapment. Direct evidence of injury to the posterior tibial nerve and its branches may be difficult with this modality due to the small size of the nerves. Tarsal tunnel syndrome is primarily a sensory neuropathy, nevertheless it may sometimes be associated with muscle denervation changes. High-frequency sonography enables high-quality and dynamic evaluation of the peripheral nerves when entrapment is suspected. However, results of US are more dependent on the skill and expertise of the operator.

## Case 27-9

A 47-year-old woman presents with increasing left foot pain and occasional numbness and tingling between her left third and fourth metatarsals. She has also noted a mass at this level that has made it very difficult for her to wear narrow shoes. Radiographs of her left foot show splaying of the third and fourth metatarsal heads with suggestion of an intervening soft tissue mass. What imaging test should be ordered next?

This scenario concerns the next study for a patient with chronic pain in the 3-4 web space with radiation to the toes and concern for Morton neuroma. Initial radiographs unremarkable or equivocal.

Sensible recommendation: MRI FOOT WO/W CONTRAST or US FOOT, region of interest

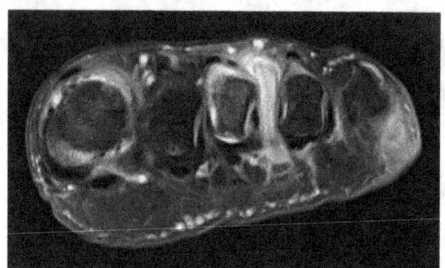

Short axis T1 FS Gd MRI of the left foot shows a dumbbell-shaped enhancing mass between the third and fourth metatarsal heads. Morton neuroma was confirmed on subsequent surgery and pathologic examination.

Morton neuroma is a non-neoplastic fibrotic nodule arising from the plantar digital nerve. It most commonly affects the second and third intermetatarsal spaces of middle-aged women and may possibly be related to footwear. MRI FOOT WO W CONTRAST and US (when appropriate operator expertise is available) are alternative methods for evaluation of Morton neuromas. In addition, US may also be used for guiding Morton neuroma injections. Morton neuromas are frequently asymptomatic, therefore, careful correlation between clinical and imaging findings is necessary before a Morton neuroma is considered to be clinically relevant.

## Case 27-10

46-year-old man presents for evaluation of chronic left foot pain. He is a longtime runner and typically does 3 to 5 half marathons a year. He has been noticing pain and stiffness along the medial aspect of his midfoot, that has been progressively getting worse. His main concern is that he has a stress fracture. Radiographs of the left foot are unremarkable. What imaging test should be ordered next?

This scenario concerns a patient who is an athlete with pain and tenderness over tarsal navicular. Radiographs unremarkable or equivocal. Clinical concern for stress injury or occult fracture.

Sensible recommendation: MRI FOOT WO CONTRAST

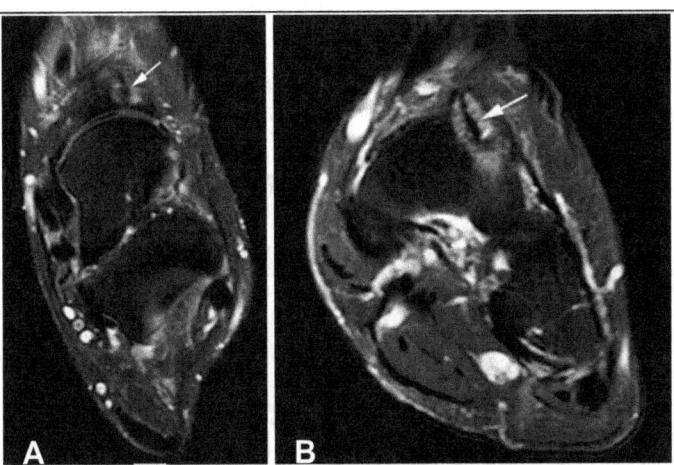

Axial (A) and coronal (B) T2 FS MRI show a nondisplaced and incomplete stress fracture of the dorsal aspect of the navicular body with surrounding bone marrow edema.

Osseous stress response is a continuum ranging from normal osseous remodeling, through accelerated remodeling with stress injury, to frank stress fracture. Stress injury can affect the majority of the ankle and foot bones. When radiographs are normal or equivocal, MRI is the most sensitive and specific modality for evaluation of suspected stress injuries. Fluid-sensitive sequences are invaluable for detection of the earlier stages of stress injury, such as periosteal or bone marrow edema. T1-weighted images are especially useful for depiction of anatomy and more advanced stress related findings. The Tc-99m bone scan is sensitive but nonspecific to the early changes of stress injury, and is the procedure of choice when MRI cannot be performed. CT is insensitive for evaluation of early stress injury. CT of the foot may be used as a problem-solving tool when there are equivocal findings on MRI or bone scintigraphy (such as differentiation of stress injury from osteoid osteoma) or especially, for follow-up of fracture healing.

## Case 27-11

A 55-year-old man presents with complain of chronic right medial foot pain. Radiographs of the right foot and ankle show soft tissue swelling laterally but are otherwise unremarkable. What imaging study should be performed next?

This scenario concerns the further imaging of the foot when radiographs are unremarkable or equivocal and there is persistent clinical concern for tendinopathy.

Sensible recommendation: MRI FOOT WO CONTRAST or US FOOT, region of interest

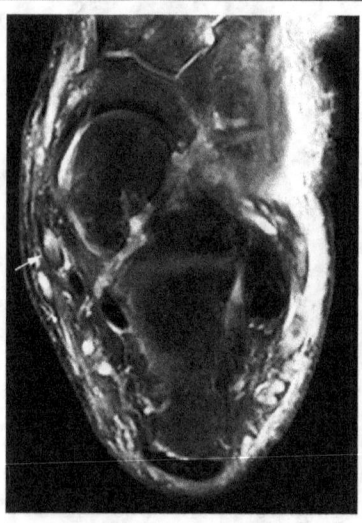

Axial T2 FS MRI of the right ankle shows tendinosis and partial thickness tear of the posterior tibial tendon (arrow). There is nonspecific subcutaneous edema laterally.

Tendon abnormalities include tendinopathy, tenosynovitis, tendon tear (partial or complete) and tendon subluxation or dislocation. MRI and US can both effectively demonstrate tendon abnormalities, although US results are more dependent on operator expertise. An exception is the significant advantage of US over MRI in the dynamic evaluation of tendon subluxation or dislocation.

# References

1. American College of Radiology. ACR Appropriateness Criteria: Chronic foot pain. American College of Radiology, revised 2020. https://acsearch.acr.org/docs/69424/Narrative/ (accessed April 24, 2021).
2. Chronic foot pain. American College of Radiology. ACR Appropriateness Criteria. el-Khoury GY, Dalinka MK, Alazraki N, et al. Radiology. 2000 Jun;215 Suppl:357-63.

# Part IV. Focal Lesions and Oncology

These patients may present in a variety of ways. Their primary care physicians may refer them for evaluation of a palpable soft tissue mass or a lesion found on radiographs, or a specialist may refer them with a diagnosis for further evaluation or staging. Radiography, MRI, CT, nuclear imaging, and the use of contrast with MRI and CT, and imaging-guided biopsy, may all have a role in the evaluation and follow-up of these patients.

# Chapter 28: Evaluation of Focal Bone Lesions

Edward Derrick, MD, Kurt Scherer, MD, Laura Bancroft, MD

Radiography is the initial exam for primary bone tumors. MRI can be used to evaluate anatomic setting, but CT offers complementary information for diagnosis. Nuclear imaging may provide physiologic information. Biopsy may be necessary.

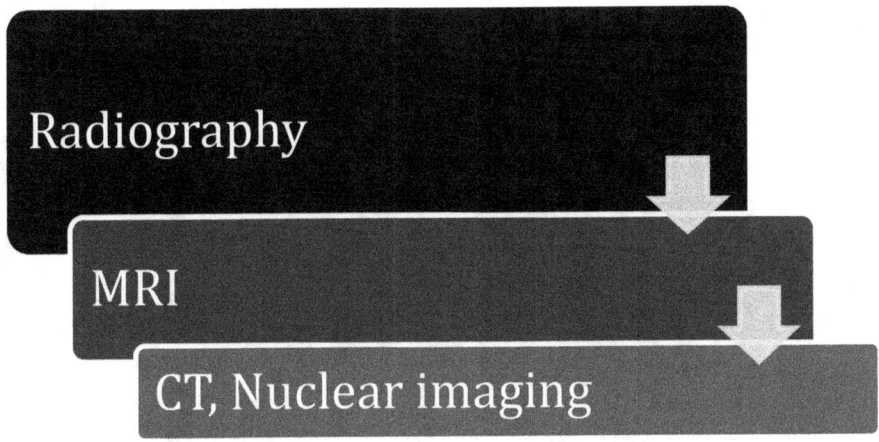

# Case 28-1

A 29-year-old woman presents for evaluation of a mass just proximal to her right knee in the inner, distal thigh. Examination of the region of interest reveals a hard, non-mobile mass without any overlying edema or erythema. Patient does not report any history of trauma. What is the most appropriate initial imaging study?

This scenario concerns the appropriate first imaging exam for a clinically apparent extremity mass.

Sensible recommendation: XR, region of interest

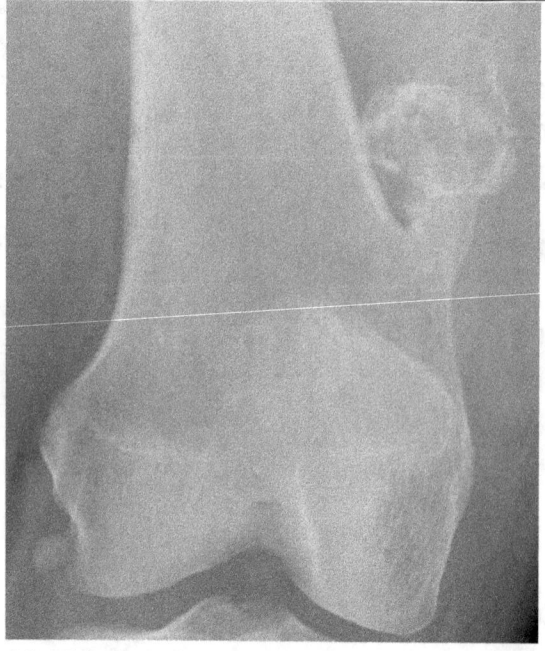

AP radiograph of the right knee demonstrates a pedunculated osseous lesion arising from the distal medial femoral metadiaphysis. The lesion demonstrates cortical and medullary continuity with the femur, classic for a pedunculated osteochondroma.

In a patient presenting for screening for a bone tumor, radiographs are the most appropriate initial imaging study. Additional imaging may be necessary if the lesion demonstrates indeterminate or aggressive features, however radiographs provide the most cost and radiation dose efficient initial screening tool in most cases as advanced imaging techniques can have misleading features that may result in unnecessary cost and procedures to the patient.

## Case 28-2

A 34-year-old woman presents with acute throbbing left hip pain for several days. She was recently diagnosed of acute leukemia, status post chemotherapy and remission. She had evening pain that was so bad she couldn't go to sleep. It also began to radiate to her knee. There is nothing that makes it feel better; she took 10 mg oxycodone several times but it did not help. It is exacerbated by movement. The pain does not radiate, although she is experiencing associated thigh and knee pain, which she attributes to limping. She denies fevers, or chills. Pelvic radiographs were negative. What is the most appropriate imaging study?

This scenario concerns the appropriate next imaging exam for a patient with positive localized or regional symptoms. Radiographs negative or findings do not explain symptoms.

Sensible recommendation: MRI WO CONTRAST, region of interest

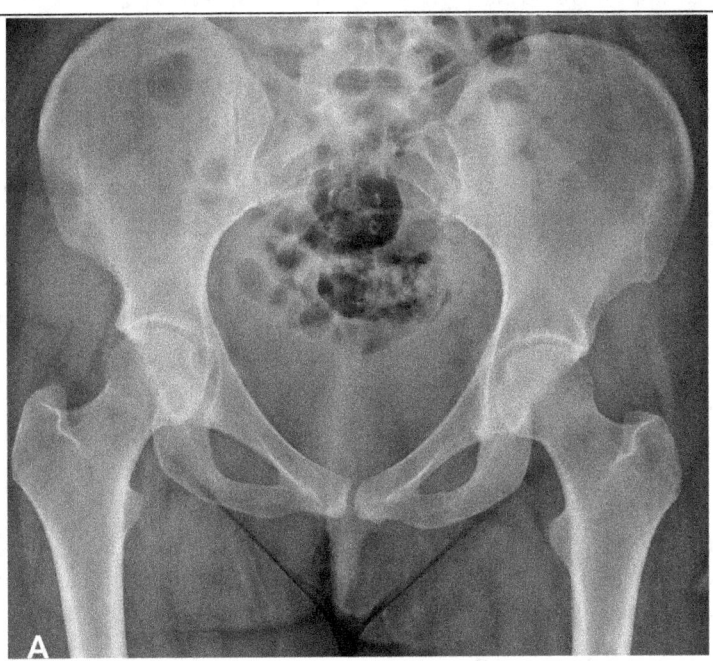

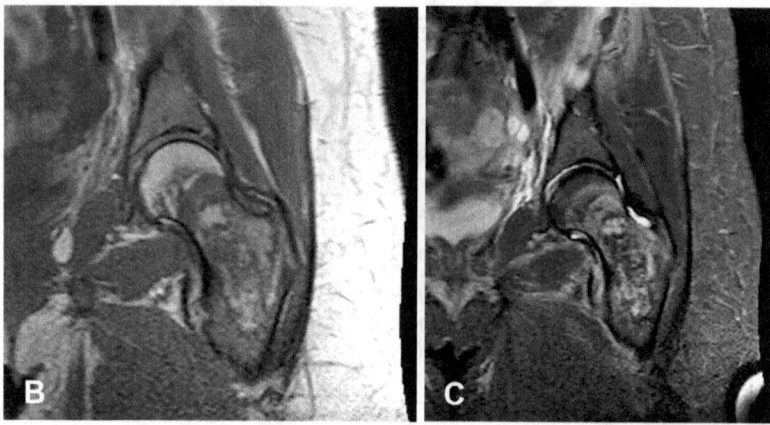

Frontal radiography of pelvis (A) shows no focal bony lesion. Coronal T1 (B) and T2 FS MRI (B) of the left hip. Within the left femoral neck there is a lesion iso-intense to muscle on T1 that demonstrates heterogeneous signal intensity on T2. Subsequent bone biopsy demonstrated the lesion to be chloroma.

There is a wide differential for symptomatic patients who either have nega-tive radiographs or have radiographs with findings that do not explain the pain. This includes injury such as stress fracture, early infection, or radio-graphically occult tumor. In any case, advanced imaging may be required based on history and degree of clinical concern. In this situation the refer-ring physician should not be confident that there is no pathology if the radiographic result is negative or nonspecific; radiographs are often insensi-tive, especially in early disease. Although CT may be performed in this setting, a radionuclide bone scan may be more useful to localize the abnor-mality. MRI can be very useful in this setting not only to identify whether a lesion is present but also to define the nature of a lesion based on the fea-tures discussed above; as a result, MRI is generally preferred.

## Case 28-3

A 46-year-old man presents for further imaging following initial evaluation for hip pain. Radiographs demonstrated a lucent, well-demarcated lesion with narrow margins and no aggressive features within the right ilium. Pa-tient has no history of malignancy. What is the most appropriate imaging study to perform next on this patient?

This scenario concerns the appropriate next imaging exam for a patient with a bone lesion on radiographs that is definitively benign (but not osteoid oste-oma).

Sensible recommendation: CT WO CONTRAST, region of interest

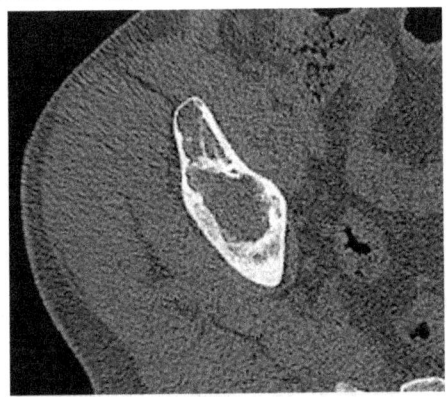

Axial non-contrast CT through the pelvis. Within the right iliac bone there is a minimally expansile, lucent lesion with a ground-glass matrix. There are no aggressive features. This is consistent with fibrous dysplasia.

In a patient with a definitely benign lesion on radiographs, there is not typically a compelling indication for further imaging. In the event that further imaging is warranted, CT or MRI examination of the region of interest is the preferred follow-up imaging method. Contrast would not likely add significant clinical value and therefore is not generally recommended. Ultrasound lacks sufficient penetration to evaluate bone lesions. Tc-99m bone scan can be abnormal but nonspecific because both benign and malignant lesions can demonstrate increased.

## Case 28-4

An 18-year-old male patient presents with left lower extremity pain which is worse at night and is relieved by NSAIDS. Recent radiographs demonstrated a sclerotic, cortical-based lesion with central lucency involving the proximal fibular diaphysis. What is the best imaging study to perform next on this patient?

This scenario concerns the appropriate next imaging exam for a patient with clinical findings and a bone lesion on radiographs suspicious for osteoid osteoma.

Sensible recommendation: CT WO CONTRAST, region of interest

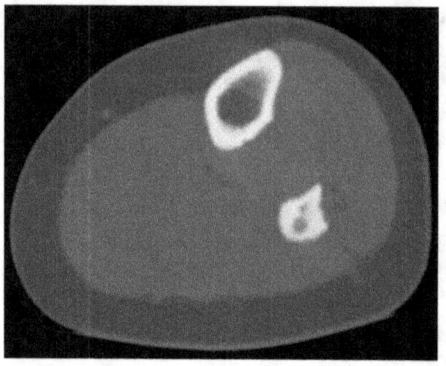

Non-contrast axial CT image trough the distal lower extremity at the level of the proximal tibia and fibula. There is sclerosis involving the posterior fibular cortex with a hypo-attenuating nidus. Within the nidus there is a faint region of calcification. These findings are classic for osteoid osteoma.

In patients with classic history and/or radiographic findings suggestive of osteoid osteoma, the best follow-up imaging exam is CT of the region of interest. CT is superior to MRI in delineating cortical anomalies and calcification. MRI has better soft tissue resolution however osteoid osteoma does not demonstrate soft tissue involvement. Ultrasound does not have sufficient penetration into the osseous structures to be useful in evaluating this entity.

## Case 28-5

A 57-year-old asymptomatic male presents after a recent visit to the ER during which he had a radiograph of the left ankle obtained for trauma. No fracture was present. The radiograph demonstrated a lesion with faint calcification, indeterminate for malignancy. What is the appropriate next imaging study?

This scenario concerns the appropriate next imaging exam for a patient with a bone lesion on radiographs that has mineralized matrix but is indeterminate for malignancy.

Sensible recommendation: MRI WO/W CONTRAST, region of interest

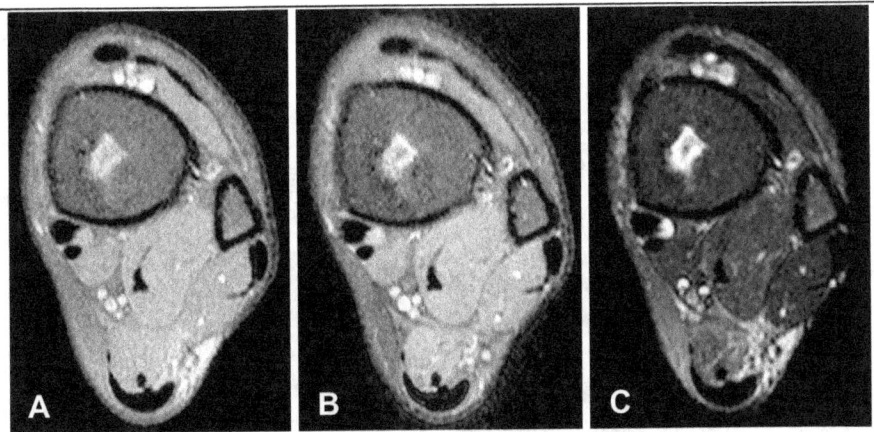

Axial T1 FS (A), T1 FS Gd (B), and T2 FS MRI (C) of the left ankle. In the distal tibia there is a medullary lesion with intermediate signal intensity which demonstrates minimal peripheral enhancement. No aggressive features are present. This is most in keeping with a benign chondroid lesion versus a bone infarct.

In a patient with an indeterminate lesion with mineralization, the next best step is an MRI examination of the region of interest wo/w contrast. MRI provides a large amount of information which often allows differentiation of benign versus malignant processes, which is facilitated by the addition of contrast. Tc-99m bone scan might be helpful to determine distribution of the lesion and presence of possible distant osseous metastases. Ultrasound has essentially no practical diagnostic role in evaluating bone lesions.

## Case 28-6

A 52-year-old man presents for follow-up imaging of her right hip. Initial radiographs of the right hip were obtained for right hip pain and demonstrated a lytic, indeterminate lesion centered in her femoral neck. No pathologic fracture was noted. Personal and family history is not contributory. What is the best imaging study for this patient to order next?

This scenario concerns the appropriate next imaging exam for a patient with a bone lesion on radiographs that appears lytic but is indeterminate for malignancy.

Sensible recommendation: MRI WO/W CONTRAST, region of interest

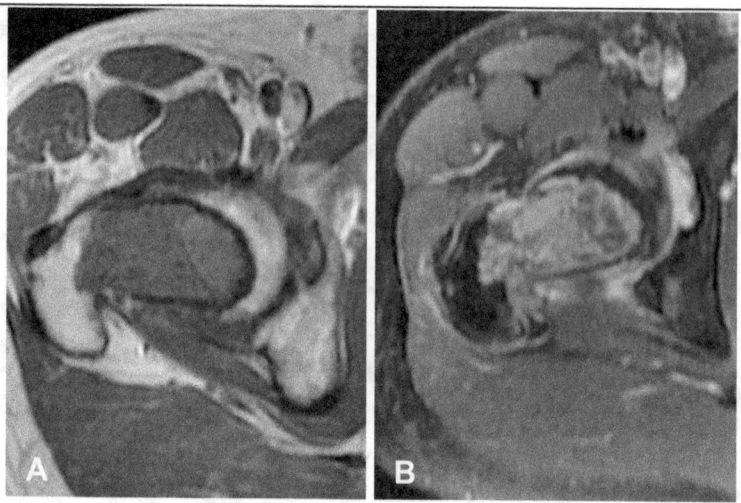

Axial T1 (A) and T1 FS Gd MRI (B) of the right hip. Within the right femoral neck there is a lesion isointense to muscle on T1 that demonstrates heterogeneous enhancement. Subsequent biopsy showed clear cell chondrosarcoma.

In a patient with an indeterminate lytic lesion, the next best step is an MRI examination of the region of interest wo/w contrast. This helps clearly identify extent of invasion and vascularity of the lesion. CT would clearly demonstrate osseous involvement; however, it has inferior soft tissue resolution compared to MRI. Tc-99m bone scan might be helpful to determine distribution of the lesion and presence of additional lesions.

# Case 28-7

A 14-year-old male patient presents for follow-up imaging for right-sided leg pain. Patient had recent radiographs of the right knee demonstrating a mixed sclerotic/lytic lesion in the distal femoral diaphysis and metadiaphysis without associated pathologic fracture. What is the appropriate imaging study for this patient?

This scenario concerns the appropriate next imaging exam for a patient with a bone lesion on radiographs that has sclerotic or mixed sclerotic and lytic features but is indeterminate for malignancy.

Sensible recommendation: MRI WO/W CONTRAST, region of interest

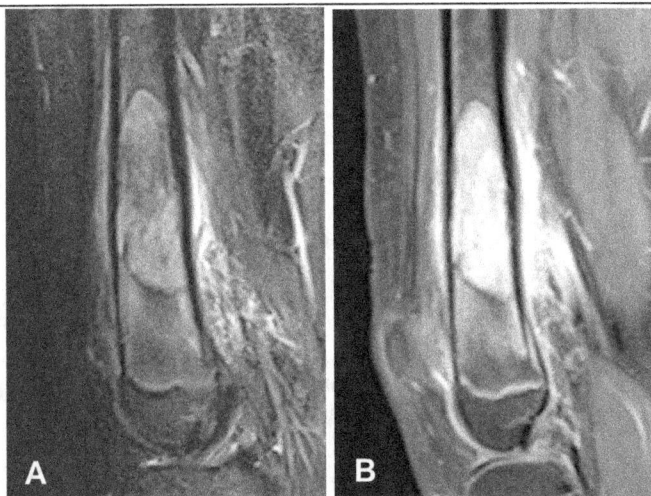

Sagittal T1 FS (A) and T1 FS Gd MRI (B) through the distal right femur. There is an intramedullary mass that enhances on post contrast enhancement. There is additional periosteal and posterior soft tissue enhancement. These findings are most suspicious for a conventional osteosarcoma.

In patients with indeterminate mixed lytic/sclerotic lesions seen on radiography, MRI wo/w contrast is the preferred imaging technique for additional imaging. MRI provides several advantages over CT including better visualization of the soft tissues, edema, and subtle tumor infiltration. CT may be obtained if MRI is contraindicated or is unavailable. CT offers better visualization of the osseous structures and is optimal to identify cortical thinning and erosion.

# Case 28-8

A 12-year-old patient presents for follow-up imaging for left thigh pain. Initial radiographs of the left knee demonstrated a sclerotic lesion involving the left femoral metaphysis with elevated periosteum and hair-on-end periosteal reaction, raising the suspicion for a malignant process. What is the most appropriate next imaging examination?

This scenario concerns the appropriate next imaging exam for a patient with a bone lesion on radiographs that appears aggressive and is suspicious for malignancy.

Sensible recommendation: MRI WO/W CONTRAST, region of interest

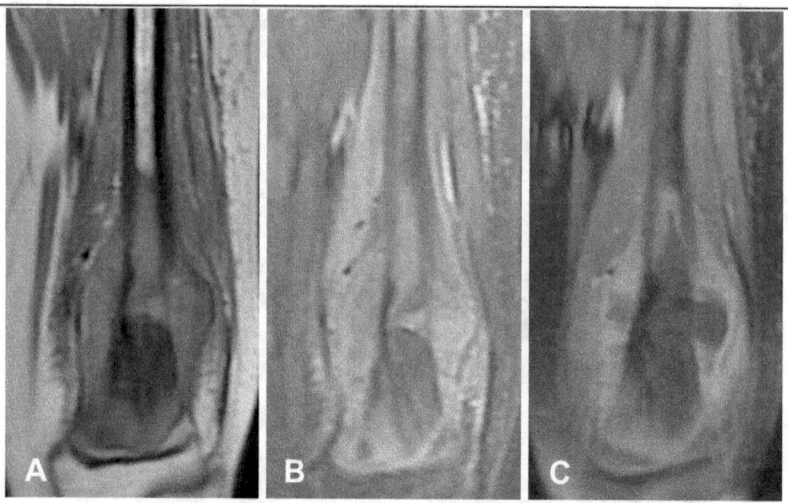

Distal femur osteosarcoma. Coronal T1 (A), T2 (B), and T1 FS Gd MRI (C) show an intramedullary lesion in the distal femur with large surrounding soft tissue mass.

In patients with aggressive-appearing lesions on radiographs, the best follow-up imaging exam is MRI wo/w contrast. MRI provides several advantages over CT including higher soft tissue contrast and visualization of edema and subtle tumor infiltration. CT may be obtained if MRI is contraindicated or is unavailable. CT offers better visualization of the osseous structures and is optimal to identify cortical thinning and erosion. Tc-99m bone scan might be helpful to evaluate for distant osseous metastases but is otherwise of limited utility in imaging of the primary lesion.

## Case 28-9

A 72-year-old woman presents with chronic, lower back pain. Recent radiograph demonstrates a compression fracture of the L3 vertebral body. She had not seen a doctor in several decades prior to this visit. What is the most appropriate imaging exam to perform next?

This scenario concerns the appropriate next imaging exam for a patient with a possible pathologic fracture on radiographs and the underlying lesion is not definitely benign.

Sensible recommendation: MRI WO/W CONTRAST, region of interest

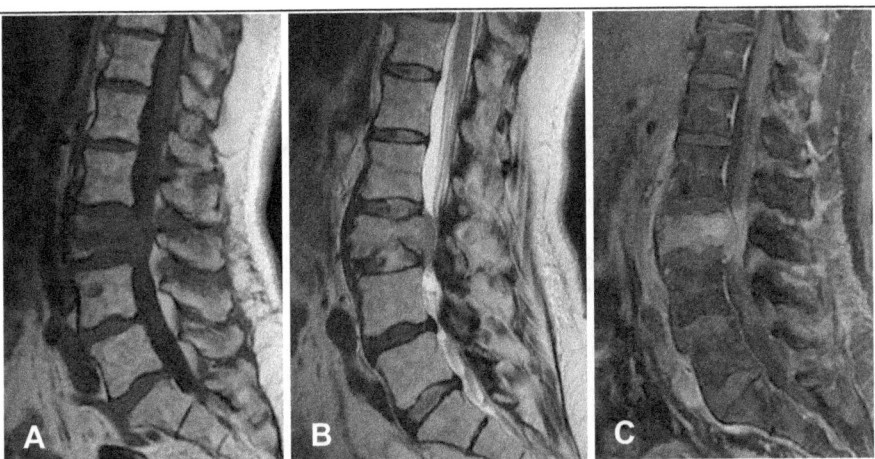

Sagittal T1 (A), T2 (B), and T1 FS Gd MRI (C) through the lumbar spine. There is height loss involving the vertebral body of L3. There is associated enhancement, raising the suspicion for a malignant process.

In a patient presenting with a pathological fracture on radiography that is not definitively benign, the best exam to perform next is an MRI of the region of interest wo/w contrast. Contrast can aid in the identification of malignant process and, if present, extent of invasion and vascularity of the lesion. Tc-99m bone scan may be helpful in evaluating the presence of multifocal disease. CT should be considered if MRI cannot be performed or is contraindicated.

# Case 28-10

A 32-year-old woman presents for follow-up imaging after a recent MRI of the pelvis for ovarian cancer in which an incidental lesion in the right proximal femur was noted. The lesion demonstrated isointensity relative to muscle on T1-weighted images and heterogeneous fat-intensity on T2-weighted images with intermixed calcified matrix. What is the best imaging exam to perform next?

This scenario concerns the appropriate next imaging exam for a patient with an incidental bone lesion found on MRI that is not definitely benign. There are no radiographs.

Sensible recommendation: XR, region of interest

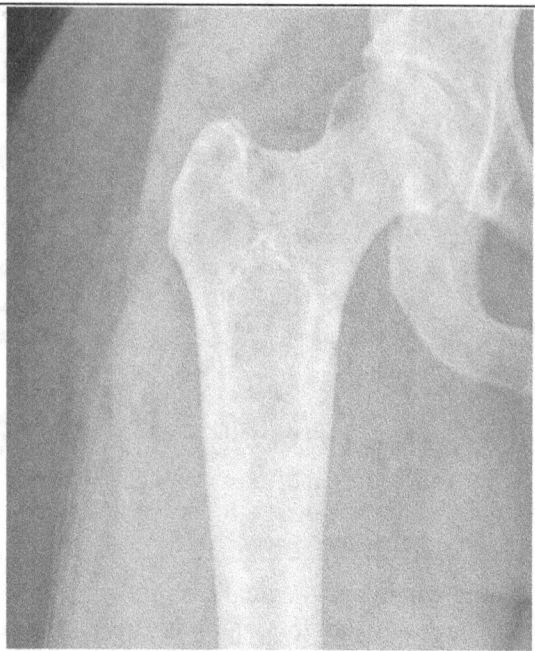

AP radiograph of the right proximal femur. In the proximal femur there is a well demarcated lucency with narrow, sclerotic borders, suggestive of a benign process.

In a patient with an incidental finding on MRI and no prior radiographs, the best follow-up imaging examination is radiography of the area of interest. Radiographs play a large role in osseous tumor diagnosis, they can identify matrix constituency, periosteal reaction, and several benign or malignant features of a lesion. Repeat MRI could be performed if the lesion was incompletely visualized on prior MRI or if sequences were not adequate to assess the lesion.

## Case 28-11

A 47-year-old woman presents for further evaluation after having an abnormal CT examination of the right knee. Initial CT was performed for knee pain and a lucent lesion was noted in the proximal tibial metaphysis. There was faint, nonspecific punctuate mineralization associated with this lesion. What is the most appropriate exam to perform next?

This scenario concerns the evaluation of an incidental bone lesion found on CT that is not clearly benign. No radiographs available.

Sensible recommendation: MRI WO/W CONTRAST, region of interest

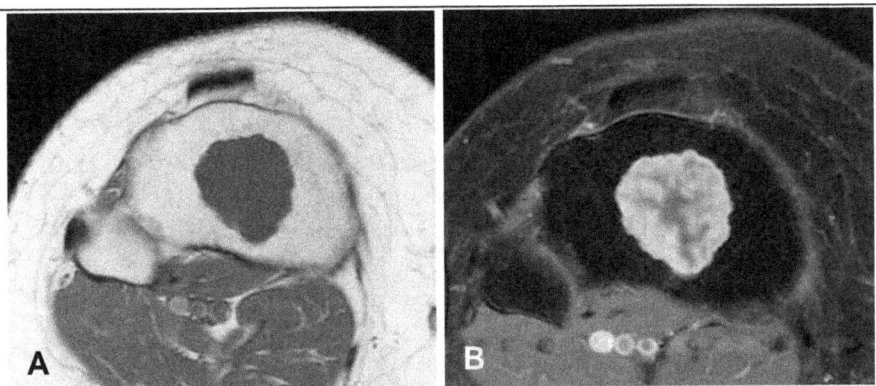

Axial T1 (A) and T2 FS MRI (B) through the proximal tibia and fibula. In the proximal tibial metaphysis, there is a lesion that is homogeneously hypointense on T1-weighted images which demonstrates peripheral hyperintensity on T2. This is a typical appearance of an enchondroma.

In patients presenting with an incidental abnormality which is not clearly benign on CT and without prior radiographs, MRI is the most appropriate exam to perform next. Repeat CT may be obtained if original CT was of suboptimal quality or otherwise inadequate. Radiographs would add little additional clinical value over a CT. Tc-99m bone scan may assist in determining activity of the lesion and additional lesions, if present, but would be a poor choice for characterizing a primary lesion.

# References

1.  American College of Radiology. ACR Appropriateness Criteria: Primary bone tumors. American College of Radiology, revised 2019. https://acsearch.acr.org/docs/69421/Narrative/ (accessed April 24, 2021).

# Chapter 29: Evaluation of Soft Tissue Masses

Edward Derrick, MD, Kurt Scherer, MD, Laura Bancroft, MD

Radiography is the initial exam for soft tissue masses, primarily to identify calcification or exclude an underlying bone lesion. US or MRI would be next to evaluate the mass, and CT and nuclear imaging could provide additional information. Biopsy may be necessary.

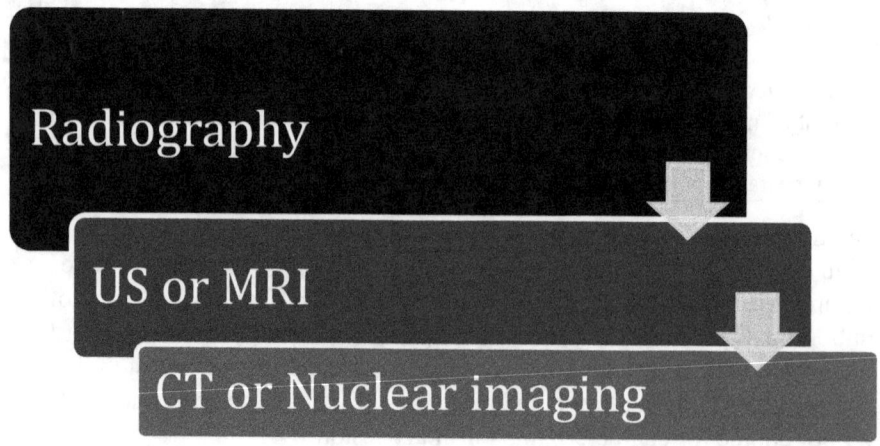

# Case 29-1

An 82-year-old man presents for evaluation of a palpable soft tissue mass in the proximal right forearm. Initial evaluation demonstrates a compressible mass in the medial soft tissues just distal to the elbow joint. What is the best initial study?

This scenario concerns the initial imaging study for a patient with a palpable soft tissue mass.

Sensible recommendation: XR, region of interest

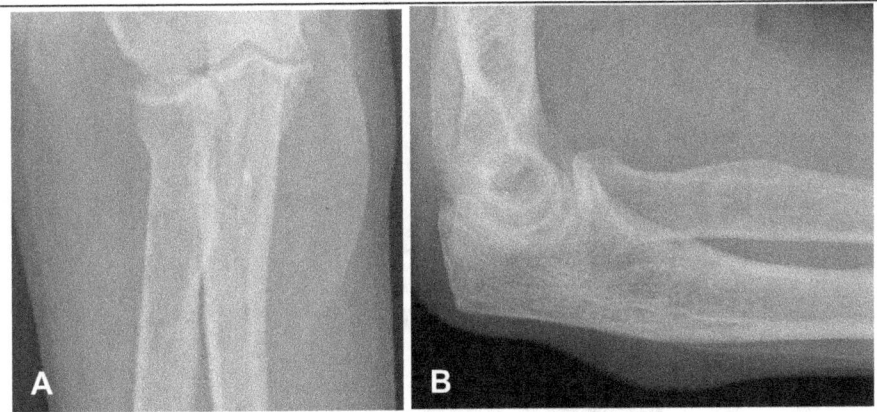

AP (A) and lateral (B) radiographs of the forearm demonstrates a well-demarcated soft tissue mass in the medial soft tissues of the proximal forearm. This finding is consistent with a diagnosis of lipoma, although imaging findings alone are not specific.

In a patient with a soft tissue mass, radiography is the best initial imaging examination as it can often delineate soft tissue masses and is good at excluding osseous complication and involvement. Cross-sectional imaging is not typically appropriate as an initial study unless there is compelling indication. Ultrasound the second line diagnostic exam of choice and can be used if there is a relative contraindication to or if radiographs cannot be performed.

# Case 29-2

A 57-year-old man presents for evaluation of a palpable mass in the right popliteal region. Exam reveals fullness involving the right popliteal fossa without erythema. The patient denies pain and any history of trauma. Distal sensation and pulses are intact. What is the best initial imaging study for this patient?

This scenario concerns the initial imaging evaluation of a patient for a soft tissue mass with non-superficial (deep) or non-specific clinical assessment or located in an area difficult to adequately evaluate with radiographs (flank, paraspinal region, groin, or deep soft tissues of the hands and feet). Initial imaging study.

Sensible recommendation: XR, region of interest

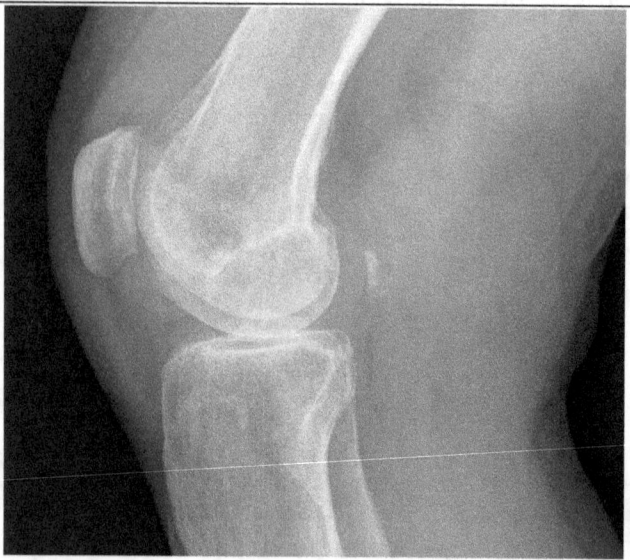

Lateral radiograph of the right knee. In the posterior soft tissues of the knee within the popliteal fossa, there is a well circumscribed soft tissue density. This is nonspecific and differential considerations would include a large popliteal cyst or a lipoma. Further imaging or clinical history is required for further diagnosis.

In a patient with a soft tissue mass with a non-specific clinical assessment, the best initial imaging study is radiography. Radiography is the most cost- and dose-effective initial exam and it may allow detection of a soft tissue mass. Radiography may yield non-specific soft tissue findings, however, it can exclude abnormality involving the underlying bone. If there is an underlying benign osseous lesion, this will often exclude he need additional for additional imaging, cost, and dose to the patient.

## Case 29-3

A 43-year-old man presents for evaluation of right knee discomfort and fullness. Exam reveals mild fullness in the popliteal region without any signs of inflammation. Patient reports a history of recurrent popliteal cysts but otherwise has not pertinent medical conditions. What is the best initial imaging study for this patient?

This scenario concerns the initial imaging evaluation of a patient for a juxta-articular soft tissue mass thought to be a ganglion or cyst.

Sensible recommendation: XR, region of interest

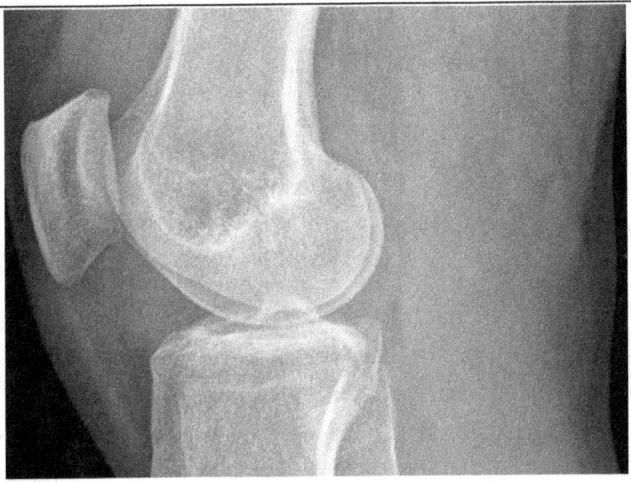

Lateral radiograph of the right knee. In the popliteal soft tissues there is a juxta-articular soft tissue mass, this is nonspecific but in the given clinical history this raises the suspicion for popliteal cyst.

In patients with a juxta-articular, soft tissue mass with clinical suspicion for a ganglion or popliteal cyst, the best initial imaging exam is a radiography of the region interest. Once again, radiography may yield non-specific abnormality involving the soft tissues however it can exclude underlying osseous involvement. MRI may be a useful problem-solving tool and can easily confirm or exclude the presence of a ganglion or popliteal cyst. Ultrasound has sufficient penetration to assess superficial lesions and may also be used but this is a more time-consuming imaging modality and may not provide definitive diagnosis.

## Case 29-4

A 37-year-old woman presents for follow-up imaging for a mass involving her left second digit. Initial radiographs demonstrate nonspecific soft tissue swelling centered about the third proximal interphalangeal joint. Laboratory values are all within normal limits. Patient has no history of malignancy and is otherwise healthy. What is the most appropriate next imaging study?

This scenario concerns the next imaging study of a patient for a soft tissue mass with nondiagnostic initial evaluation (ultrasound and/or radiograph). Next imaging study.

Sensible recommendation: MRI WO/W CONTRAST, region of interest

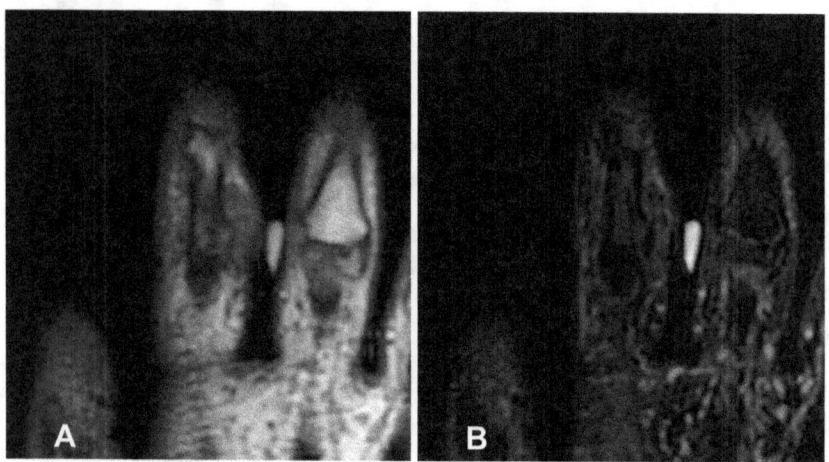

Coronal T1 (A) and STIR MRI (B) of the left hand focused around the area of abnormality. T1-weighted images demonstrate a small mass of intermediate signal intensity. There is no significant fluid signal associated with this mass. This is nonspecific and could represent pigmented villonodular synovitis, giant cell tumor, neuroma, or gout.

In a patient with a soft tissue mass with negative radiographs, the best examination to perform next is MRI of the region of interest. MRI is the best imaging modality for evaluation of the soft tissues. Contrast may be used if there is suspicion of malignancy or infection to assess for vascularity and spread of disease. Ultrasound has sufficient penetration to evaluate superficial soft tissues but findings are often non-specific.

## Case 29-5

67-year-old woman presented to the ER for a painful, palpable mass in her left thigh. Initial radiographs demonstrated a nonspecific density in the posterior soft tissues of the thigh. Patient denies any trauma or history of malignancy. What is the best follow-up imaging examination for this patient? Soft tissue mass. Nondiagnostic initial evaluation (ultrasound and/or radiograph). Next imaging study.

This scenario concerns the next imaging study of a patient presenting with spontaneous hemorrhage, suspicion of vascular mass. Negative radiography.

Sensible recommendation: MRI WO/W CONTRAST, region of interest

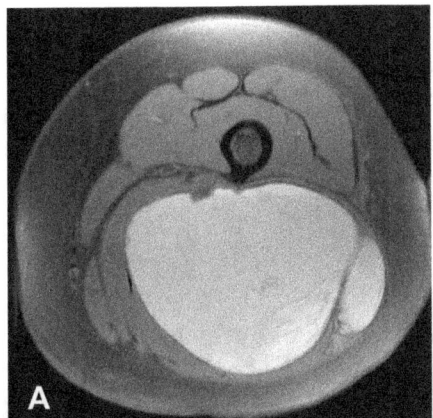
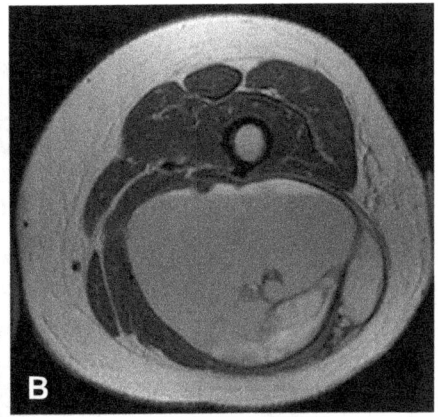
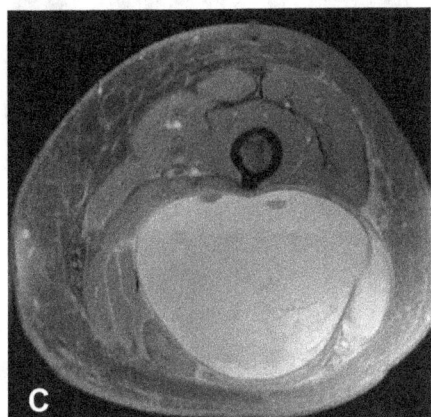

Axial T1 FS (A), T2 (B), and T1 FS Gd MRI (C) through the left thigh. In the posterior thigh, in the region of the hamstrings there is a large collection demonstrating increased signal on T1 and intermediate signal on T2. There is layering within the lesion. Additionally, there is peripheral nodular enhancement. This raises the suspicion for a hemorrhagic collection associated with a malignancy. Biopsy subsequently confirmed this lesion to be dedifferentiated sarcoma.

In patients presenting with a soft tissue mass suspicious for spontaneous hemorrhage or suspicion of vascular mass and negative radiography, MRI wo/w contrast is the next best imaging study. MRI provides superior soft tissue contrast when compared to all other imaging modalities. The addition of contrast can assist in locating and diagnosing suspicious lesions, assessing vascularity, and determining extent of invasion, if present. Ultrasound can be useful for real time evaluation of soft tissue lesions however it provides significantly less information than MRI. CT is the imaging method of choice to evaluate for osseous involvement of disease, however it has inferior soft tissue resolution compared to MRI.

# Case 29-6

A 68-year-old-man presents for follow-up imaging of his left shoulder. Initial imaging demonstrated a calcified mass in the soft tissues anterior to the scapula. Patient reports having long-standing left shoulder pain. Patient denies history of trauma, malignancy, or prior surgery. What is the most appropriate next imaging exam for this patient?

This scenario concerns the next imaging study of a patient for a soft tissue mass with prominent calcifications on radiographs.

Sensible recommendation: MRI WO/W CONTRAST, region of interest

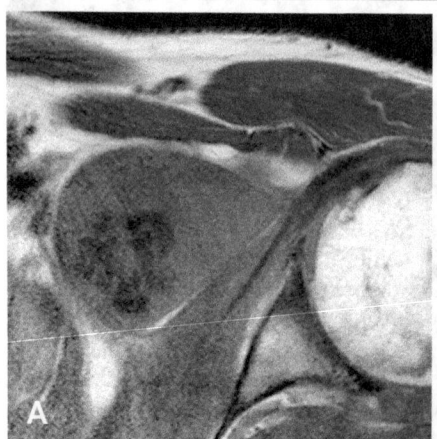
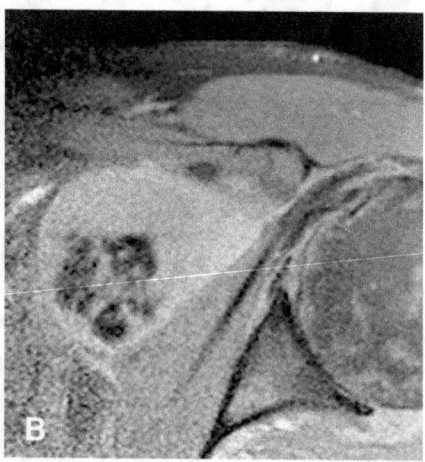

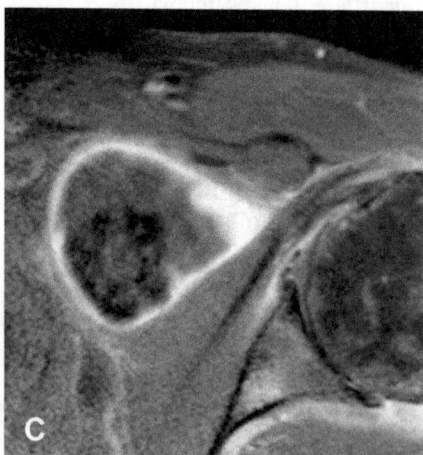

Axial T1 (A), T1 FS(B), and T1 FS Gd MRI (C) of the left shoulder. There is a synovial cyst containing multiple hypointensity foci. There is normal synovial enhancement. These findings are consistent with synovial osteochondromatosis.

In a patient with a soft tissue mass with prominent calcification on radiography, the next best imaging exam is MRI wo/w contrast. MRI is superior in the evaluation of the soft tissues when compared to CT. Contrast should be used in these patients. CT is superior for visualization of mineralization and osseous involvement. Ultrasound may be limited by the lesion's calcifications, which could produce significant shadowing, thus limiting the examination.

## Case 29-7

A 35-year-old man presents with to the ER with acute right thigh pain. Examination demonstrated marked tenderness to palpation of the anterior tissues of the thigh. No palpable mass was noted. Comparison to the contralateral leg demonstrated asymmetric swelling of the right thigh. Initial radiographs did not demonstrate any osseous abnormality. What is the most appropriate imaging exam to perform next?

This scenario concerns the next imaging study for a patient presenting with spontaneous hemorrhage, no palpable mass, and negative radiographs.

Sensible recommendation: MRI WO/W CONTRAST, region of interest

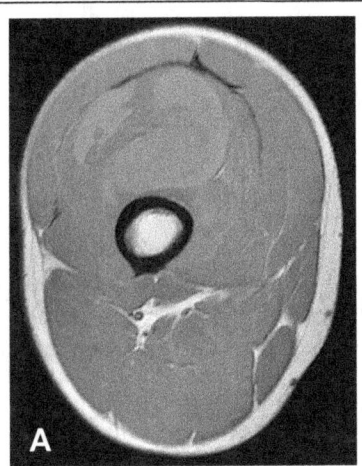 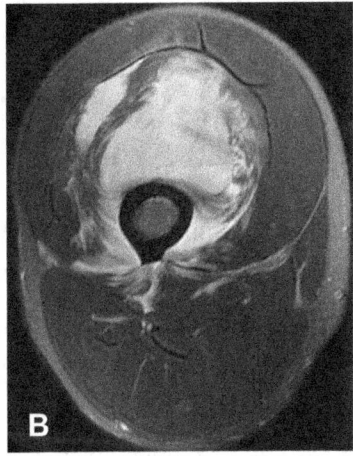

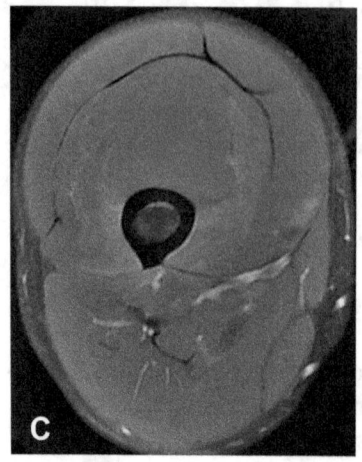

Axial T1 (A), T2 FS (B), and T1 FS Gd MRI (C) through the right mid-thigh. There is abnormal signal involving the vastus intermedius muscle demonstrating iso-intensity on T1-weighted and hyper-intensity on T2-weighted images. There is minimal peripheral enhancement. There is a small amount of abnormal signal on fluid sensitive images in the surrounding soft tissues. These findings are most indicative of an acute, spontaneous hemorrhage in the vastus intermedius muscle.

In patients presenting without a palpable mass suspicious for spontaneous hemorrhage and a negative radiograph, MRI wo/w contrast is the next best imaging study. As previously discussed, MRI provides superior soft tissue contrast when compared to all other imaging modalities. Ultrasound examination would not be particularly useful in the absence of a palpable abnormality. CT is inferior to MRI in evaluation of soft tissues and hemorrhage has a nonspecific appearance on CT.

## Case 29-8

31-year-old man presents with a right posterolateral distal thigh mass. He reports it has been painless. Over the year, the mass has grown significantly in size, but has remained painless. It does not affect running, walking, or any other activities. He denies any weight loss, fevers, chills otherwise. Radiographs of right femur was non-diagnostic. Patient has a non-MRI compatible cardiac pacer. What is the most appropriate next imaging?

This scenario concerns the next imaging study for a patient presenting with a soft tissue mass. Nondiagnostic initial evaluation. Patient non-MRI compatible or with metal limiting MRI evaluation. Next imaging study.

Sensible recommendation: CT WO/W CONTRAST or CT WO CONTRAST, region of interest

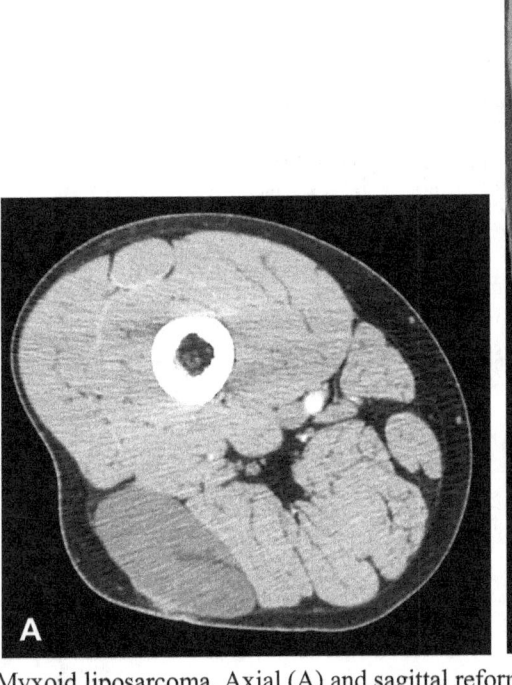

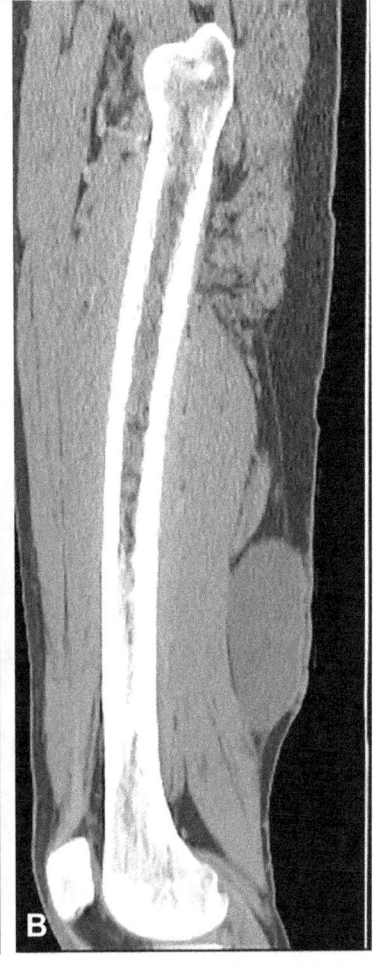

Myxoid liposarcoma. Axial (A) and sagittal reformatted images (B) of CT of right high with IV contrast. There is a well-defined soft tissue mass centered in the sub-cutaneous fat and displaces but does not clearly invade the adjacent biceps femoris muscle. It is predominantly of low attenuation with central areas of lower attenuation and a posterior lateral region of high attenuation. No surrounding fat stranding is present.

CT has become a useful technique for the evaluation of patients who cannot undergo MRI. In the evaluation of suspected tumors, contrast imaging is especially useful in distinguishing vascularized from potentially necrotic regions of the tumor. Pre-contrast imaging is also important to differentiate calcification from vascular enhancement. Dual-energy CT is a relatively new technology that has proved itself as a useful adjunct in evaluation of soft- tissue masses. Using the differences in energy attenuation of soft tissue at 80 kVp and 140 kVp, this technique has proven to be a useful method to evaluate metal implants by generating images acquired by monoenergetic high- energy quanta, reducing metal artifact. Use of this technique can significantly reduce metal artifact in the assessment of metal implants, improving the diagnostic value of imaging.

# References

1. Kransdorf MJ, Murphey MD, Wessell DE, Cassidy RC, Czuczman GJ, Demertzis JL, Lenchik L, Motamedi K, Pierce JL, Sharma A, Walker EA, Ying-Kou Yung E, Beaman FD. ACR Appropriateness Criteria(®) Soft tissue Masses. J Am Coll Radiol. 2018 May;15(5S):S189-S197. doi: 10.1016/j.jacr.2018.03.012. PMID: 29724421.
2. American College of Radiology. ACR Appropriateness Criteria: Soft tissue masses. American College of Radiology, revised 2017. https://acsearch.acr.org/docs/69434/Narrative/ (accessed April 24, 2021).

# Chapter 30: Metastatic Bone Disease

Edward Derrick, MD, Kurt Scherer, MD, Laura Bancroft, MD

The bone scan is the initial exam to screen for metastatic bone disease from a known primary. Any unexplained abnormalities or symptomatic sites should be further evaluated with radiography and sometimes with MRI or CT. PET/CT may be useful for evaluation of metabolic activity.

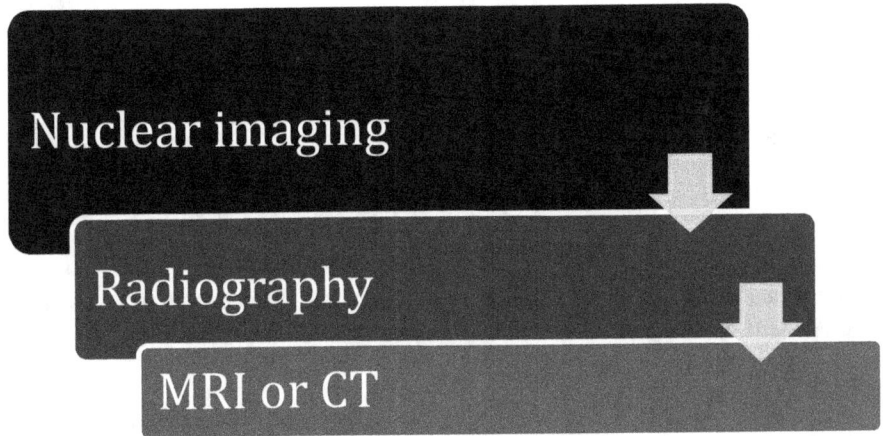

# Case 30-1

A 36-year-old woman with stage 1 breast cancer presents with no current complaints. She states she feels well and denies any history of metastatic disease. What is the most appropriate initial imaging examination for this patient?

This scenario concerns screening for metastatic bone disease in an asymptomatic patient with Stage 1 carcinoma of the breast.

Sensible recommendation:  NO IMAGING

In an asymptomatic patient with stage 1 breast cancer without metastases, there is no clear indication for further imaging. Nuclear studies are unlikely to yield clinically relevant diagnostic information and would expose the patient to radiation.

# Case 30-2

A 36-year-old woman presents for initial evaluation of back and hip pain. Patient has stage 2 breast cancer with no prior imaging comparisons available. Patient has no history of back or hip surgeries. What is the most appropriate first imaging examination for this patient?

This scenario concerns screening for metastatic bone disease in a patient with Stage 2 carcinoma of the breast and complaints of back and hip pain.

Sensible recommendation: Tc-99m BONE SCAN

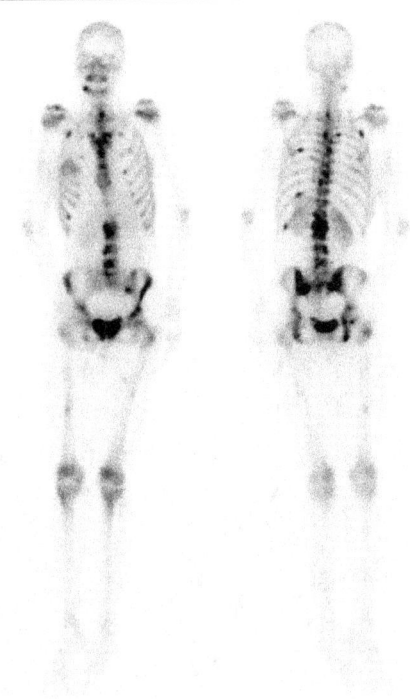

Anterior and posterior views from Tc-99m bone scan. There is multifocal abnormal radiotracer uptake throughout the axial and appendicular skeleton. This is suspicious for diffuse osseous metastases.

In a patient with known stage 2 breast cancer without history of metastatic disease who presents with back and hip pain, the best initial imaging examination is a Tc-99m bone scan. A Tc-99m bone scan is very sensitive in detecting metabolically active lesions which would raise the suspicion for metastatic disease. Radiographs can be obtained after the bone scan to further characterize lesions. In the absence of abnormal uptake and radiographic abnormality, one can generally exclude metastasis with a fairly high degree of confidence. PET/CT may also be used if it will influence systemic therapy.

## Case 30-3

A 35-year-old woman with a history of small cell lung cancer presents with new left hip pain. Radiographs are normal. Bone scan demonstrates increased uptake in the left femoral neck, with differential considerations that include both fracture and metastasis. What study would be most appropriate to help establish a more definitive diagnosis?

This scenario concerns further imaging to distinguish fracture from metastasis in the long bone of a patient with a known primary malignancy. Initial radiographs normal, bone scan hot but nonspecific.

Sensible recommendation: MRI WO/W CONTRAST, region of interest

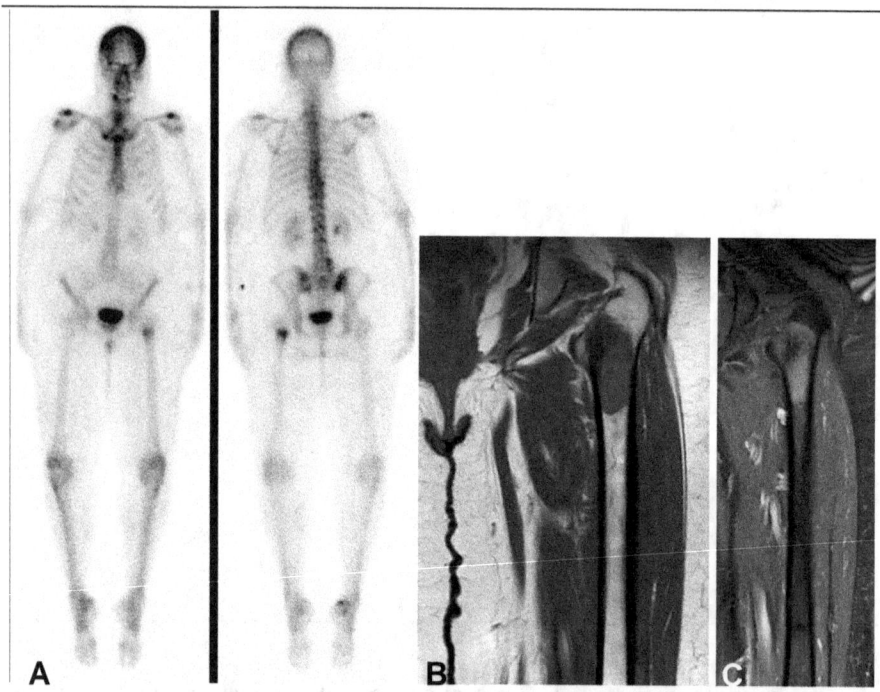

Whole body bone scan (A) demonstrates abnormal activity within the left proximal femur with a differential diagnosis including both stress fracture and metastasis. Coronal T1 MRI (B) demonstrates a hypointense focal lesion within the proximal left femur concerning for metastasis. Contrast was given for further evaluation. Coronal T1 FS Gd MRI (C) shows enhancement within this lesion. The combination of multi-modal findings indicates metastasis.

When the differential diagnosis includes stress fracture versus metastasis in a long bone, and a bone scan is positive but non-specific, and radiographs are non-contributory, MRI of the area of interest is considered most appropriate. Contrast could be administered in those cases where preliminary findings are ambiguous, such as the presence of a soft tissue mass. MRI of the long bone often shows the fracture line itself, making the modality both sensitive and specific.

## Case 30-4

A 60-year-old man with history of prostate cancer and new rising PSA. Bone scan demonstrates multifocal uptake in the skeleton with several foci in the sacrum and pelvis concerning for insufficiency fracture and/or metastases. What modality is considered the most appropriate to help separate these two entities?

This scenario concerns the imaging differentiation of insufficiency fracture from metastasis in sacrum. Initial radiographs normal, bone scan hot but nonspecific.

Sensible recommendation: CT WO CONTRAST, region of interest

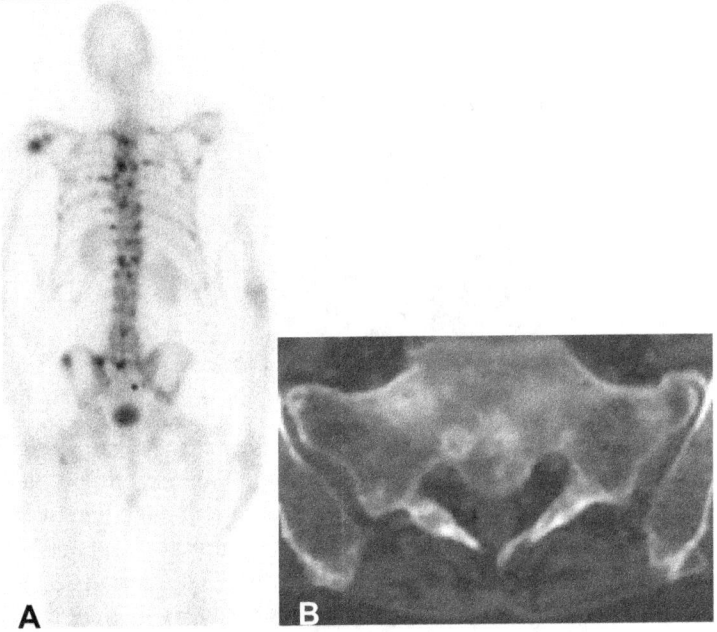

**A**   **B**

Whole body Tc-99m bone scan (A) demonstrates numerous regions of abnormal bone marrow activity, including within the sacrum. Follow-up CT of the sacrum (B) demonstrates multiple sclerotic osseous metastases.

When a normal radiograph and hot, but non-specific bone scan findings result in a differential diagnosis that includes stress fracture and metastasis at the sacrum, CT of the sacrum is considered most appropriate. There are particular sites for which CT is particularly well suited for the diagnosis of stress fracture, such as the sacrum and tarsal navicular. Multiplanar reformatting is recommended to make the diagnosis, demonstrating periosteal reaction, sclerosis, or discrete fracture lines when stress fracture is present. MRI of the sacrum is an alternative choice that may demonstrate other causes for pain.

## Case 30-5

An 83-year-old woman with a history of breast cancer treated several years prior presents for follow-up imaging after a Tc-99m bone scan. Tc-99m bone scan demonstrated a single hot lesion in the sternum. What is the most appropriate imaging examination to perform next?

This scenario concerns the next imaging exam for a patient who has been treated for breast carcinoma but now has a single hot lesion in the sternum on bone scan.

Sensible recommendation: CT WO CONTRAST, region of interest

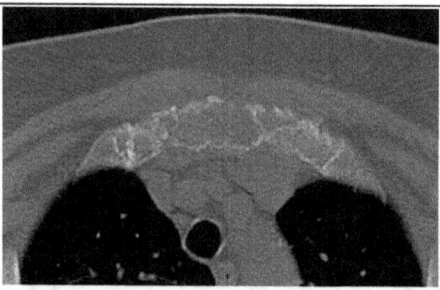

Axial non-contrast CT image through the sternum. There is a lytic lesion involving the sternum with cortical destruction. This is suspicious for metastatic breast cancer.

In a patient with history of treated breast carcinoma presenting with a single hot lesion in the sternum revealed by bone scan, the main concern is metastatic breast cancer to the sternum. The most appropriate imaging examination to perform next is CT of the sternum. The sternum is very difficult to image well using only radiography. CT is favorable over MRI in this scenario given the higher spatial resolution and better visualization of cortical structures on CT. Contrast may be useful to assess soft tissue extension and for biopsy planning. PET/CT may also be used if it will influence systemic therapy.

## Case 30-6

A 65-year-old woman with a history of metastatic breast cancer presents for further imaging after a recent radiograph of the left femur which demonstrated a pathological fracture. What is the most appropriate imaging exam to perform next?

This scenario concerns the next imaging exam for a patient with known metastatic bone disease who presents with a pathological fracture of the femur on radiography.

Sensible recommendation: Tc-99m BONE SCAN

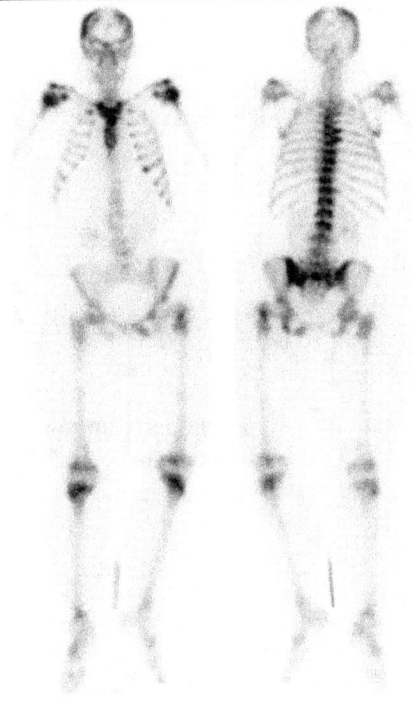

Anterior and posterior views from whole-body Tc-99m bone scan. There is multifocal abnormal radiotracer uptake throughout the axial and appendicular skeleton consistent with metastatic disease. Additionally, there is focal abnormal activity in the left hip. This was confirmed to be a pathologic fracture on radiography.

In a patient with known metastatic disease who is presenting for pathological fracture involving a femur, the most appropriate imaging exam to perform next is a Tc-99m bone scan. MRI or CT wo/w contrast of the region of interest is not likely to contribute significant clinical information. PET/CT may also be used if the Tc-99m bone scan is negative or if the results will influence systemic therapy.

## Case 30-7

An 85-year-old male is found to have a prostatic nodule on exam but is otherwise asymptomatic. Biopsy demonstrated the nodule to be a well differentiated carcinoma. Serum analysis revealed a PSA of 12 mg/ml. What is the best initial imaging examination for this patient?

This scenario concerns an asymptomatic patient with prostate nodule found on physical examination proven to be a well- or moderately differentiated carcinoma and PSA less than 20 mg/ml. Screening for metastatic bone disease.

Sensible recommendation: NO IMAGING

In an asymptomatic patient with a prostate nodule on physical examination which is proven to be a well- or moderately differentiated carcinoma and a PSA less than 20 mg/ml, there is no clear indication for further imaging. This patient is at low risk of metastasis and further imaging is unlikely to affect prognosis and clinical course.

# Case 30-8

An 85-year-old man is found to have a prostatic nodule on exam but is otherwise asymptomatic. Biopsy demonstrated the nodule to be a poorly differentiated carcinoma. Serum analysis revealed a PSA of 78 mg/ml. What is the best initial imaging examination for this patient?

This scenario concerns an asymptomatic patient with prostate nodule found on physical examination proven to be a poorly differentiated carcinoma and PSA of 20 mg/ml or higher. Screening for metastatic bone disease.

Sensible recommendation: Tc-99m BONE SCAN

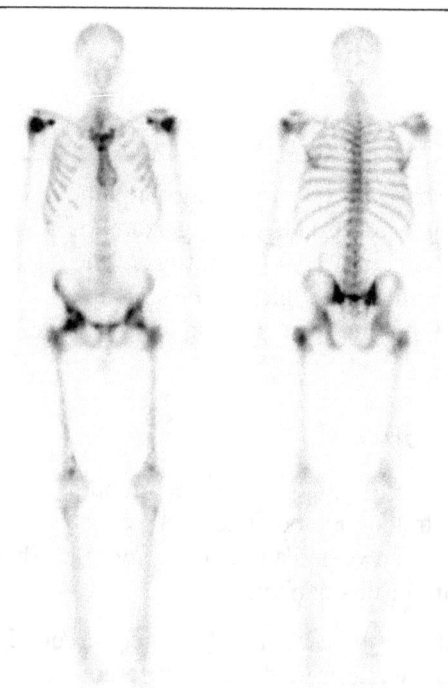

Anterior and posterior whole-body Tc-99m bone scan. There is multifocal abnormal uptake throughout the axial and appendicular skeleton, consistent with diffuse osseous metastasis.

In an asymptomatic patient with a prostate nodule on physical examination which is proven to be a poorly differentiated carcinoma or PSA of 20 mg/ml or higher, Tc-99m bone scan is the best initial imaging exam. This patient is at high risk for metastasis therefore, even in the absence of symptoms, there is clear indication for search for metastases. Prostatic carcinoma has a propensity for metastasizing to osseous structures, therefore a bone scan is a cost and time effective method for initial evaluation.

## Case 30-9

A 74-year-old male with known malignancy presented initially for back pain. History is otherwise non-contributory. Radiographs demonstrated partial collapse of two thoracic vertebrae. What is the most appropriate imaging examination to perform next?

This scenario concerns the next imaging exam for a patient with known malignancy, back pain, and partially collapsed vertebra on radiography.

Sensible recommendation: MRI WO CONTRAST, region of interest

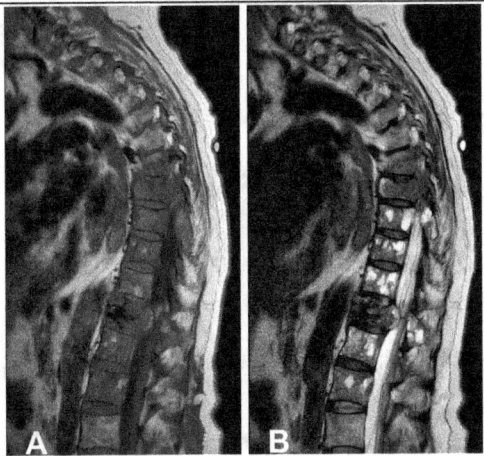

Sagittal T1 (A) and T2 MRI (B) through the thoracic spine. There are compression deformities involving the T3 and T7 vertebral bodies. Additionally, there are multifocal bone marrow signal abnormalities, raising the suspicion for metastasis with pathologic compression fractures. There is marked vertebral retropulsion at the T7 level with resultant compression of the anterior thecal sac and severe central canal stenosis raising the concern for spinal cord injury.

In an otherwise healthy patient with known malignancy who is presenting with back pain and a partially collapsed vertebra on radiography, the most appropriate imaging examination to perform next is MRI thoracic spine. The main concern in this patient would be differentiating between osteoporotic pathologic fracture versus collapse secondary to a destructive lesion, which can be done on non-contrast MRI examination of the spine. Tc-99m bone scan may be helpful in assessing for additional lesions but would provide little additional information of the abnormality in question. PET/CT may also be used if Tc-99m bone scan is negative or if it will influence systemic therapy.

# Case 30-10

A 58-year-old male smoker was found to have a 1 cm lung nodule on CT examination of the chest. Subsequent biopsy demonstrated the lesion to be non-small cell carcinoma. The patient now presents for staging and resection. What is the most appropriate imaging exam?

This scenario concerns a patient with a 1 cm lung nodule proven to be small-cell carcinoma on needle biopsy. Screening for metastatic bone disease.

Sensible recommendation: PET/CT, from skull base to thigh

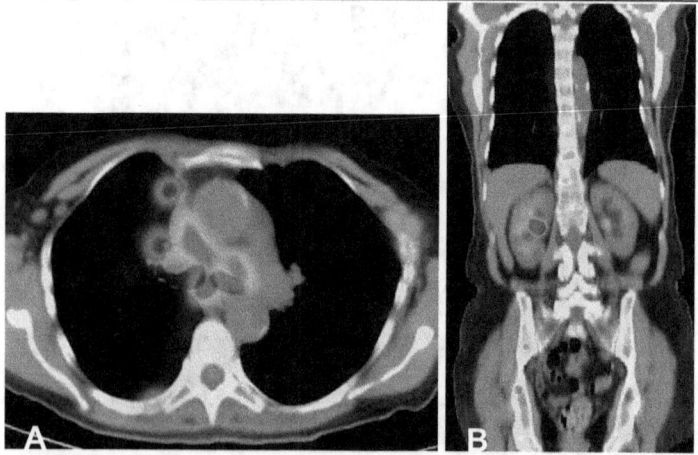

Axial (A) and coronal reformations (B) of a PET/CT examination from the skull base to the thigh. There is focal hypermetabolism associated with a 1-cm lung nodule in the peripheral anterior segment of the right upper lobe. There are also multiple foci of hypermetabolism in the mediastinum and the axial skeleton, including the ribs bilaterally, the thoracic and lumbar spine, and the right iliac and ischial bones, suspicious for metastasis.

In a patient with a 1 cm lung nodule confirmed to be non-small cell carcinoma, the most appropriate staging examination is PET/CT from the skull base to the thigh. PET/CT is an excellent imaging modality for staging of most malignancies. FDG-PET provides superior spatial resolution over most other radionuclide imaging and the CT component provides anatomic correlation that allows for very accurate lesion localization. A bone scan could be performed to assess for osseous metastases in this patient but this is obviated if PET/CT is performed.

## Case 30-11

A 68-year-old woman with history of multiple myeloma presents with lower back pain. Patient denies any radiating pain. Exam does not reveal neurologic symptoms. Radiographic bone survey 5 months prior did not demonstrate any lytic or blastic lesions and no fractures. Surgical history is negative. What is the most appropriate initial exam?

This scenario concerns the appropriate imaging exam for a patient with multiple myeloma who presents with acute low back pain.

Sensible recommendation: XR, region of interest, and MRI WO CONTRAST, region of interest

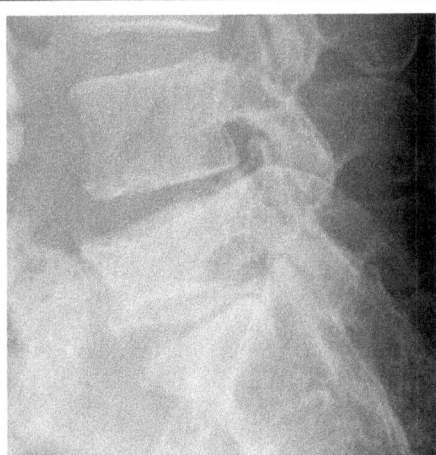

Lateral radiograph of the inferior lumbar spine. There is height loss and deformity involving the L5 vertebral body, consistent with a compression fracture. No lytic lesion is observed.

In a patient with multiple myeloma presenting with acute low back pain, the most appropriate initial imaging examination is radiography of the lumbar spine. This is a cost and dose effective method to assess for structural damage and presence of lesions. MRI is very well suited to differentiate malignant from benign fractures, as discussed previously. Additionally, presence of neurologic symptoms should also prompt MRI examination, however it is seldom the most appropriate study initial study in a patient with focal symptoms. Radiographic skeletal survey is a worthwhile consideration if there has been a long time interval from the prior bone survey.

# Case 30-12

A 15-year-old male with osteosarcoma of the right distal femur presents for staging. CT chest is negative for metastasis. What is the most appropriate imaging exam to perform next?

This scenario concerns a young patient with osteosarcoma of a long bone being imaged for initial staging. Chest CT normal. Screening for metastatic bone disease.

Sensible recommendation: Tc-99m BONE SCAN

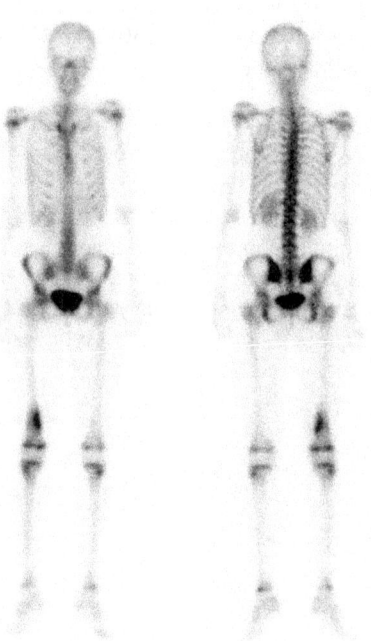

Anterior and posterior Tc-99m bone scan. There is focal increased uptake in the distal right femur consistent with known osteosarcoma. There is no abnormal uptake to suggest metastasis.

In a young patient presenting for staging for osteosarcoma in a patient with a negative CT of the chest, Tc-99m bone scan is the best exam. MRI examination of the primary tumor is indicated in these patients and should be ordered if not already performed. Contrast can be used to evaluate extent and presence of soft tissue involvement and vascularity of the lesion. CT has limited application in staging when imaging the primary tumor. PET/CT scan can be performed if the bone scan is negative or if MRI examination of the primary and the adjacent tissues is equivocal.

## Case 30-13

A 17-year-old male with history of osteosarcoma of the right femur status post resection and chemotherapy presents for six-month follow-up after completion of treatment. Patient denies any symptoms. What is the most appropriate imaging exam?

This scenario concerns surveillance for metastatic bone disease in an asymptomatic patient treated for an osteosarcoma (resected clear margins, chemotherapy). Six-month follow-up after completion of treatment.

Sensible recommendation: Tc-99m BONE SCAN

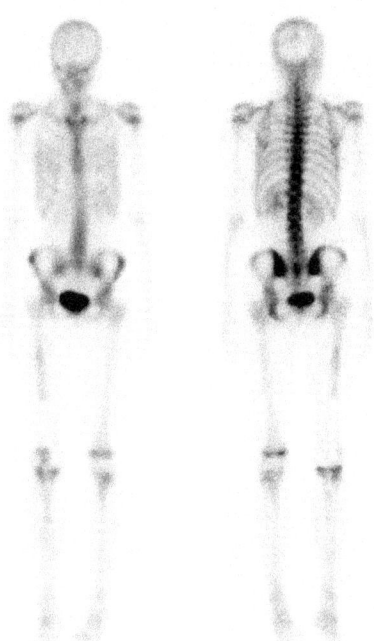

Anterior and posterior Tc-99m bone scan. There is focal photopenia in the distal right femur consistent with prior resection. In the proximal diaphysis of the femur, there is mild increased radiotracer uptake, this is likely related to stress changes. There is no abnormal uptake suspicious for metastasis.

In an asymptomatic patient with osteosarcoma status post resection with clear margins, and chemotherapy who is presenting for six-month follow-up after treatment to exclude bone metastases, the most appropriate study to perform is Tc-99m bone scan. In the absence of clinical suspicion for recurrence, CT and MRI of the region of interest provide little utility. To assess for local recurrence, radiography is the preferred initial imaging exam.

# Case 30-14

A 46-year-old pregnant woman patient with known breast cancer presents for left hip pain. She is currently 8 weeks pregnant and wants to continue the pregnancy. What is the most appropriate exam?

This scenario concerns the appropriate imaging for a pregnant patient (8 weeks) with known primary cancer, now suspected of having bone metastasis. She wants to continue with the pregnancy.

Sensible recommendation: XR, region of interest

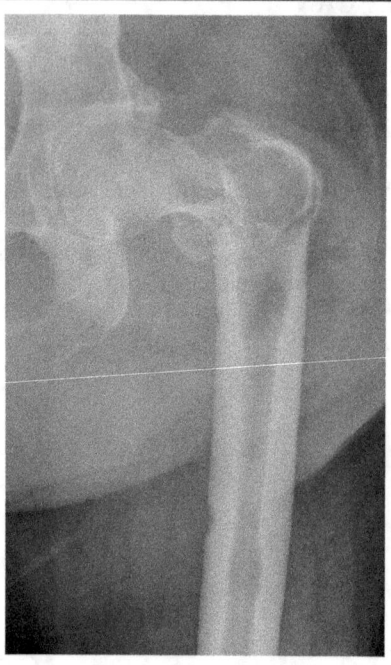

AP radiograph of the left hip. There are multiple lytic osseous metastases in this patient. There is an acute, displaced intertrochanteric fracture of the left proximal femur suspicious for a pathologic fracture.

In a pregnant patient with known primary malignancy and suspected metastasis, the best option is radiography of the area of interest. Ideally, MRI whole body could be performed but this technique is not common practice. Radiography generally has a low dose however fetal dosing remains a concern therefore measures should be taken to minimize dose via shielding. If the abnormality involved the extremity, CT can be performed with proper shielding.

# References

1.  Roberts CC, Daffner RH, Weissman BN, Bancroft L, Bennett DL, Blebea JS, Bruno MA, Fries IB, Germano IM, Holly L, Jacobson JA, Luchs JS, Morrison WB, Olson JJ, Payne WK, Resnik CS, Schweitzer ME, Seeger LL, Taljanovic M, Wise JN, Lutz ST. ACR appropriateness criteria on metastatic bone disease. J Am Coll Radiol. 2010 Jun;7(6):400-9. doi: 10.1016/j.jacr.2010.02.015. Erratum in: J Am Coll Radiol. 2010 Sep;7(9):e1. PMID: 20522392.

# Chapter 31. Suspected Infection

Lindsay Stratchko, DO, Eric Walker, MD, Jonelle Petscavage-Thomas, MD, Hyojeong Lee, MD, Felix S. Chew, MD

Radiography is the initial exam for suspected infection of any musculoskeletal site, followed by MRI or CT. Consider nuclear imaging if further evaluation is needed. Biopsy or aspiration may be necessary.

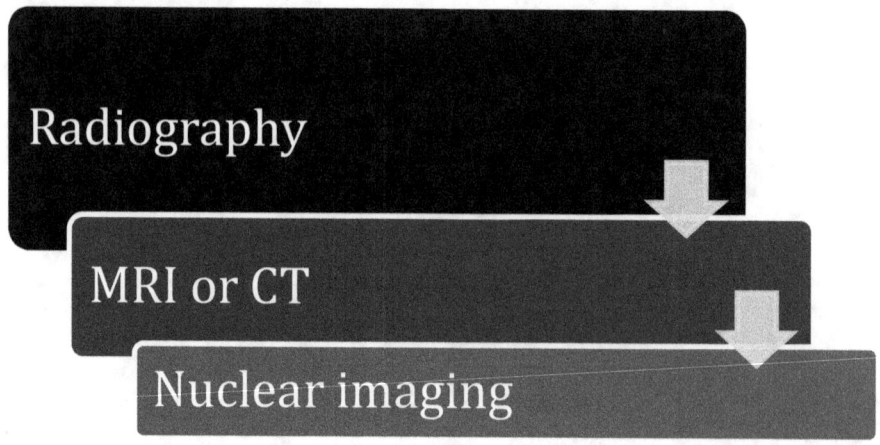

# Case 31-1

A 51-year-old diabetic male presents for further evaluation of right foot swelling that has worsened over the past 10 days. He has a known history of Charcot arthropathy and a navicular fracture of his right foot. The patient states he otherwise feels well. On examination, the patient is found to have decreased sensation in his right foot with abnormal monofilament test. He has plantar soft tissue swelling and deformity of his right foot, but no ulcers were identified. What is the most appropriate first imaging study?

This scenario concerns the first imaging of a diabetic patient with suspected osteomyelitis.

Sensible recommendation: XR, region of interest

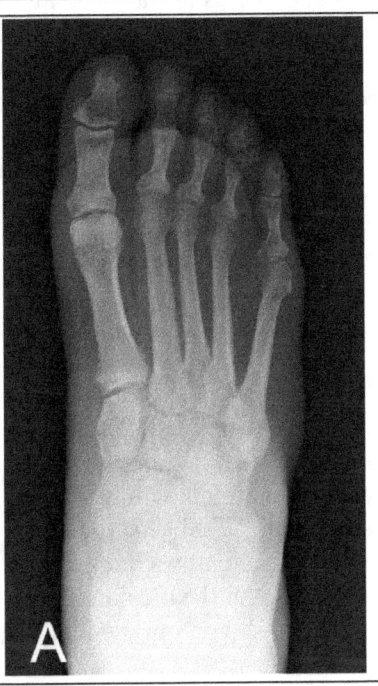

AP (A) and Lateral (B) left foot radiographs demonstrate findings of neuropathic change with dense bones, degeneration, destruction of the navicular, deformity, debris, and dislocation of the midfoot.

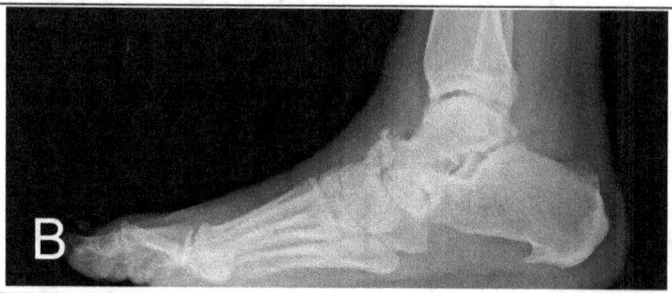

Neuropathic arthropathy (Charcot joint) results from the effects of long-standing diabetic neuropathy and microvascular change. The incidence of osteomyelitis in the neuropathic foot without an ulcer is low, but radiographs and MRI are indicated as complimentary studies to further evaluate for sources of infection (soft tissue infection, osteomyelitis, or septic joint). Radiographs are useful as the initial screening examination. They evaluate anatomic detail and previous surgeries and are useful to evaluate for other causes of pain, such as radiopaque foreign body, soft tissue gas, fracture, degenerative changes, neuropathic arthropathy, or tumor. Early bony changes of osseous infection include periosteal reaction, lytic bone destruction, endosteal scalloping, osteopenia, loss of trabecular architecture, and new bone apposition. Radiographs are insensitive in the detection of early stages of acute osteomyelitis. Soft tissue swelling and obscuration of the fat planes will precede osseous changes. Osseous changes may take 10 to 12 days to develop in adults.

## Case 31-2

72-year-old woman presents to the emergency department with left posterior elbow pain, swelling, and erythema. Her symptoms have been worsening over the past 3 days and she has developed fever and chills. On examination, there is edema, warmth, erythema and fluctuance over the olecranon process. Range of motion is preserved. What is the most appropriate imaging study to order once radiographs are obtained?

This scenario concerns evaluation of patients with soft tissue or juxta-articular swelling. Suspected soft tissue infection. Additional imaging following radiographs.

Sensible recommendation: MRI WO/W CONTRAST, region of interest

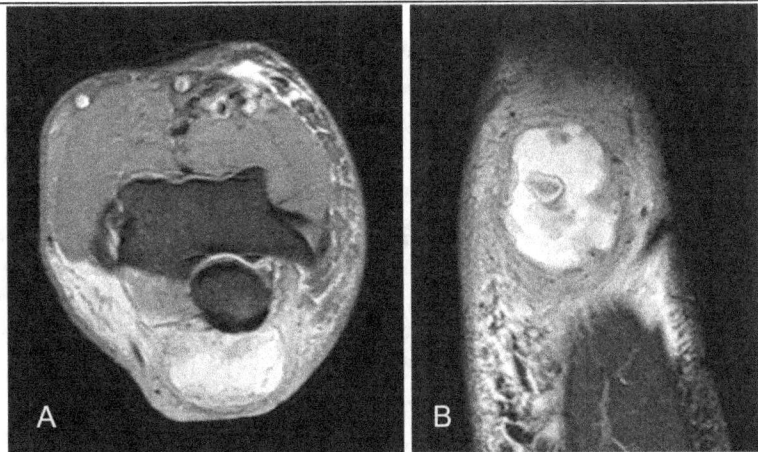

Axial (A) and coronal (B) T2 FS MRI at the level of the olecranon process reveals a complex collection at the olecranon bursa with significant adjacent inflammation and edema. This patient underwent arthrocentesis and subsequent irrigation and debridement of her septic olecranon bursitis with cultures positive for staphylococcus aureus.

Once radiographs are obtained, MRI is the most appropriate imaging study to further evaluate inflammatory arthritis or bursitis. MRI can determine complexity of effusion, degree of synovitis and can identify osseous erosions. Intravenous contrast aids in detecting active synovial inflammation and is the preferred imaging protocol. There are several bursae about the elbow that may become inflamed and contribute to chronic pain. These bursae are readily evaluated with MRI but may also be assessed with ultrasound. Tc-99m bone scan can show increased radiotracer uptake in inflammatory arthritis; however, the finding is non-specific and accurate localization is difficult secondary to poor spatial resolution.

# Case 31-3

41-year-old man presents with acute pain, erythema and swelling of his right elbow. He was recently discharged from hospital that he was admitted for his right lower leg infection. He has type II diabetes, and history of intravenous drug use. He reports that he had intravenous catheter on his right antecubital fossa while he was in hospital. Radiographs of his elbow were negative. The clinician is concerned about a foreign body. What imaging should be ordered next?

This scenario concerns the next appropriate imaging study for a patient with soft tissue or juxta-articular swelling with a history of puncture wound. Suspected foreign body. Negative radiographs.

Sensible recommendation: US, region of interest

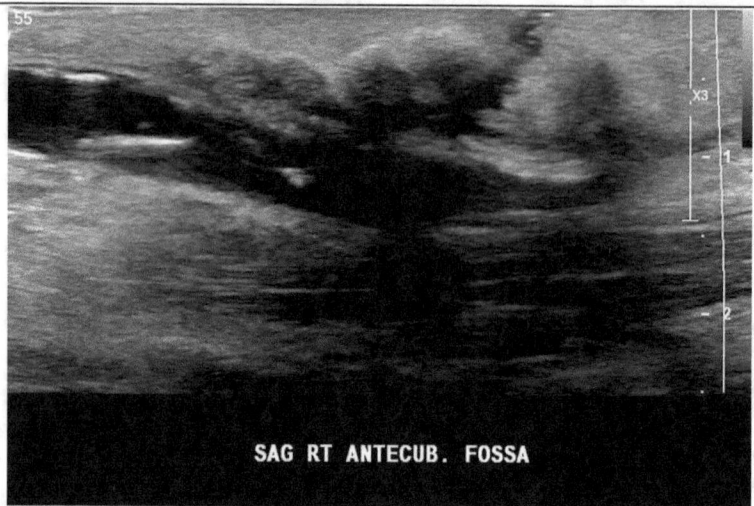

SAG RT ANTECUB. FOSSA

US of right antecubital fossa, longitudinal image shows linear echogenic material in the antecubital vein, that was broken catheter tip. There is low echoic area along the superficial fat in keeping with a phlegmon.

In patients with a puncture wound, any imaging evaluation should determine presence or absence of a retained foreign body. Such retained material in the soft tissue triggers a granulomatous reaction, and subsequently a soft- tissue infection can develop. Radiographs are indicated for initial imaging, especially if the composition of the material is unknown, and are well suited in the detection of radiodense foreign bodies such as metal, graphite, and stone. Glass is inconsistently visible radiographically, particularly if fragments are small or obscured by adjacent osseous structures. Optimal imaging for radiolucent (eg, plastic or wood) material is US. Both US and CT allow for precise foreign body localization. CT is favored over MRI for identification of foreign bodies, being well suited for detection of radiodense bodies and wood.

# Case 31-4

A 19-year-old man with hand pain and swelling that has become progressively worse since "punching a wall" with his closed fist 5 days ago. Initial radiographs show a fifth metacarpal neck fracture with soft tissue swelling and skin lacerations. What imaging study should be performed to establish the diagnosis of infection?

This scenario concerns a patient with soft tissue or juxta-articular swelling with cellulitis and a skin lesion, injury, wound, ulcer, or blister. Suspected osteomyelitis. Additional imaging following radiographs.

Sensible recommendation: MRI WO/W CONTRAST, region of interest

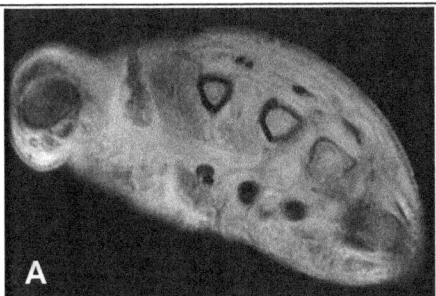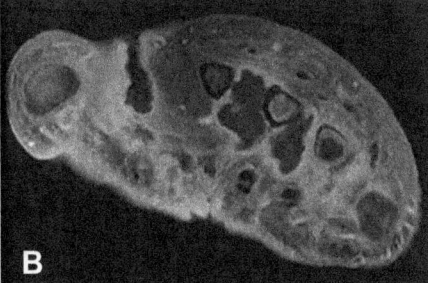

Axial T2 MRI (A) and T1 FS Gd MRI (B) through the metacarpal shafts show diffuse edema, abscess formation, and the first web space soft tissue wound.

If infection is suspected, MRI wo/w contrast may be obtained. If MRI is not available, CT w/ contrast may be obtained. If nuclear imaging is desired, an In-111 leukocyte scan would be a better choice than a Tc-99m bone scan because of the presence of the fracture.

# Case 31-5

56-year-old woman presents with left knee pain and swelling for two weeks. She first noted general redness with increased redness and heat over time. She had left femur fracture about 7 years ago, had metal rod, screws and plate placement. With regards to her ulcers on her knee, she says they heal on and off and get them frequently. Radiographs of left knee show dislodgement of interlocking screws with suspected soft tissue lesion. What is the most appropriate next imaging study?

This scenario concerns a patient presents with soft tissue or juxta-articular swelling with a history of prior surgery. Suspected osteomyelitis or septic arthritis. Additional imaging following radiographs.

Sensible recommendation: MRI WO/W CONTRAST, region of interest

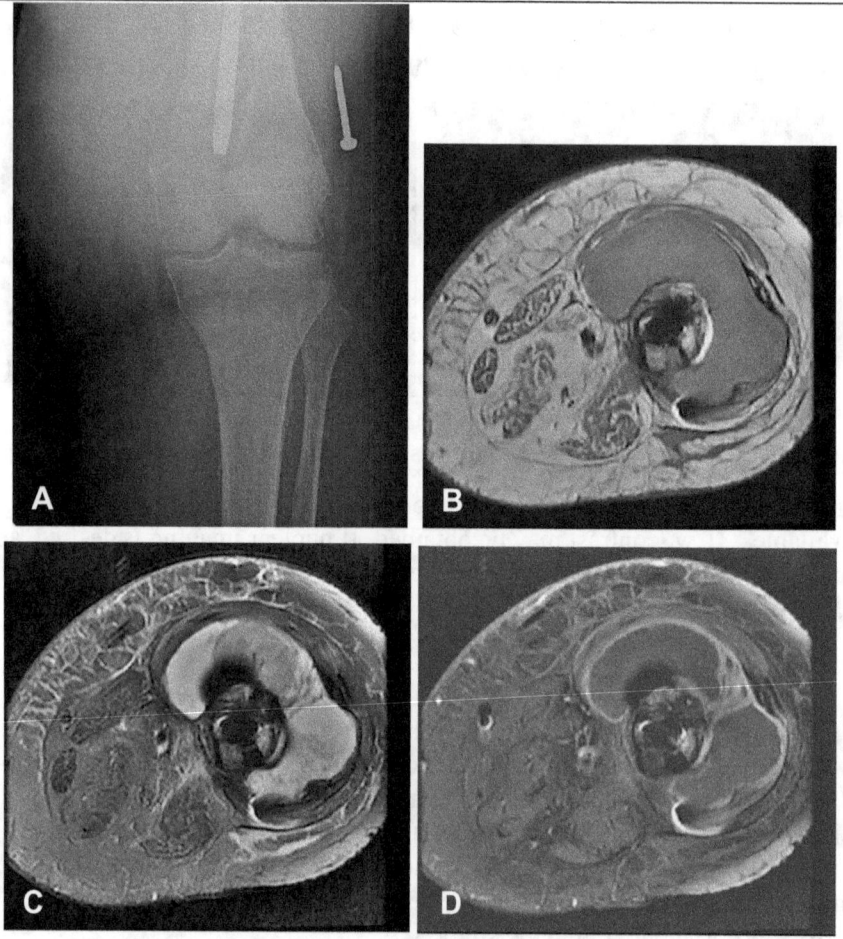

Frontal radiograph of left knee shows a dislodged distal interlocking screw of femoral intramedullary nail. There is perihardware lucency about the distal stem of the rod. There is soft tissue swelling about the medial distal thigh. Axial images of distal femur with T1 (A), STIR (B), and post-contrast T1 FS (D) images demonstrate multiloculated fluid collection with rim enhancement surrounds the distal femur, encircling approximately 270 degrees anterolaterally (confined by the anterior muscle compartment). There is increased STIR signal with enhancement and a periosteal reaction in the distal femur suggesting osteomyelitis.

Radiographs reveal information about hardware and bone fractures, such as evidence of hardware loosening or fracture, degree of bone fracture healing or nonunion, and presence of heterotopic ossification. Chronic osteomyelitis occurs if residual infection is inadequately treated or refractory to therapy and can result from continuous infection or reactivation. Radiographs depict bone sclerosis and areas of destruction. Although complementary, radiography should not be the sole or primary imaging modality. Although MRI is exceptional in the detection of acute osteomyelitis, detecting acute osseous changes in the setting of chronic post-traumatic osteomyelitis is challenging in the setting of bone altered by prior trauma or surgery. Marrow signal heterogeneity following trauma or surgery limits detection of superimposed infection, as reparative fibrovascular scar tissue in the bone marrow and soft tissues can persist following surgical intervention, mimicking infection. Both CT and MRI are susceptible to hardware artifact, although technological advances with the development of artifact-reducing protocols mitigate this shortcoming.

## Case 31-6

A 73-year-old man presents with a swollen, painful knee. He has been receiving treatment for multifocal methicillin-resistant staphylococcal infections elsewhere in his body. The obvious concern is for infection. Radiography of the knee shows a large joint effusion, but no other pathology. What imaging exam should be ordered next?

This scenario concerns the next appropriate imaging study for a patient with soft tissue or juxta-articular swelling. Suspected osteomyelitis or septic arthritis. Additional imaging following radiographs.

Sensible recommendation: MRI WO/W CONTRAST, region of interest, and JOINT ASPIRATION, region of interest

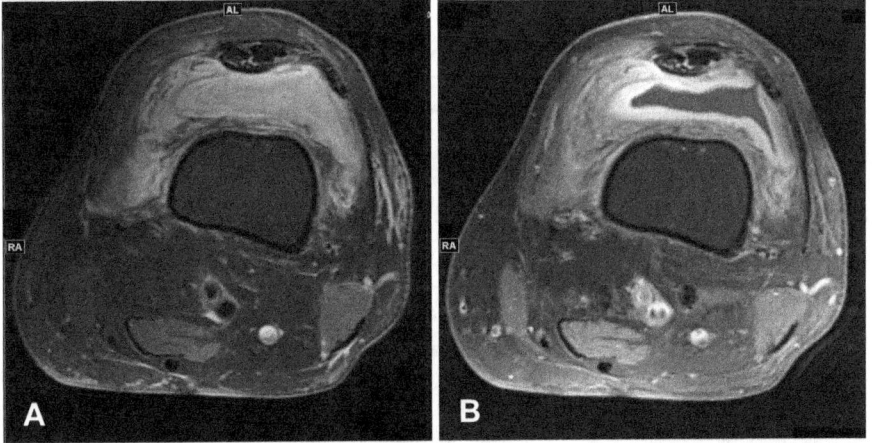

Septic knee without osteomyelitis. Axial T2 MRI (A) and axial T1 FS Gd MRI (B) show a large, complex knee effusion with synovitis and surrounding cellulitis. There was no intramedullary abnormality to suggest concurrent osteomyelitis.

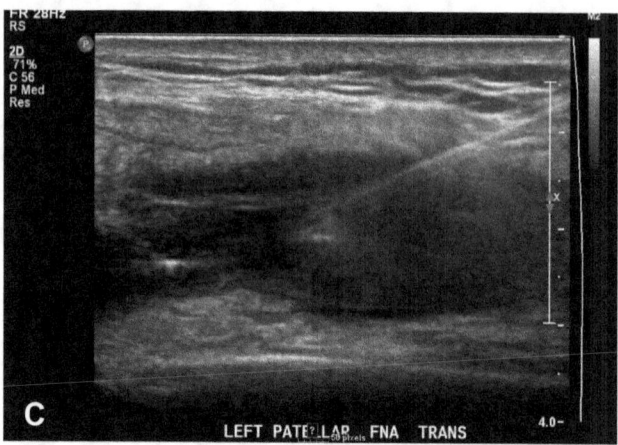

US knee transverse at the level of the suprapatellar recess (C) shows a large compled joint effusion. Arthrocentesis produced 3 ml of grossly purulent fluid. Cultures were positive for Staphylococcus.

In the adult patient with suspected septic arthritis, the final diagnosis often requires culture of aspirated joint fluid. Imaging has a role in identifying the presence of joint fluid, if it is not evident on physical exam, and in identifying accompanying cellulitis, myositis, soft tissue abscess, or osteomyelitis. MRI wo/w contrast is more sensitive and specific than CT for the diagnosis of acute osteomyelitis.

# Case 31-7

A 27-year-old man presents for evaluation of ischial decubitus ulcers. The patient has paraplegia from a spinal cord injury sustained several years ago. He has a draining sinus into the decubitus ulcer. Radiographs of pelvis demonstrate sclerosis and periostitis of right ischial tuberosity suspected chronic osteomyelitis. Patient has a non-MRI compatible cardiac pacer. What imaging exam should be ordered next?

This scenario concerns a patient with a draining sinus (not associated with a joint prosthesis). Suspected osteomyelitis. Additional imaging following radiographs.

Sensible recommendation: CT W CONTRAST, region of interest

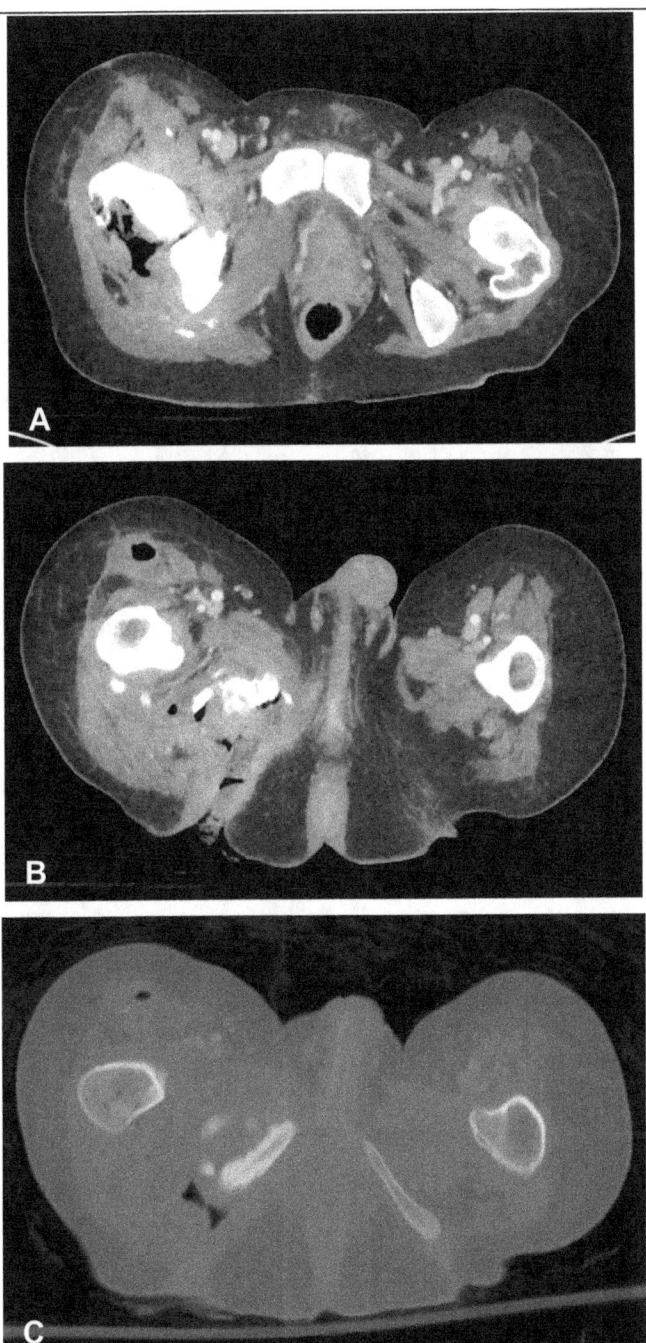

Consecutive CT axial images of pelvis with intravenous contrast (A, B, and C from top to bottom) demonstrate decubitus ulcers with underlying chronic osteomyelitis.

A draining sinus should prompt a high clinical suspicion for chronic infection. While a well-described complication of chronic osteomyelitis, sinuses also can be secondary to abscess formation from a retained foreign body. Persistent bone infection results in continuous infection of the overlying soft tissue, with consequent formation of a sinus tract to allow pus drainage through the skin. Initial imaging typically includes radiographs of the affected bone or joint. Both MRI and CT are sensitive in the diagnosis of chronic osteomyelitis, revealing cortical thickening, cortical destruction, and soft tissue involvement. CT will show effusions and soft tissue fluid collections, with depiction of bone erosions more striking than on radiographs. MRI is superior in delineating the extent of involved versus uninvolved bone marrow, as well as intraosseous abscess. CT better depicts sequestrum, cloaca, and osseous erosion.

# Case 31-8

A 62-year-old man presents with gangrene of the left foot. On physical exam demonstrates soft tissue crepitus. The clinician is concerned about necrotizing soft tissue infection. What is the most appropriate initial exam?

This scenario concerns about necrotizing soft tissue infection. Clinical examination suggesting crepitus. Suspected soft tissue gas. First study.

Sensible recommendation: XR, region of interest

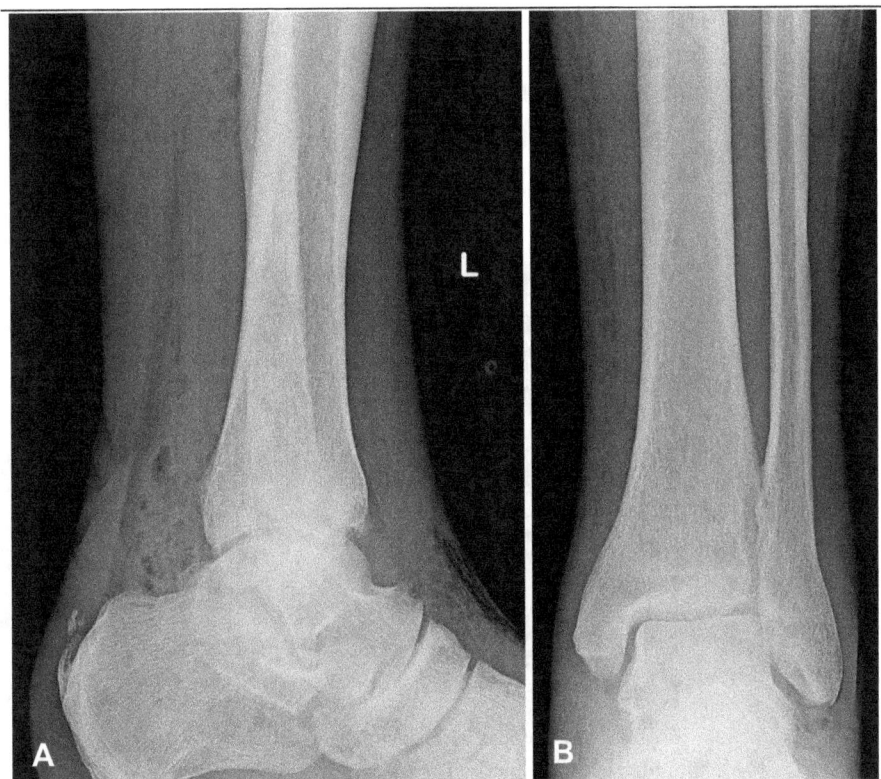

Necrotizing soft tissue infection. (A) lateral radiograph and (B) AP radiograph of the ankle show small collections of soft tissue gas extending from the foot into the ankle and lower leg.

Articular crepitus—joint grating or popping—most commonly is associated with arthritis. Conversely, extremity soft tissue crepitus could represent soft tissue gas, so a history of recent surgical intervention, trauma (subcutaneous emphysema), or puncture wound should be sought. Necrotizing fasciitis is rapidly progressive, can be life-threatening, and when suspected should be treated with surgical debridement. Radiographs are well suited for the detection of soft tissue gas in the extremities or juxta-articular tissues but are limited in evaluation of deep fascial gas. CT is the most sensitive means of detection of soft tissue gas and can delineate extent and compartmental location.

## Case 31-9

44-year-old man presents with a left arm swelling and abscess. He reports that he has had the abscess for at least two months, and it has increasing in size. He has had recent fevers and chills and the site of his abscess has been very painful. He denies any history of injury. Radiographs of left shoulder demonstrate soft tissue gas around his left shoulder. What is the most appropriate next imaging study?

This scenario concerns about necrotizing soft tissue infection. Initial radiographs showing soft tissue gas in absence of puncture wound.

Sensible recommendation: CT W CONTRAST, region of interest

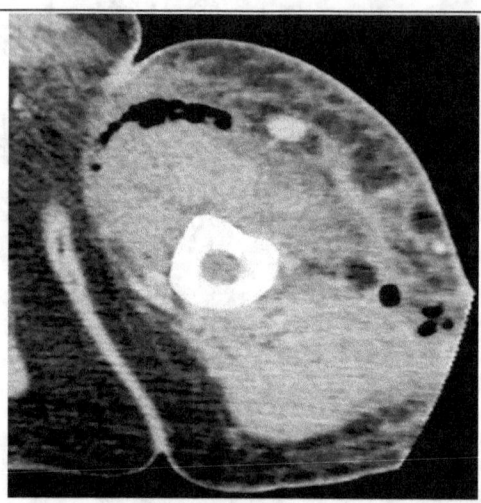

Axial CT of left shoulder was obtained with IV contrast. There is soft tissue gas along the superficial and intermuscular deep fascia. Also, there is fluid along the deep fascia associated with less enhancement of the flexor muscles suggestive ov necrotizing soft tissue infection.

In the absence of recent surgery, trauma, or puncture wound, soft tissue gas is a reliable indication of infection. Gas in the deep fascial planes is a hallmark of necrotizing fasciitis and can be diagnosed radiographically. However, this infection can be difficult to diagnose early or when soft tissue gas is not present; thus, cross-sectional imaging can play a vital role in early recognition. Fascial thickening, fluid collections along the deep fascial planes, and intermuscular septal edema are MRI and CT features of deep fascial inflammation. Postcontrast imaging is favored, as lack of enhancement confirms tissue necrosis, distinguishing necrotizing from non-necrotizing fasciitis. CT remains the most sensitive modality for identification of soft tissue gas and is preferred in some situations due to rapid acquisition.

# Case 31-10

A 62-year-old woman presents to the Emergency Department with left foot pain and swelling for the past week. The patient denies trauma to her foot and is otherwise in her usual state of health. Her past medical history includes hypertension, hyperlipidemia and type II diabetes (last hemoglobin A1C of 9.1 mg/dL). On examination, she has mild soft tissue swelling of the plantar aspect of her left forefoot without identifiable ulcer. Radiographs do not demonstrate underlying osseous change. What is the most appropriate next imaging examination?

This scenario concerns the imaging of a diabetic patient with soft tissue swelling of the foot without ulcer. Suspected osteomyelitis or early neuropathic arthropathy changes of the foot. Additional imaging following radiographs.

Sensible recommendation: MRI WO/W CONTRAST, region of interest

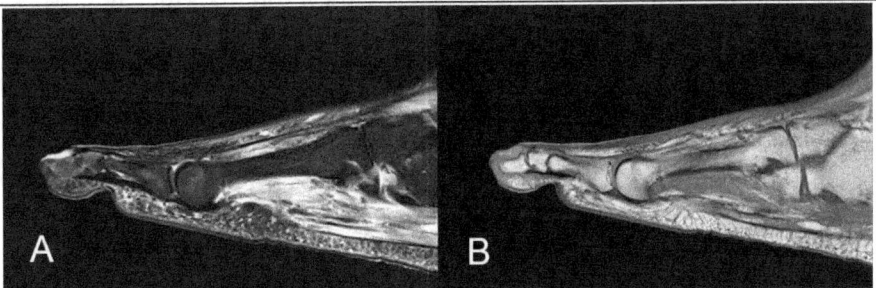

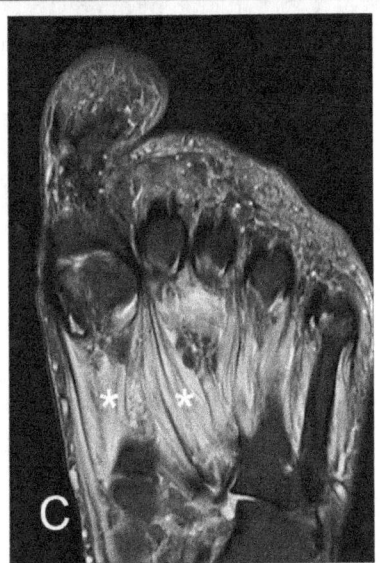

Sagittal STIR MRI (A) and T1 MRI (B) at the level of the second metatarsal demonstrate mild edema within the plantar soft tissues of the forefoot consistent with cellulitis. No identifiable ulcer or fluid collection to suggest abscess. There is normal high T1 marrow signal throughout the second digit, excluding osteomyelitis by established criteria. There is diffusely increased STIR signal within the intrinsic muscles (asterisks) of the foot correlating with denervation change, which is a common finding in diabetic patients. These muscle findings are well-depicted on the long axis STIR image (C).

Osteomyelitis is the principal concern in diabetic patients presenting with foot swelling and an abnormal physical examination. In the absence of a soft tissue ulcer, the likelihood of osteomyelitis is extremely low; however, imaging is often indicated to identify the rare cases of osteomyelitis as well as to define the extent of soft tissue infection and diagnose neuropathic arthropathy. Radiographs are the most appropriate initial imaging study, but radiographs are insensitive in the early stages of infection. MRI is the most appropriate complimentary examination to radiographs.

## Case 31-11

A 42-year-old poorly controlled type I diabetic presents to his primary care provider for evaluation of an ulcer along the plantar aspect of his left first metatarsophalangeal joint. On examination, the ulcer extends to the bone with associated mild purulent drainage. The surrounding soft tissues are edematous and erythematous. Radiographs show a soft tissue defect involving the plantar aspect of the left first MTP with underlying destructive changes of the first metatarsal head. What is the most appropriate imaging study to order to further delineate the degree and extent of infection?

This scenario concerns the imaging of a diabetic patient with soft tissue swelling of the foot and associated ulcer. Suspected osteomyelitis of the foot with or without neuropathic arthropathy. Additional imaging following radiographs.

Sensible recommendation: MRI WO/W CONTRAST, region of interest

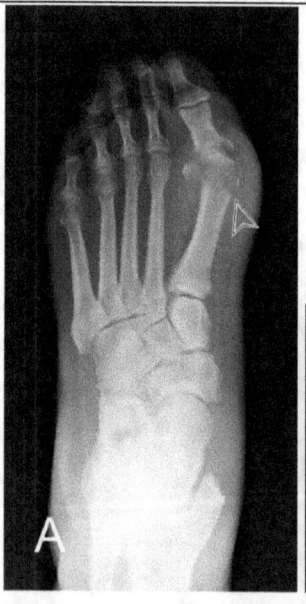
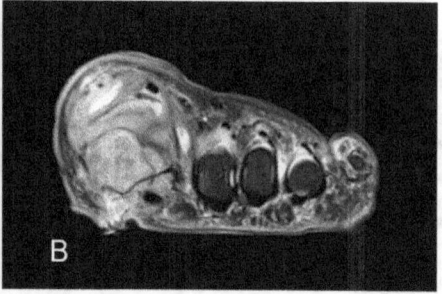

AP left foot radiograph (A) demonstrates marked soft tissue swelling centered at the first metatarsophalangeal joint with focal osteopenia and lytic destructive changes at the first metatarsal head (arrowhead).

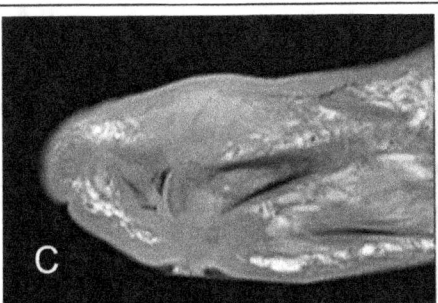
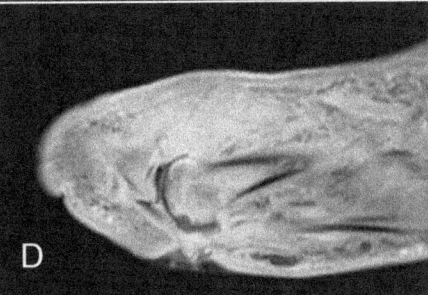

Axial T2 FS MRI (B) and sagittal T1 MRI (C) reveal an ulcer along the plantar aspect of the first metatarsal head with diffuse edema within the soft tissues extending to the level of the bone. Note the abnormal low T1 marrow signal within the distal first metatarsal and first proximal phalanx. There is marked enhancement within the marrow and soft tissues on sagittal T1 FS Gd MRI (D). Findings are consistent with osteomyelitis. Scrolling through the forefoot images will allow evaluation of the extent of forefoot involvement.

The likelihood of osteomyelitis in the diabetic patient presenting with foot swelling and ulcer is high, particularly if the ulcer extends to bone. MRI compliments radiographs by confirming the presence of osteomyelitis and detailing the extent of infection. Intravenous contrast plays a helpful role not only in identifying osteomyelitis, but also in recognizing potential complications (i.e. abscess, devitalized/ischemic tissue). Impaired renal function is not uncommon in this patient population and intravenous contrast may be omitted in the setting of low glomerular filtration rate to avoid the rare but potentially fatal complication of nephrogenic systemic fibrosis (NSF) associated with gadolinium-based contrast. When MRI is contraindicated, nuclear medicine labeled leukocyte scan is helpful in excluding osteomyelitis when negative; however, results are non-specific if positive.

# Case 31-12

A 43-year-old diabetic male presents to the clinic for evaluation of the left foot with purulent drainage from skin ulcer. When questioned, the patient stated he does not routinely check his blood glucose levels, but when he remembers to check, his levels are typically in the high 200's mg/dL when fasting. He is currently maintained on oral agents. On examination, there is soft tissue swelling and deformity of the patient's left foot. A 2 x 2 cm ulcer is noted along the lateral plantar aspect of the patient's midfoot.

Radiographs show findings of neuropathic (Charcot) arthropathy involving the left midfoot and hindfoot. What is the most appropriate next imaging examination to order?

This scenario concerns the imaging of a diabetic patient with soft tissue swelling of the foot and associated ulcer. Suspected osteomyelitis of the foot with or without neuropathic arthropathy. Additional imaging following radiographs.

Sensible recommendation: MRI WO/W CONTRAST, region of interest

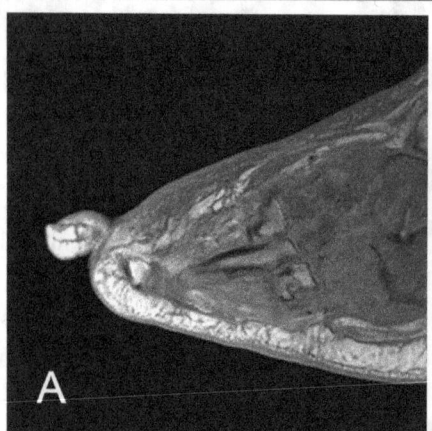
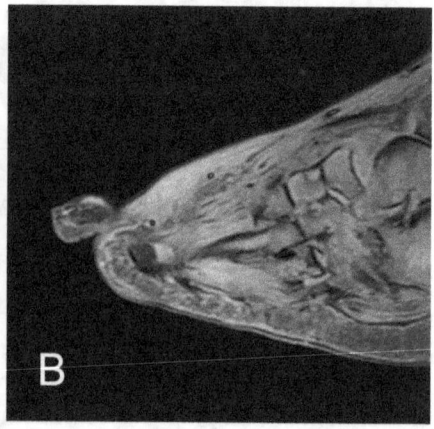

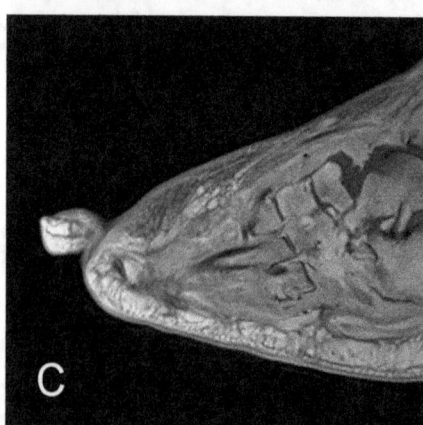

Sagittal T1 MRI (A), T2 FS (B), and T1 FS Gd MRI (C) reveal extensive edema and abnormal enhancement about the Charcot midfoot. Note the poor definition of the midfoot bones on the T1 sequence. Findings are compatible the ghost sign which is indicative of neuropathic osteoarthropathy with superimposed osteomyelitis. The ghost sign refers to poor definition of the margins of a bone on T1, which become clear on T2 or after Gd. There was also deep lateral plantar ulceration extending to bone on short axis images (not shown).

Similar to the previous scenario, the risk of osteomyelitis is relatively high in a diabetic patient with neuropathic arthropathy and soft tissue ulcer. MRI compliments radiographs by delineating the extent of involvement as well as identifying associated complications. Superior soft tissue detail and spatial resolution makes MRI the preferred diagnostic modality when compared to other imaging options. Nuclear medicine labeled leukocyte scan and marrow scan can identify osteomyelitis; however, it does not accurately determine the anatomic extent of infection. CT will detail the neuropathic changes but will not help in determining the presence of active osteomyelitis.

# References

1.  Beaman FD, von Herrmann PF, Kransdorf MJ, Adler RS, Amini B, Appel M, Arnold E, Bernard SA, Greenspan BS, Lee KS, Tuite MJ, Walker EA, Ward RJ, Wessell DE, Weissman BN. ACR Appropriateness Criteria(®) Suspected Osteomyelitis, Septic Arthritis, or Soft Tissue Infection (Excluding Spine and Diabetic Foot). J Am Coll Radiol. 2017 May;14(5S):S326-S337. doi: 10.1016/j.jacr.2017.02.008. Review. PMID: 28473089.
2.  Walker EA, Beaman FD, Wessell DE, Cassidy RC, Czuczman GJ, Demertzis JL, Lenchik L, Motamedi K, Pierce JL, Sharma A, Ying-Kou Yung E, Kransdorf MJ. ACR Appropriateness Criteria® Suspected Osteomyelitis of the Foot in Patients with Diabetes Mellitus. J Am Coll Radiol. 2019 Nov;16(11S):S440-S450. PMID: 31685111
3.  American College of Radiology. ACR Appropriateness Criteria: Chronic Foot Pain. American College of Radiology, revised 2019. https://acsearch.acr.org/docs/69340/Narrative/ (accessed April 24, 2021).
4.  American College of Radiology. ACR Appropriateness Criteria: Suspected Osteomyelitis, Septic Arthritis, or Soft Tissue Infection (Excluding Spine and Diabetic Foot). American College of Radiology, 2016. https://acsearch.acr.org/docs/3094201/Narrative/ (accessed April 24, 2021).
5.  Baker JC, Demertzis JL, Rhodes NG, Wessell DE, Rubin DA. Diabetic musculoskeletal complications and their imaging mimics. Radiographics. 2012 Nov-Dec;32(7):1959-74. doi: 10.1148/rg.327125054. PMID:23150851.
6.  Collins MS, Schaar MM, Wenger DE, Mandrekar JN. T1-weighted MRI characteristics of pedal osteomyelitis. AJR Am J Roentgenol. 2005 Aug;185(2):386-93. PMID: 16037509.
7.  Donovan A, Schweitzer ME. Use of MR imaging in diagnosing diabetes-related pedal osteomyelitis. Radiographics. 2010 May;30(3):723-36. doi:10.1148/rg.303095111. PMID: 20462990.

# Part V. Imaging After Treatment or Surgery

These patients will typically be obvious in their presentation, although the reason for their visit may not be. In general, for patients with previous treatment or surgery, the recommended initial imaging is radiography. Whenever possible, previous radiographs should be obtained for comparison. The next recommendations would be CT, MRI or US.

# Chapter 32. Imaging After Trauma Treatment

Felix S. Chew, MD

Radiography is the appropriate exam after treatment of fractures and dislocations. CT is often the next step if complications are suspected. MRI and the bone scan may be helpful in some circumstances.

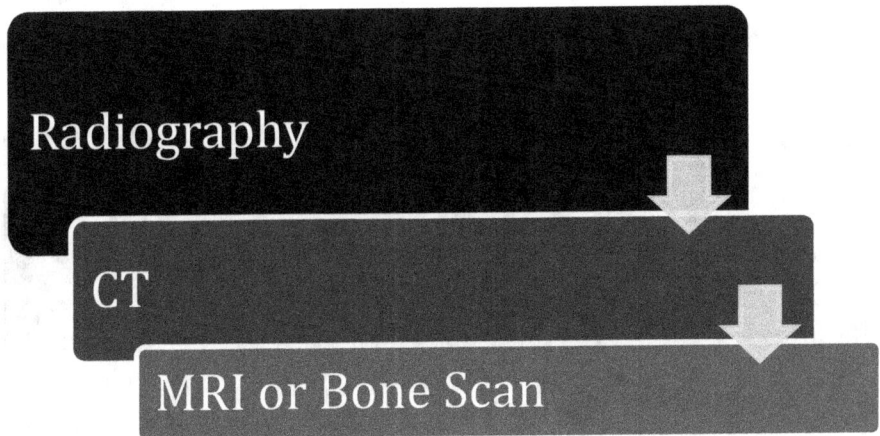

# Case 32-1

49-year-old man who injured his left humerus in a motorcycle crash. The intial radiographs showed a comminuted fracture of the proximal shaft, without dislocation. Because of the lack of displacement and the status of his other injuries, it was elected to treat his humerus fracture with closed reduction. He now returns for follow-up at 3 months without specific complaints. What is imaging exam should be performed to evaluate for fracture healing?

This scenario concerns routine follow-up of closed fracture treatment.

Sensible recommendation: XR, region of interest

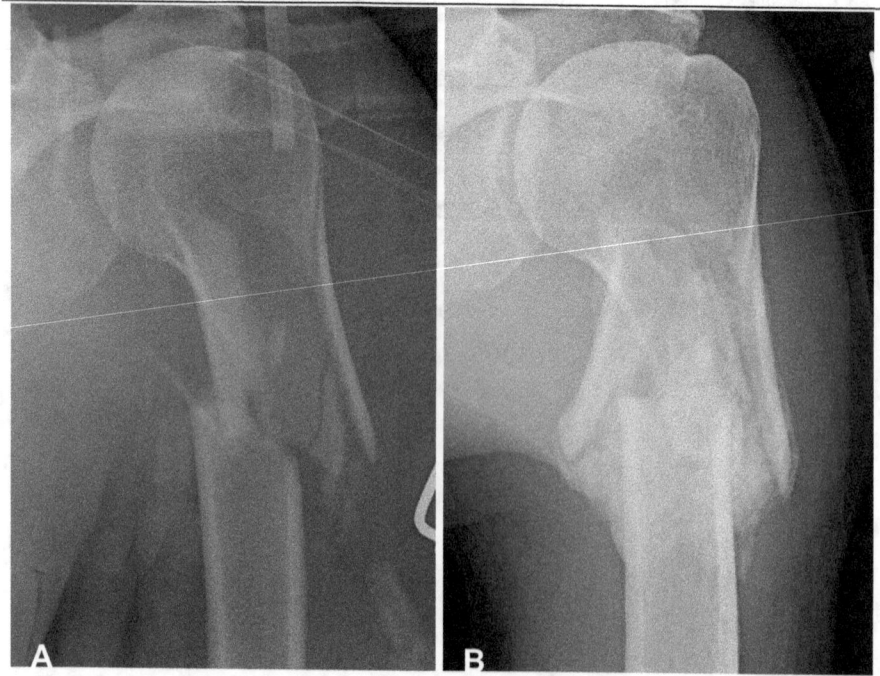

AP radiograph of the right shoulder at the time of injury (A) and at the 3-month follow-up visit (B) demonstrates healing of the comminuted proximal shaft fracture without significant change in position or alignment and without complication.

Although all of the imaging modalities listed would demonstrate fracture healing, radiography is routinely used to document fracture healing and to screen for possible complications. If there are specific clinical issues or abnormalities on the radiographs that require further evaluation, CT is typically the next step.

# Case 32-2

76-year-old woman who sustained an intertrochanteric fracture of her left proximal femur in a ground-level fall. She was noted to have osteopenia at the time of surgical fixation of her fracture. She returns for follow-up after 2 months. What imaging procedure should be performed?

This scenario concerns routine follow-up of a patient with surgical treatment of a fracture.

Sensible recommendation: XR, region of interest

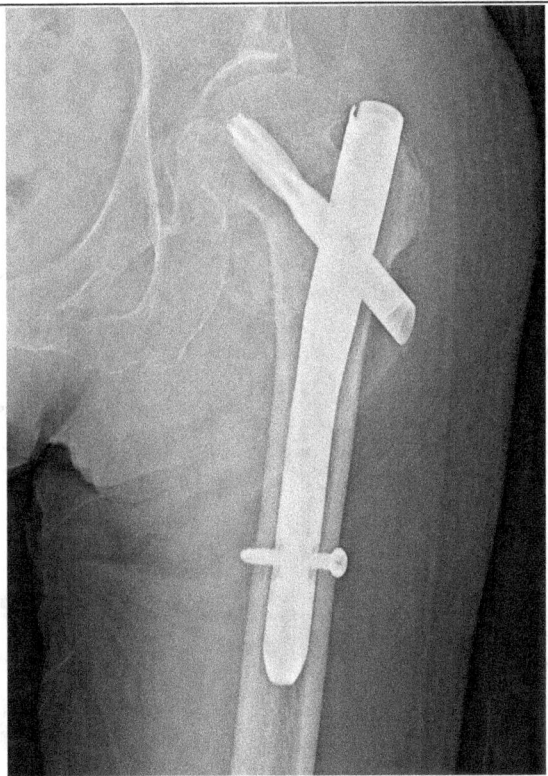

AP radiograph of the left hip demonstrates a healing intertrochanteric proximal femur fracture with fixation by a short intramedullary rod with interlocking hip screw.

Radiography is the initial study for follow-up of fracture patients with hardware. Radiographs document progress towards healing and screen for possible complications. Although this patient presumably has osteoporosis, DXA of a hip with hardware implant should not be performed.

# Case 32-3

33-year-old man who suffered a comminuted humeral shaft fracture two years ago that was treated with open reduction and internal fixation. He presents with worsening arm pain but no clinical findings that suggest infection. What imaging procedure should be obtained initially?

This scenario concerns a patient with pain and previous internal fixation for fracture, without clinical findings of infection.

Sensible recommendation: XR, region of interest

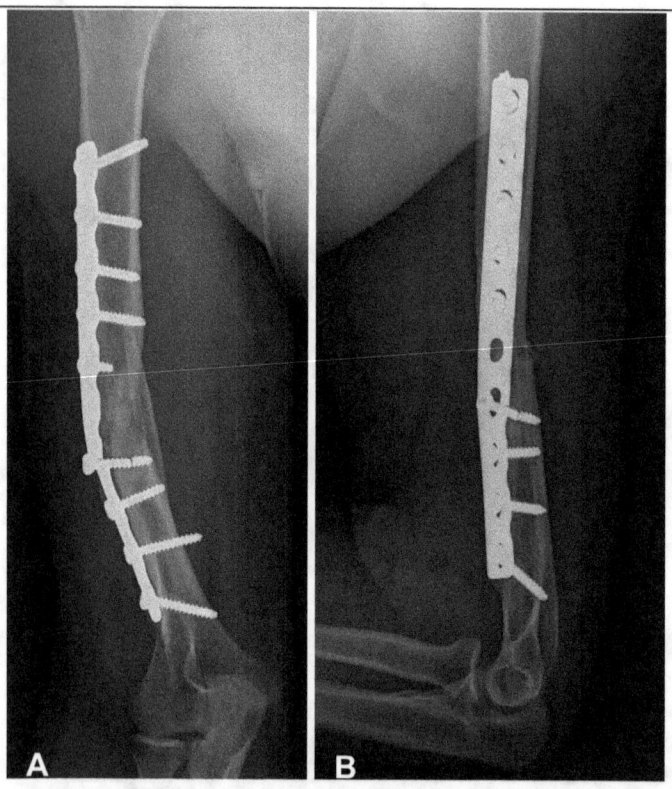

(A-B) AP and lateral radiographs of the right humerus demonstrates previous internal fixation of comminuted shaft fractures. The plate is bent, one screw is broken, and the fracture has only partially healed. There are no findings to suggest infection.

The initial evaluation for hardware is radiography, if only to identify the type of hardware and its condition. Comparison with previous radiographs would be helpful but often are not available. If additional imaging is necessary for diagnosis or surgical planning, CT is the recommended next step. If radiographs show intact hardware and healed bone, the search for the underlying causes should be focused by clinical exam.

# Case 32-4

57-year-old man who sustained an open spiral fracture of the distal tibial that extended to the articular surface two years prior. The fracture was treated with open reduction and internal fixation but an infection developed, and the wound was debrided and the hardware was removed. Radiographs were obtained to assess healing and were suggestive but not definitive for nonunion. What should the next imaging procedure be to evaluate for fracture nonunion?

This scenario concerns a patient with possible fracture nonunion.

Sensible recommendation: CT WO CONTRAST, region of interest

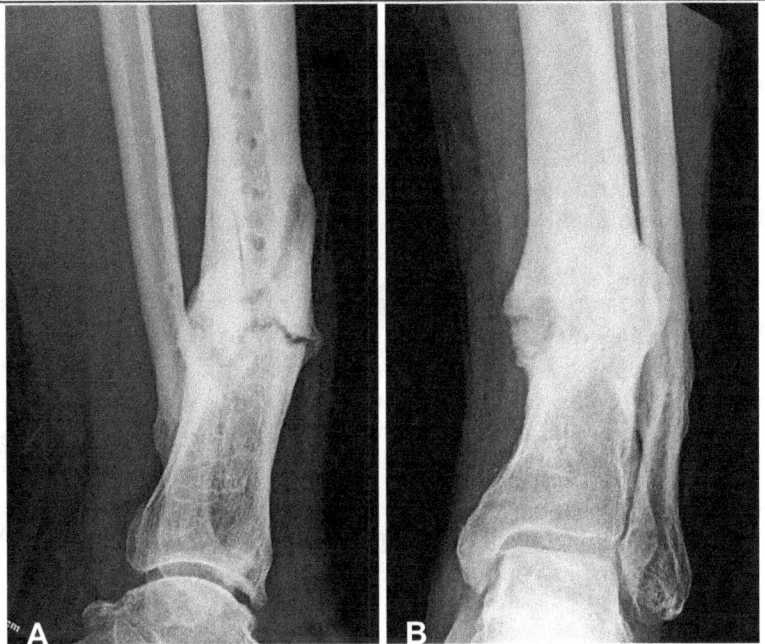

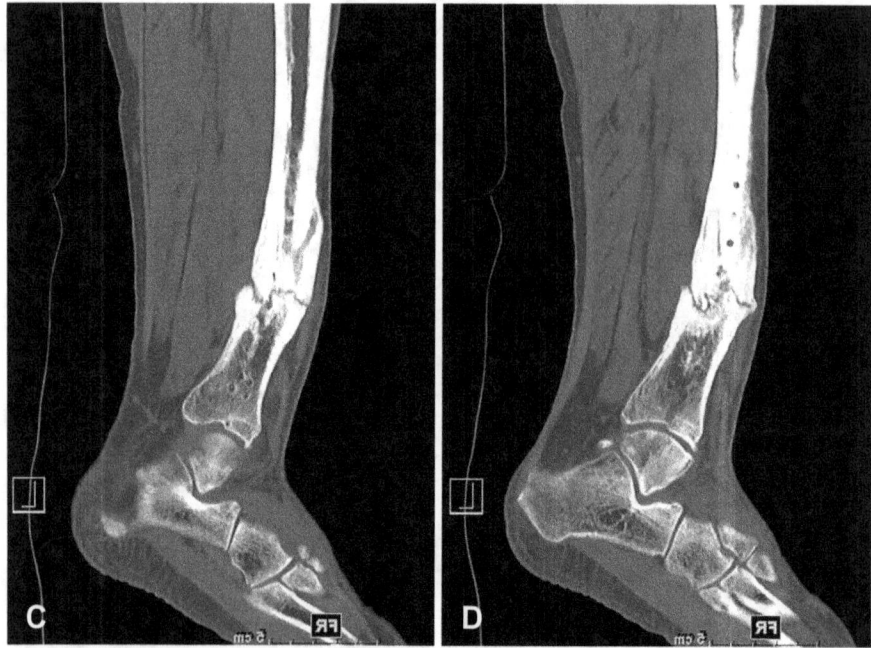

(A-B) Lateral and AP radiographs of the lower leg show a partially visible fracture line across the tibial shaft, with deformity and healed fracture fragments. (C-D) Sagittal CT images show sclerosis and persistent fracture line traversing the shaft, indicative of nonunion.

Radiography is the initial imaging for the evaluation of possible fracture nonunion. If there is sclerosis and a fracture whose morphology does not allow an unobscured view of the site, CT is the recommended modality to identify whether nonunion is present. Multiplanar reformations are necessary, but 3D reconstructions are generally not helpful. Even though hardware may have been removed, MRI often has severe artifacts at surgical sites and is not recommended for this purpose. Repeat radiographs in 10 days, while possibly appropriate in the acute setting, are not appropriate in this setting.

## References

1. Chew FS. Imaging of Fracture Treatment and Healing. In: Chew FS (ed). Musculoskeletal Imaging: The Essentials. Philadelphia: Lippincott Williams & Wilkins, 2018:62-80.

# Chapter 33. Imaging After Small Joint Arthroplasty

Felix S. Chew, MD, Jack Porrino, MD, Erin Flaherty, MD, Jennifer Favinger, MD

Radiography is the appropriate exam after small joint arthroplasty. CT or MRI are often the next step if complications are suspected. The bone scan or US may be helpful in some circumstances.

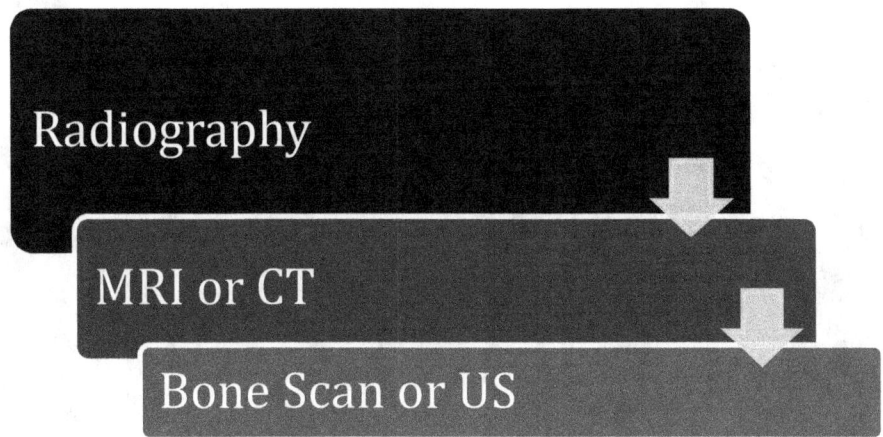

Radiography

MRI or CT

Bone Scan or US

## Case 33-1

61-year-old woman status-post replacement arthroplasty of the second through fifth MCP joints with Silastic implants for underlying rheumatoid arthritis. She presents for routine 6-week post-surgical follow-up without specific complaints. What imaging exam should be obtained to evaluate her hand and document the status of the implants?

This scenario concerns routine follow-up for a patient with Silastic MCP arthroplasty and no particular complaints.

Sensible recommendation: XR HAND 3 VIEW

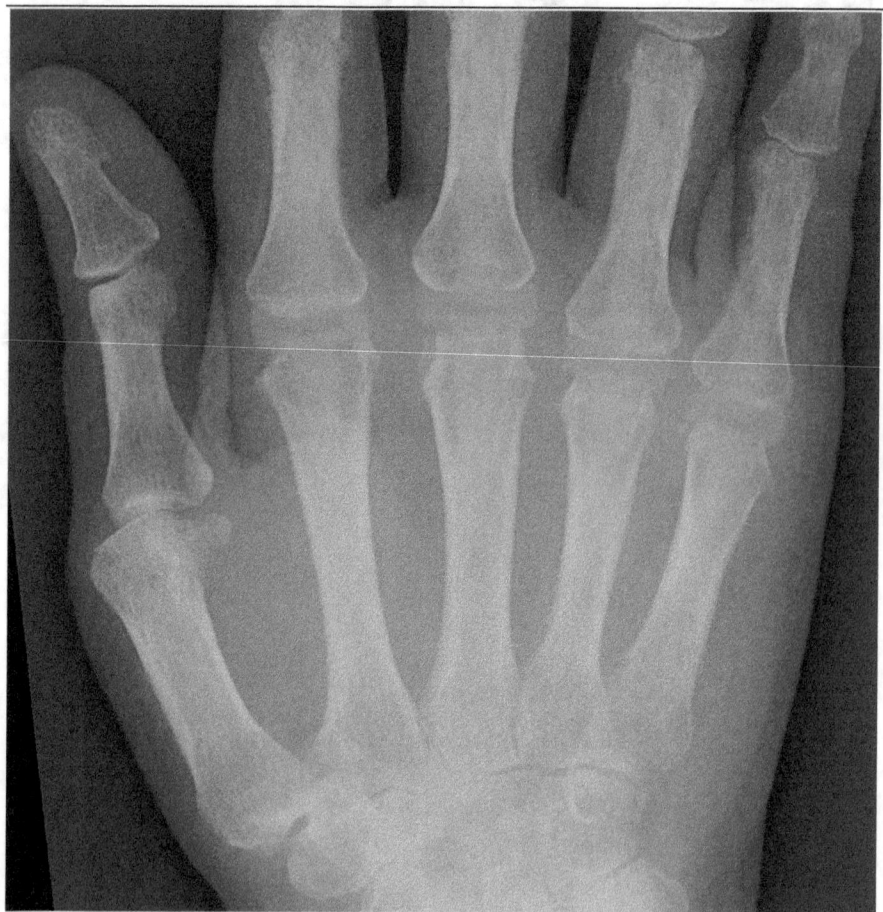

PA radiograph of the right hand shows Silastic implants at the second through fifth MCP joints without evidence of complication.

Radiography should be routinely obtained in patients with joint prostheses when they present for follow-up in order to document the status of the implants and screen for complications. Other imaging modalities may be applicable if specific issues are raised by clinical presentation or the radiographs. Silastic implants do not create artifacts on MRI, should that modality be contemplated.

## Case 33-2

35-year-old woman status-post left total elbow arthroplasty with linked prosthesis for underlying rheumatoid arthritis. She presents for routine annual post-surgical follow-up. What imaging procedure should be obtained to evaluate her elbow?

This scenario concerns a patient with routine follow-up for a patient with elbow arthroplasty. First imaging.

Sensible recommendation: XR ELBOW 2 VIEW

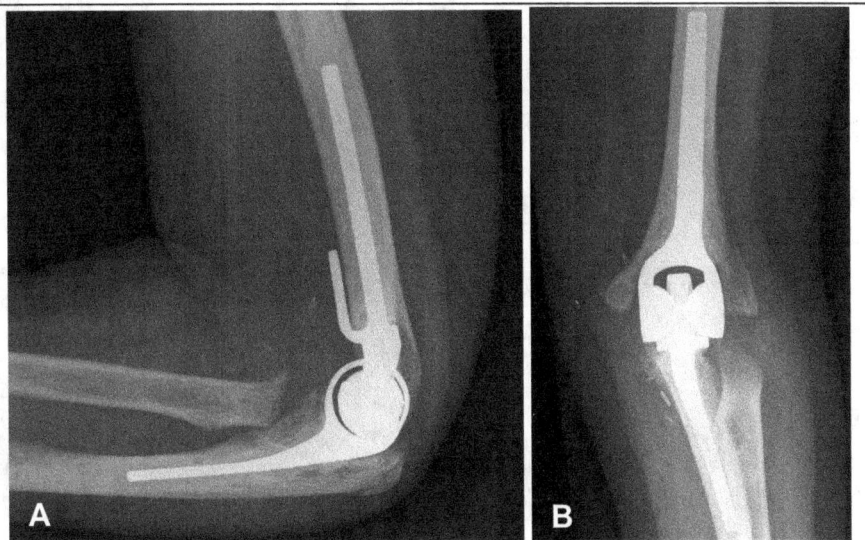

(A-B) Lateral and AP radiographs of the left elbow show post-surgical changes of total elbow arthroplasty with linked prosthesis. No complications are present.

Radiography and clinical exam provide the information typically needed for follow-up. Previous radiographs are important for comparison. If there are specific problems that require further evaluation, CT, MRI, US, or bone scan may be helpful.

# Case 33-3

63-year-old woman status-post left total ankle arthroplasty two years prior. She presents for her second annual check-up complaining of pain and swelling about the ankle. Radiographs from her visit one year earlier are available. What imaging exam should be performed?

This scenario concerns a patient with ankle pain of unknown etiology and previous total ankle arthroplasty.

Sensible recommendation: XR ANKLE 3 VIEW

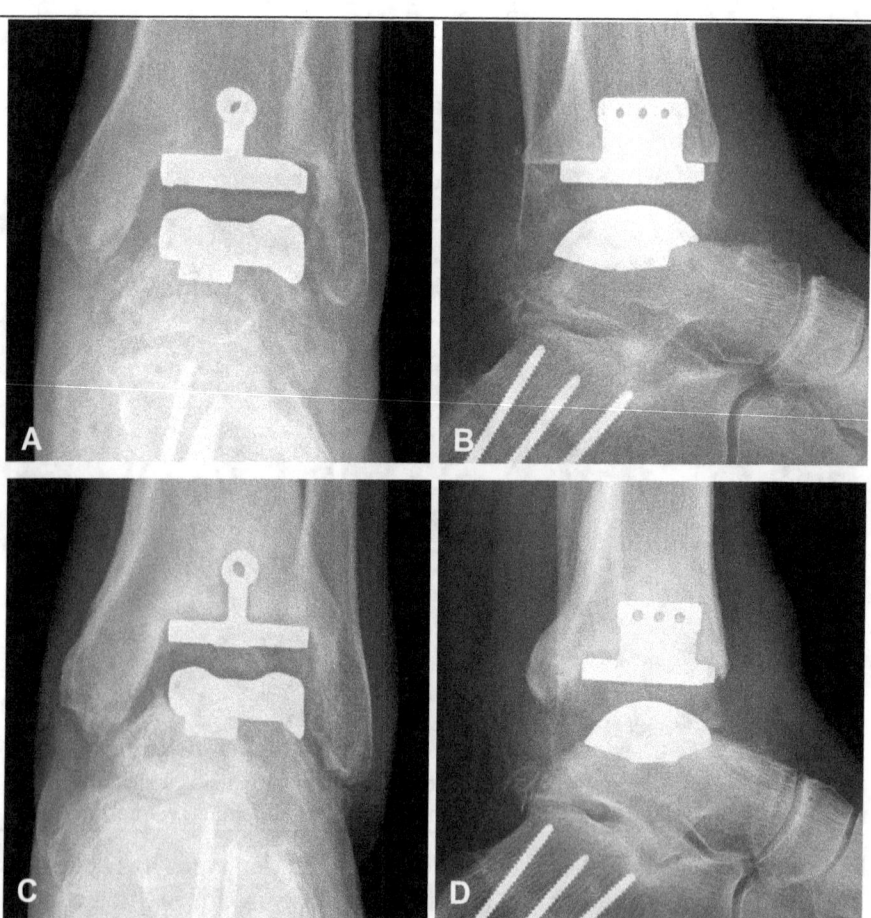

(A-B) AP and lateral radiographs of the left ankle one year ago show a normal postoperative appearance of a Salto Talaris total ankle replacement. (C-D) Current AP and lateral radiographs demonstrate lucency at the bone-metal interfaces and diffuse sclerosis of the surrounding bone, suggestive of loosening.

Pain after total ankle arthroplasty has many possible causes, including complications directly related to the prosthesis, fractures, arthritis of neighboring joints, and muscle and tendon disease. Radiography is generally the starting point for imaging evaluation, and its accuracy is greatly improved when radiographs shortly after surgery are available for comparison. Further evaluation of the bones and joints may be performed with CT or MRI, although both will be degraded by metal artifact, and further evaluation of the muscles and tendons may be performed with ultrasound.

# Case 33-4

74-year-old woman sustained trauma to her elbow in a motor vehicle crash nine months earlier. Fractures of the proximal ulna were reduced and internally fixed with plate and screws. A displaced radial head fracture was treated with a radial head hemiarthroplasty. She presents now with worsening elbow pain. What imaging exam should be performed to evaluate her elbow?

This scenario concerns a patient with elbow pain and previous fracture treatment with internal fixation and radial head replacement.

Sensible recommendation: XR ELBOW 2 VIEW

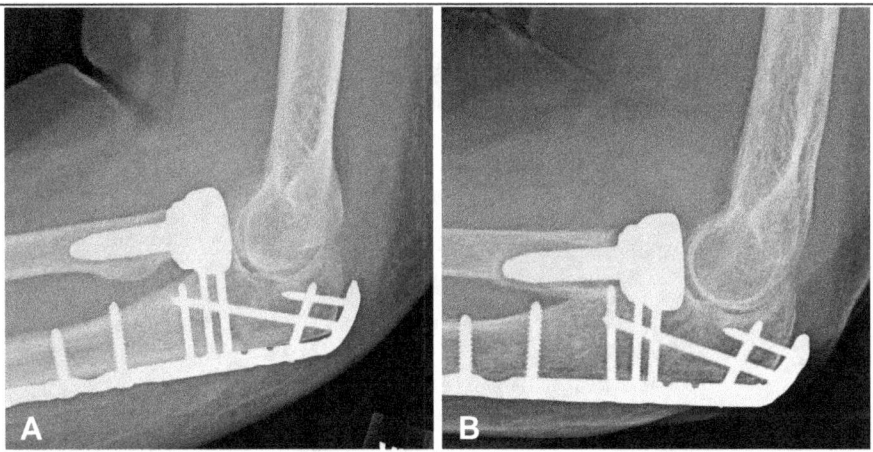

Lateral radiographs of the elbow after trauma surgery (A) and nine months later (B). The initial radiographs show no complications. The subsequent radiographs show loosening of the stem of the radial head prosthesis and healed fractures of the ulna.

Radiography is the initial imaging exam for the evaluation of orthopedic hardware. If further imaging evaluation is necessary, CT, MRI, US, or nuclear imaging may be considered, depending on which direction the clinical presentation suggests.

# References

1. Gyftopoulos S, Rosenberg ZS, Roberts CC, Bencardino JT, Appel M, Baccei SJ, Cassidy RC, Chang EY, Fox MG, Greenspan BS, Hochman MG, Jacobson JA, Mintz DN, Newman JS, Shah NA, Small KM, Weissman BN. ACR Appropriateness Criteria Imaging After Shoulder Arthroplasty. J Am Coll Radiol. 2016 Nov;13(11):1324-1336. doi: 10.1016/j.jacr.2016.07.028. PMID: 27814833.
2. Wise JN, Daffner RH, Weissman BN, Bancroft L, Bennett DL, Blebea JS, Bruno MA, Fries IB, Jacobson JA, Luchs JS, Morrison WB, Resnik CS, Roberts CC, Schweitzer ME, Seeger LL, Stoller DW, Taljanovic MS. ACR Appropriateness Criteria® on acute shoulder pain. J Am Coll Radiol. 2011 Sep;8(9):602-9. doi: 10.1016/j.jacr.2011.05.008. PMID: 21889746.

# Chapter 34. Imaging After Hip Arthroplasty

Hyojeong Lee, MD

Radiography is the appropriate exam after hip arthroplasty. CT or MRI are often the next step if complications are suspected. The bone scan or US may be helpful in some circumstances. If infection is suspected, arthrocentesis would be appropriate.

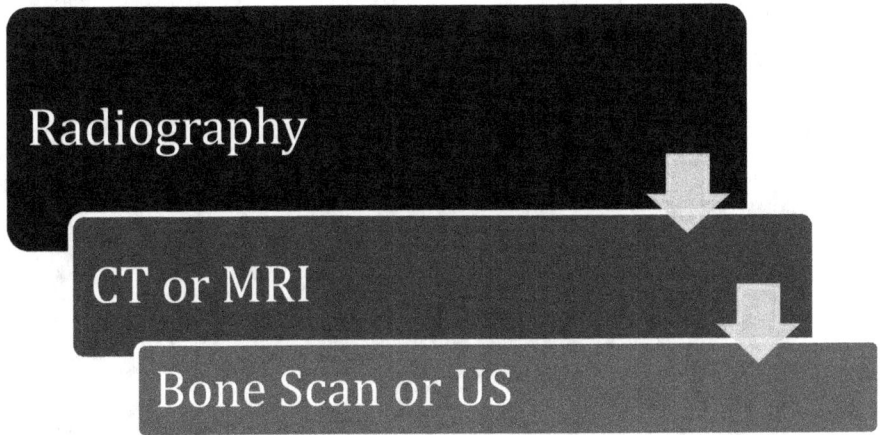

## Case 34-1

A 60-year-old woman for an annual routine check-up for her hips. She had bilateral total hip arthroplasties several years ago, and currently has no specific complaints. Which imaging test should be ordered?

This scenario concerns the routine follow-up imaging after total hip arthroplasty in an asymptomatic patient.

Sensible recommendation: XR PELVIS AND HIP

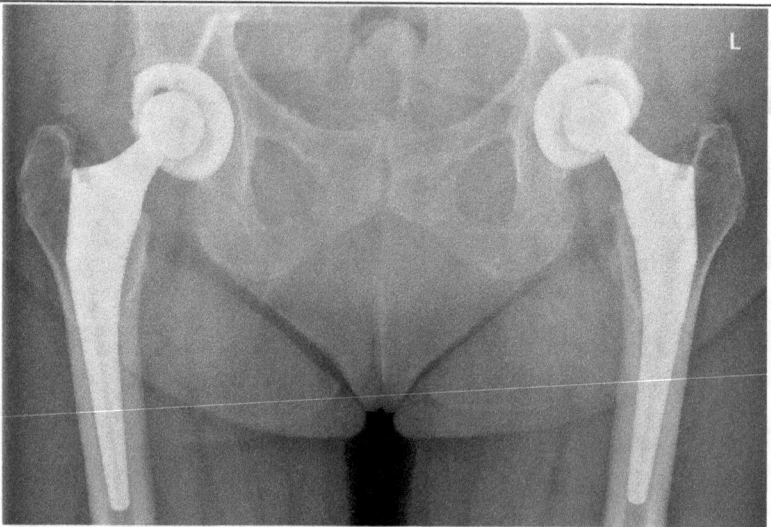

Anterior-posterior (AP) radiograph of pelvis demonstrates normal appearance of total hip arthroplasty. Both femoral prostheses are metal-on-polyethylene bearings with cementless fixation. Both acetabular components are augmented with derotational screws. The femoral heads are seated in the center of the acetabular cups. There is no periprosthetic lucency around the prostheses.

The number of primary total hip arthroplasties (THAs) performed in the United States was 220,000 in 2003 and this number is expected to rise to 572,000 by 2030. Results are often long lasting, with approximately 87% survival after 10 years. Revisions are most often due to instability/dislocation, mechanical loosening, or infection. Metal-on-metal prostheses can be associated with additional complications, including tissue hypersensitivity reaction.

Radiography is the standard first examination for evaluating total hip arthroplasties. Radiographs shortly after surgery are usually recommended to identify surgical complications and provide a baseline for future evaluation. They are particularly important after revision surgery. Late radiographic follow-up is usually advocated to identify osteolysis or loosening. The value of postoperative radiographs generally has been questioned. One reason is their limited sensitivity for detecting osteolysis. Another is based on cost-benefit analysis. Bolz et al evaluated 3 follow-up strategies for 7 years after primary total hip replacement: 2 yearly routine follow-ups; Arthroplasty Society of Australia strategy of a minimum follow-up after 3 months, at 1 to 2 years, and then no follow-up for 7 years; and a third strategy of no follow-up. The no follow-up strategy costs were lower and health benefits slightly higher at 7 years. Patients with metal-on-metal prostheses may need a different schedule. Regarding clinical follow-up, the United States Food and Drug Administration recommends that if the patient is asymptomatic and has a well-functioning hip, follow-up should occur periodically (typically 1 to 2 years).

# Case 34-2

A 40-year-old woman presents with left hip pain. She had her left hip replacement outside of the United States 4 years ago. She denies fever, chills or warmth around the left hip. What imaging test should be ordered?

This scenario concerns imaging of total hip arthroplasty patients when there is suspected component malposition.

Sensible recommendation: XR PELVIS AND HIP

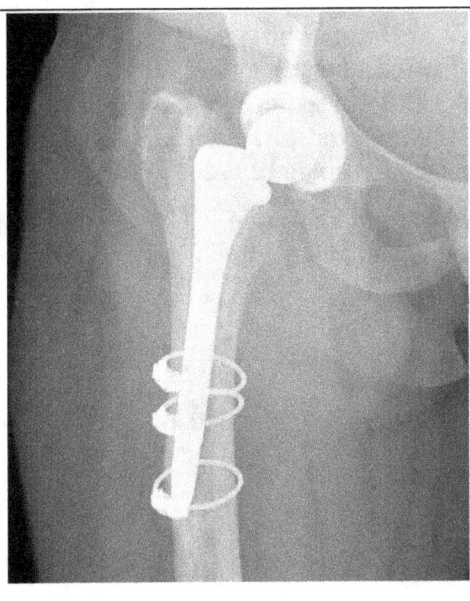

Component malposition. AP radiograph of the right hip demonstrates THA with a non-modular femoral component. The femoral stem is not aligned with the axis of the femoral shaft and its tip abuts to lateral cortex.

After THA, patients with loosening or infection usually (but not always) have pain, whereas those with particle disease and resulting osteolysis or with metal hypersensitivity can be asymptomatic. Pain patterns can suggest the correct diagnosis, but complications can be difficult to identify clinically. Therefore, understanding the use of imaging is of particular importance. All symptomatic patients should undergo radiography. Availability of old radiographs to compare to new ones facilitates the diagnosis of subtle changes such as can occur in loosening, particle disease, or infection.

Radiographs are the usual method for evaluating component positions. The initial placement of prosthetic components should correspond with the expected anatomic site of each. In the initial evaluation of a patient who has undergone THA, leg length, vertical and horizontal centers of rotation, lateral acetabular inclination, acetabular anteversion, and femoral stem position should be assessed. Specialized projections have been suggested for some assessments and positioning for radiographic examination may be difficult. A CT scan, or fluoroscopy can augment assessment in patients who are unable to position.

# Case 34-3

A 35-year-old woman presents with right hip pain. She has a complicated history of spondylitis, and hemiarthroplasty of right hip. AP radiograph of the right hip shows periprosthetic lucency around the femoral stem and greater trochanter. Her ESR and CRP are high (CRP: 70.1 mg/L, ESR: 27 mm/hr). What imaging test should be ordered next?

This scenario concerns further imaging of hip arthroplasty patients when there is a painful primary total hip arthroplasty and infection is possible.

Sensible recommendation: XR JOINT ASPIRATION HIP

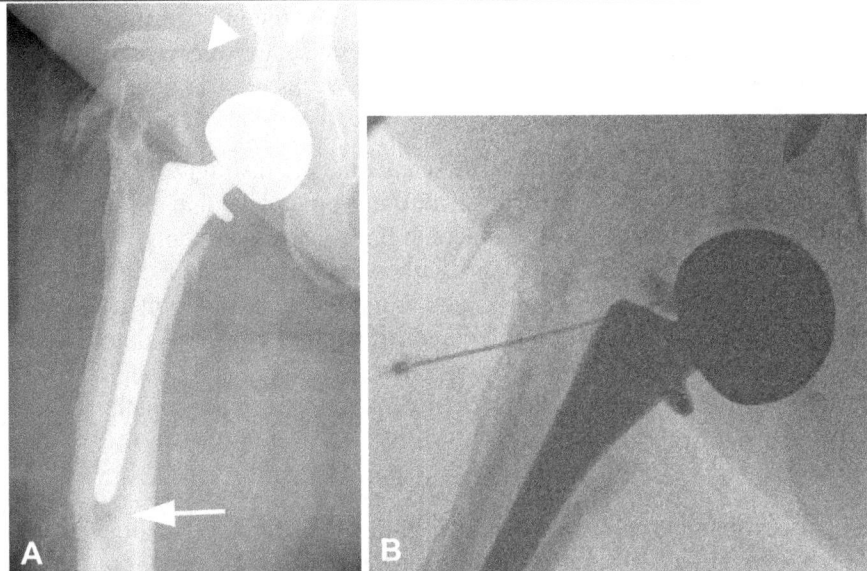

Infected hip prosthesis. AP radiograph of the right hip (A) demonstrates hemiarthroplasty with a bipolar femoral component. Prominent periprosthetic lucency is noted around the femoral stem (arrow). Also, prominent globular lucency is present at greater trochanter (arrowhead). A spot fluoroscopic image obtained during hip arthrocentesis (B). 30 ml of yellowish turbid fluid was aspirated and the culture was positive for *S. aureus*.

Infection occurs in 1-2% of primary total hip arthroplasties and is even more frequent after revision procedures. Confirmation of infection of failed hip prostheses can be difficult since organisms may be inaccessible, residing in a biofilm.

Radiographic findings can vary from completely normal to frank bone destruction mimicking loosening or particle disease. A distinction between septic and aseptic loosening often cannot be made on a single radiograph. Usually, previous radiographs are necessary for comparison. Aseptic loosening usually takes a slowly progressive course, whereas infection usually occurs with a rapid time course and an aggressive appearance.

Arthrocentesis is probably the most useful test for confirming of the presence or absence of infection. The sensitivity of preoperative arthrocentesis ranges from 40% to 93% and the specificity from 82% to 100%. In 2010, the American Academy of Orthopedic Surgeons recommended a selective approach to arthrocentesis of the hip based on the patient's probability of periprosthetic joint infection and the results of the erythrocyte sedimentation rate and C-reactive protein. In cases where there is a discrepancy between the probability of periprosthetic joint infection and the initial arthrocentesis culture result, repeat arthrocentesis was suggested. They recommend that patients be off antibiotics for a minimum of 2 weeks prior to obtaining intra-articular culture.

Combining marrow scans with WBC scans can help distinguish WBC up-take due to variations in marrow distribution from uptake due to infection. Both radiopharmaceuticals accumulate in bone marrow but only WBCs accumulate in infection. CT in patients with infection can demonstrate periprosthetic fluid collections, acetabular malposition, and joint effusion. MRI in patients with infection can demonstrate joint effusion, edema and enhancement of synovial and extra-capsular soft tissues and bone, the presence of extra-capsular collections, bone destruction, and adenopathy.

# Case 34-4

A 23-year-old male comes with left hip pain. He had left THA about 6 months ago. He reports that the hip is constantly painful. When asked to specify where he has pain, he localizes it to the lateral aspect of the hip. It does not appear to be worse with any particular activity. The patient denies fevers, chills, night sweats, or other signs of systemic infection. On exam, he demonstrates a bilateral abductor weak gait. What imaging test should be ordered?

This scenario concerns imaging of a total hip arthroplasty patient with painful primary total hip arthroplasty where aseptic loosening is suspected but not infection.

Sensible recommendation: XR PELVIS AND HIP

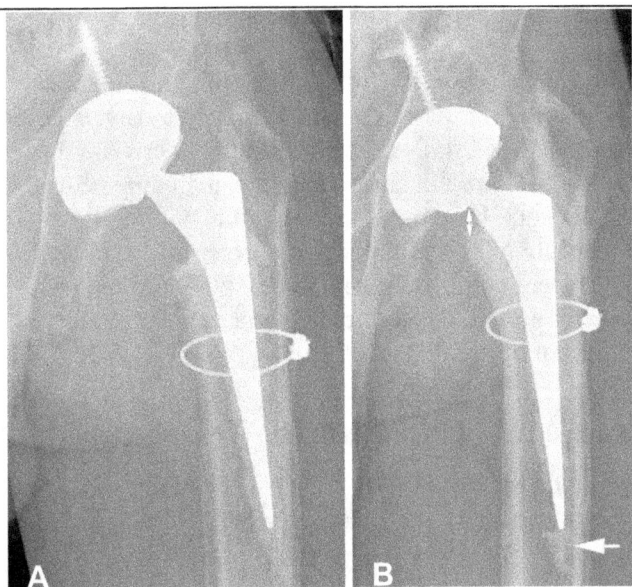

Serial AP radiographs (three months apart) of the left hip (A, B) demonstrate THA with loosening and subsidence of the cemented femoral component. There is subsidence of the femoral stem (double headed arrow in B), and distally migrated broken cement along the tip of the stem (arrow in B).

Loosening (complete failure of fixation of an implant at surgery) is usually evaluated on radiographs. Mechanical or aseptic loosening is inferred if an infection work-up is negative and no wear-induced synovitis is present. Up to 60% of arthroplasties are revised due to loosening. Membrane formation and bone resorption along interfaces can precede loosening. On radiographs and CT, linear radiolucencies are seen along the interface. Loosening may only be diagnosed with certainty on imaging if there is implant displacement, progressive subsidence, contrast material surrounding an implant entirely at arthrography, or a 2 degree or more difference of version angles on CT images obtained in maximum external and internal rotation. The role of MRI in detecting component loosening is not yet established. Intra-articular injection of anesthetic that results in pain relief indicates an articular cause for the symptoms. Arthrography is still occasionally performed to evaluate suspected loosening of an implant. The arthrographic criterion of loosening of either the femoral stem or acetabular cup is the presence of contrast in either the metal-cement interface or the cement-bone interface, although the criteria and results are very variable.

# Case 34-5

A 53-year-old woman presents with left hip pain. She has a history of left total hip arthroplasty. She states she has continued to have significant symptoms with regard to her left hip. She can stand with crutches but is significantly impaired. Inflammatory markers, including ESR, CRP, and white blood cell count, have been normal. Initial cultures of left hip arthrocentesis were negative. The patient denies fevers, chills, night sweats, or other signs of systemic infection. AP radiograph of left hip (A) demonstrates globular lucencies around the acetabulum and acetabular protrusio. What imaging test should be ordered next?

This scenario concerns total hip arthroplasty patients when radiographs show suspected particle disease (osteolysis) but not infection. Next imaging.

Sensible recommendation: CT HIP WO CONTRAST

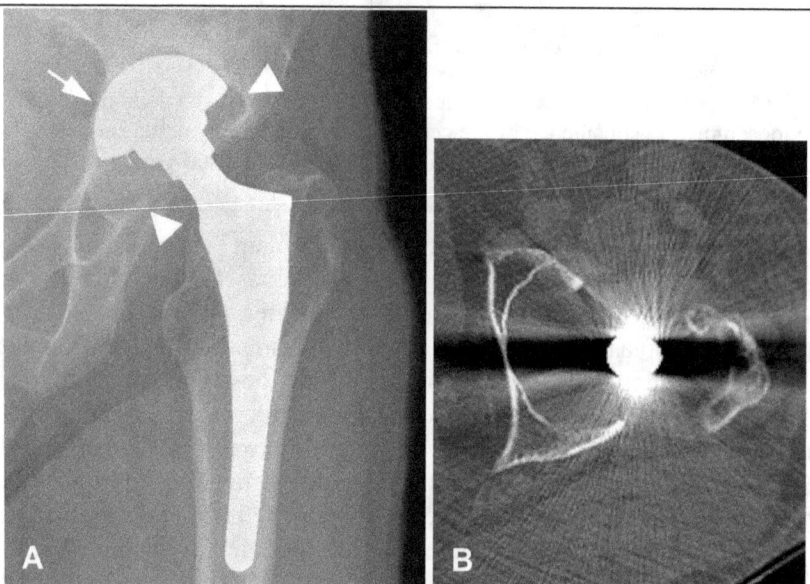

Osteolysis. AP radiograph of the left hip (A) demonstrates cementless THA. There is globular lucency around the acetabular component (arrowheads) with acetabular protrusion (arrow). Axial CT image (B) demonstrates osteolysis of left acetabulum.

Localized areas of bone resorption around total hip arthroplasties occur as a response to the release of small particles of cement, polyethylene, or metal. Osteolysis increases as component wear increases. Osteolysis has been a more frequent complication than infection, dislocation, or extensive heterotopic bone formation, although improvements in polyethylene are likely to decrease the rate of this complication. Loosening may or may not accompany granulomatous disease. With continued particle shedding, the lesions progress over time. The condition may be clinically silent, emphasizing the need for imaging.

Radiographs are typically the first method of identifying these areas of bone resorption. Judet views can be used to supplement the AP radiograph for this assessment. However, particularly in the acetabulum, considerable bone loss is necessary before lesions are identified with certainty on radiographs. Focal osteolysis is seen on CT as multiple expansile oval or round radiolucencies that form a multilobular shape. Improved CT scanning techniques enable better demonstration of bone adjacent to prostheses and provide a more sensitive method than radiography for determining the extent and location of areas of osteolysis. Stulberg et al found the prevalence of osteolysis without clinical or radiographic findings (silent osteolysis) to be 48% on CT scans and 24% on radiographs in 80 young, active patients who had undergone bone- ingrowth total hip replacement at least 7 years before. In MRI, focal periprosthetic intraosseous masses of intermediate to slightly increased signal with a low signal rim have been described in cases of aggressive granulomatous disease. Peripheral and some internal enhancement of these granulomas have been noted after intravenous gadolinium injection. There are few data on the role of FDG-PET in the evaluation of particle disease. Increased FDG uptake in a mass due to aggressive granulomatous disease has been described.

## Case 34-6

A 49-year-old woman presents with concerns about her hips. She has a history of bilateral hip arthroplasties using metal-on-metal (MoM) bearings that are under recall from the manufacturer. She has numbness in the left lateral thigh. She had metal ion testing; her chromium was 41.1 micrograms/L (upper normal is 5 micrograms/L) and her cobalt was 169 micrograms/L (upper normal is 1.0 micrograms/L). She is here to see whether she needs hip revision. Pelvic radiograph of both hips demonstrates normal bilateral THAs. Which imaging test should be ordered next?

This scenario concerns imaging patients after total hip arthroplasty when there is a painful primary metal-on-metal total hip prosthesis and possible aseptic lymphocyte-dominated vasculitis-associated lesion.

Sensible recommendation: MRI HIP WO CONTRAST

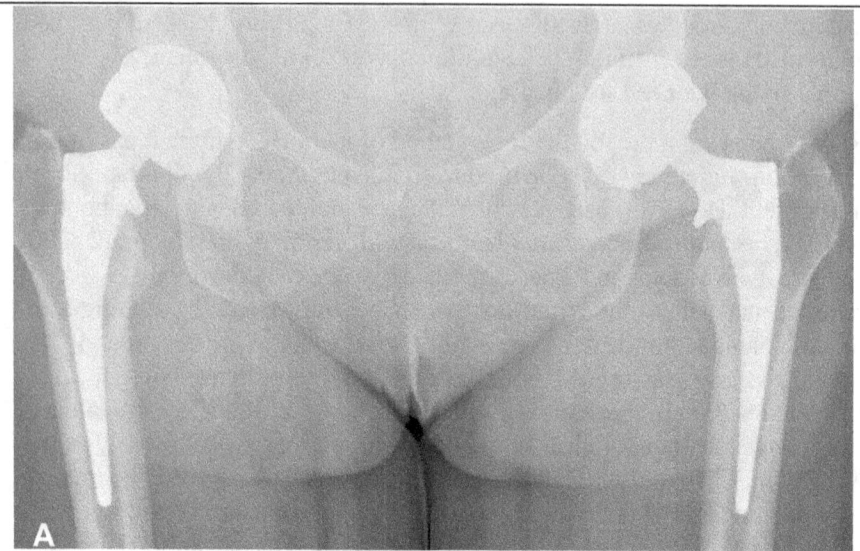

AP radiograph of the pelvis (A) demonstrates bilateral THA's with metal-on-metal bearing.

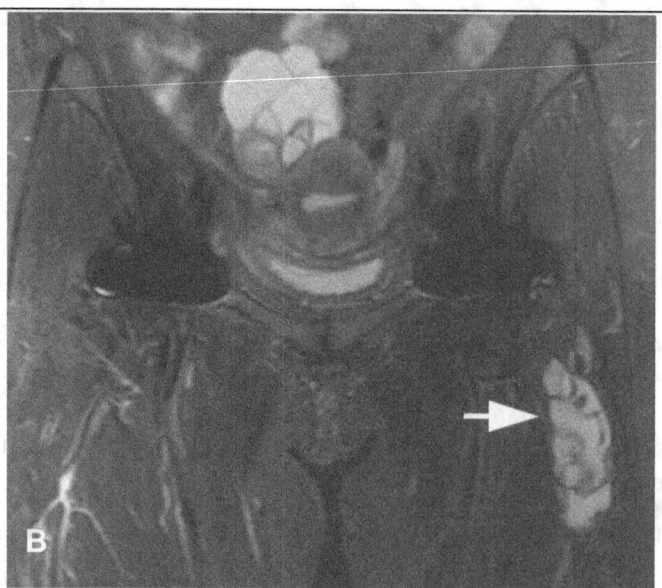

Coronal T2 FS MRI (B) shows a lobulated fluid collection along the anterior lateral aspect of the left thigh (arrow). It is consistent with a cystic ALVAL.

Newer MoM prostheses have been reintroduced in an effort to reduce wear and osteolysis associated with metal-on-polyethylene articulations. MoM prostheses can be conventional total hip replacements or resurfacing prostheses. Adverse local tissue reactions seen in patients with MoM prostheses include wear-induced metallosis (macroscopic staining of soft tissues) and a metal-induced hypersensitivity reaction variously termed metal hypersensitivity reaction, pseudotumor, or aseptic lymphocyte-dominated vasculitis-associated lesion (ALVAL). Although ALVAL is thought to be due to a local hypersensitivity response to the metal component alloys, the cause remains uncertain. The characteristic histologic feature of ALVAL is the presence of a dense perivascular infiltrate. Masses are formed that can contain areas of necrosis. Anterior lesions tend to be solid, whereas posterior and lateral lesions can be more cystic.

Radiographs in cases of ALVAL are often normal, although early osteolysis may be present. Using metal artifact reduction techniques, MRI can demonstrate ALVAL pseudotumors after MoM prostheses even in asymptomatic individuals and the relation of the soft tissue masses to symptoms is variable. Findings including fluid collections, synovitis, periprosthetic soft tissue masses, proximal femoral bone marrow edema, surrounding muscular and soft tissue edema, tendon avulsions, bone loss, periosteal stripping, neurovascular involvement, and periprosthetic fractures have been described after MoM hip replacement. US has been helpful in detecting reactive masses as this technique is not compromised by the presence of metal components. It can be used in patients who cannot have MRI or when MRI is not available. Although US has been noted to be limited in its ability to detect deep fluid collections and osseous abnormalities.

## Case 34-7

A 68-year-old woman with a pacemaker presents with left hip weakness and pain. She underwent a left total hip replacement for degenerative change three years ago. She notes she was weak after that in her left hip and her gait never really normalized at all. She has pain in the lateral aspect of her hip. On exam, her gait is notable for marked Trendelenburg. Radiograph of the left hip shows normal THA with metal-on-metal prosthesis (not shown). What imaging test should be ordered next?

This scenario concerns imaging patients after hip arthroplasty when there is trochanteric pain and suspected abductor injury or trochanteric bursitis. Radiographs non-diagnostic. Next imaging study.

Sensible recommendation: US HIP or MRI HIP WO CONTRAST

---

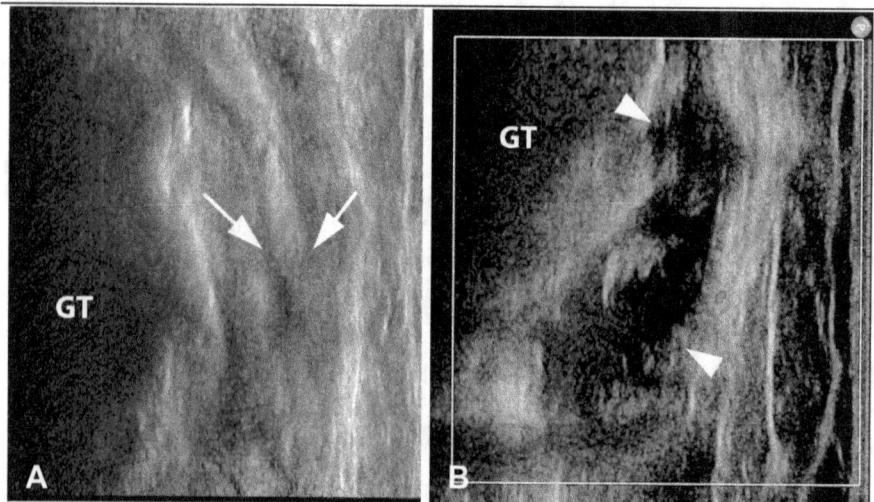

Gluteus medius avulsion. Longitudinal US images at left greater trochanter (GT in A, B). There is a discontinuity of gluteus medius tendon avulsed from the greater trochanter (arrows in A). Colored US image shows an associated avascular hypoechoic lesion, consistent with a hematoma (arrowheads in B). GT= Greater Trochanter

Radiographic examination is usually the first test in patients presenting with trochanteric pain after hip arthroplasty to help identify trochanter fractures or heterotopic bone formation. Surface irregularities of the trochanter may suggest abductor tendon abnormality. MRI has been shown to be an effective method for evaluating postoperative gluteal muscle atrophy and tendon tears. Sonography can identify and characterize hip abductor tendon abnormalities even in postoperative THA patients. US findings are best correlated with the clinical site of pain. This technique can be used to separate patients with abductor tendon avulsion from those with other causes of postoperative insufficiency of the abductor muscles (such as decreased femoral offset or denervation).

Arthrography in cases of tendon disruption can demonstrate a capsular defect with contrast extending to the region of the trochanteric bursa. Development of a fibrous capsule can lead to false- negative studies, however. Thus, a positive arthrographic study is helpful but a negative study does not exclude tendon avulsion. Trochanteric bursitis can be identified on US, MRI, or CT.

## Case 34-8

A 48-year-old woman presents with right hip and groin pain. She has a longstanding right hip pain that has persisted despite right THA. She has a distinct pain that she has with active hip flexion. The pain is only caused by active flexion and not by passive range of motion. It will happen every time when she flexes past 90 degrees. She denies pain while going uphill or up stairs unless there is a sharp incline. She does have pain when she is sitting and stands up. She denies numbness/tingling. AP radiograph of her right hip shows normal THA (not shown). Which imaging test should be ordered next?

This scenario concerns imaging patients after hip arthroplasty when there is suspected iliopsoas bursitis or tendinitis. Radiographs non-diagnostic. Next imaging study.

Sensible recommendation: MRI HIP WO CONTRAST or US HIP

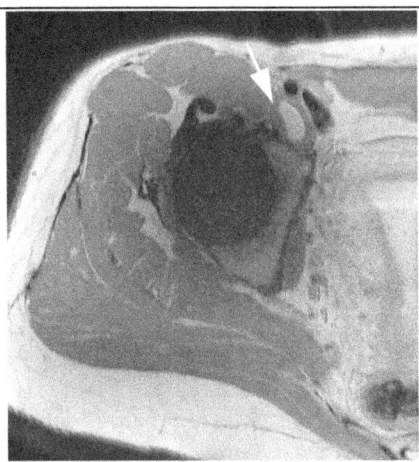

Iliopsoas bursitis. Axial T2 MRI shows a small, hyperintense fluid collection near the iliopsoas tendon, consistent with iliopsoas bursitis (arrow).

Anterior iliopsoas impingement may lead to postoperative groin pain and functional disability. Impingement can occur as a result of protrusion of the acetabular cup past the anteromedial edge of the acetabulum, protruding bone graft, acetabular fixation screws, anterior cement, an acetabular cage or reinforcement ring, prominence of the femoral head-neck junction, or osteophytes of the femoral neck.

Radiographs, CT, MRI, US, or diagnostic injection can be used to confirm the diagnosis. MRI can be used to evaluate the iliopsoas tendon. Abnormal findings include deviation of the tendon from an oversized acetabular component, tendinopathy, tear, or bursitis. Snapping of the tendon over the anterior acetabular component can be demonstrated on US. Injection of the tendon with anesthetic, with or without corticosteroid, can be confirmatory and alleviate symptoms.

Iliopsoas bursitis can be demonstrated by MRI, US, or CT. At US the iliopsoas bursitis appears as well-defined, thin-walled, cystic lesion. At CT the iliopsoas bursa appears as hypodense, well-defined cystic structures with clear enhancement of the bursal wall after contrast agent administration. At MRI the iliopsoas bursitis presents as homogeneously hypointense mass on T1 that was homogeneously hyperintense on T2. Contrast enhancement of the wall of the bursa is seen.

# Case 34-9

A 51-year-old woman presents with weakness in her right lower extremity. She has a history of right hip replacement about 10 months ago for hip osteoarthritis. She had weakness in her right lower extremity that has not significantly improved over the last 10 months. She notes that her right hip pain has resolved. An electromyography (EMG) and electrodiagnostic studies show severe nerve injury to the common peroneal nerve. What imaging test should be ordered?

This scenario concerns imaging patients after hip arthroplasty when there is suspected nerve damage.

Sensible recommendation: MRI HIP WO CONTRAST

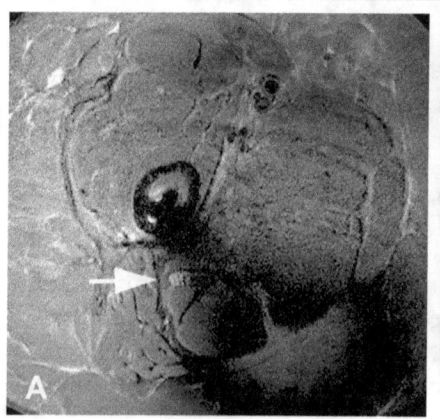
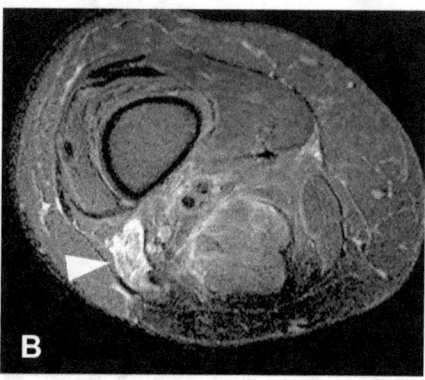

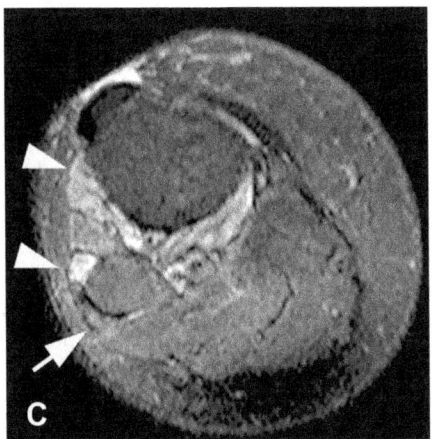

Sciatic nerve injury. Axial STIR MRI. From the proximal thigh to the proximal calf (A-C). The image at the level of proximal thigh (A) shows hyperintense signal of the right sciatic nerve (arrow). There is limited evaluation of the proximal aspect of the nerve to the hardware from associated right hip arthroplasty. The image at the level of the knee (B) shows hyperintense signal within the hamstring muscles, predominantly the biceps femoris (arrowhead). The image at the level of the proximal calf (C) shows high signal within the common peroneal nerve (arrow), and high signal in the muscles innervated by the common peroneal nerve (arrowheads).

The overall prevalence of nerve palsy following THA is 1%. The sciatic nerve or the peroneal division of the sciatic nerve is involved in nearly 80% of cases. The inferior division of the superior gluteal nerve is the main nerve supplying the abductor muscles and can be damaged during a direct lateral approach to hip replacement. Poorly positioned acetabular screws, extravasated cement, heterotopic ossification, scar tissue, synovial expansion, and osteolytic lesions, as well as hematomas and fluid collections, can compress nerves.

MRI has been used successfully to evaluate nerves around the hip, including the sciatic nerve. US is less satisfactory than MRI for detecting subtle nerve lesions in this region, especially in obese patients or when evaluating lesions at the level of the piriformis.

# Case 34-10

A 69-year-old man presents with weakness of his left hip although he does not report any significant pain or mechanical symptoms. He has history of a left hip replacement 7 years ago that was complicated by a proximal femoral fracture, which was treated. He has not had any recent trauma or additional procedures on the hip. His mobility is limited to household distances and occasionally the grocery store with a walker. He denies any systemic symptoms including fevers, chills or night sweats. What imaging test should be ordered?

This scenario concerns imaging after hip arthroplasty for the evaluation heterotopic bone.

Sensible recommendation: XR PELVIS AND HIP

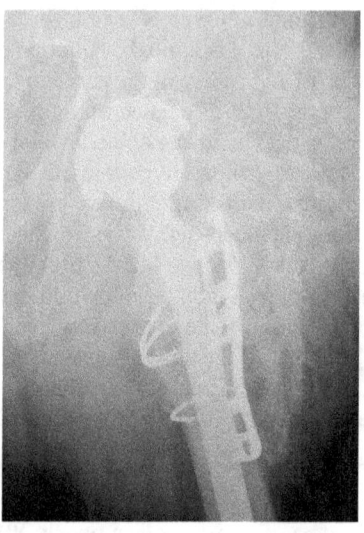

AP radiograph of left hip shows cementless THA with plate and cable fixation at the proximal femur. There is marked heterotopic ossification around the proximal femur extending to the pelvis (Brooker grade 4). The hardware is in anatomic alignment without evidence of loosening.

Heterotopic new bone formation occurs in 15 to 50% of patients, but a clinically significant limitation of motion is rare (1 to 5% of patients) Predisposing factors include infection, posttraumatic arthritis, ankylosing spondylitis, and previous hip surgery.

Radiographs are the standard method for evaluating and grading heterotopic bone. A lateral view can be helpful. Heterotopic bone is usually visible within 6 weeks postoperatively and generally does not increase after 6 months. The radiographic description of heterotopic ossification is performed on the AP view utilizing the Brooker classification: grade 0, no heterotopic ossification; grade 1, one or two foci of heterotopic ossification less than 1 cm each; grade 2, ossification or osteophytes occupying less than half the space between the femur and pelvis; grade 3, ossification or osteophytes occupying more than half the space between the pelvis and femur; and grade 4, ossification that bridges the pelvis and femur.

CT can be used to identify and determine the volume of heterotopic bone and its relationship to neurovascular structures. MRI can also be used to evaluate the relation of heterotopic bone to vessels, nerves, and the joint. Three-phase bone scanning is reported to be the most sensitive test for detecting heterotopic ossification. Serial bone scans can be used to determine the maturity of the heterotopic bone and aid in the timing of surgical resection. However, in practice, performance of bone scanning for determination of the maturity of heterotopic ossification for surgical resection after THA is not often done.

# Case 34-11

A 58-year-old woman presents with severe right hip pain and inability to bear weight. She had right THA for severe arthritis and activity-limiting pain 5 days ago. After discharge, the patient fell in her bathroom and noted the immediate onset of inability to bear weight. What imaging test should be ordered?

This scenario concerns the imaging evaluation of a patient after hip arthroplasty where there is suspicion for periprosthetic fracture.

Sensible recommendation: XR PELVIS AND HIP

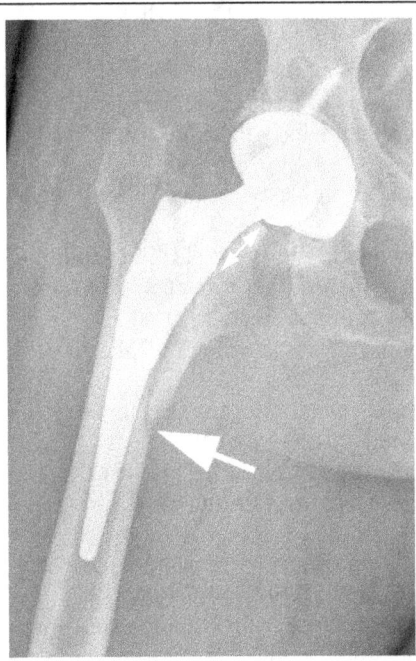

AP radiograph of the right hip shows cementless THA. There is a periprosthetic fracture along the medial aspect of the femoral stem (arrow) associated with subsidence of femoral component (double headed arrow).

Periprosthetic fractures occur more often around the femoral than the acetabular components. Postoperative femoral fractures may also occur any time after the surgery, typically at the level of the tip of the femoral stem because of stress risers at this level caused by the difference in stiffness between the metal stem and bony shaft. The cause of postoperative periprosthetic femoral fractures is most often a minor episode of trauma.

Most cases of suspected fracture are diagnosed on radiographs. CT is thought by some authors to be more helpful than MRI in evaluating fractures of the acetabular bone.

# References

1. American College of Radiology. ACR Appropriateness Criteria: Imaging after total hip arthroplasty. American College of Radiology, last review 2015. https://acsearch.acr.org/docs/3094200/Narrative/ (accessed April 24, 2021).
2. Bolz KM, Crawford RW, Donnelly B, Whitehouse SL, Graves N. The cost-effectiveness of routine follow-up after primary total hip arthroplasty. J Arthroplasty. 2010;25(2):191-196.
3. FDA Safety Communication: Metal-on-Metal Hip Implants. 2013; Available at: http://www.fda.gov/MedicalDevices/Safety/AlertsandNotices/ucm335775.htm. (accessed Jun 21, 2016).
4. Mulcahy H, Chew FS. Current concepts of hip arthroplasty for radiologists: part 1, features and radiographic assessment. AJR Am J Roentgenol. 2012;199(3):559-569.
5. The diagnosis of periprosthetic joint infections of the hip and knee guideline and evidence report 2010. American Academy of Orthopedic Surgeons. 2010; Available at: http://www.aaos.org/research/guidelines/PJIguideline.pdf. (accessed Jun 21, 2016).
6. Fritz J, Lurie B, Miller TT. Imaging of hip arthroplasty. Semin Musculoskelet Radiol. 2013;17(3):316- 327.
7. Stulberg SD, Wixson RL, Adams AD, Hendrix RW, Bernfield JB. Monitoring pelvic osteolysis following total hip replacement surgery: an algorithm for surveillance. J Bone Joint Surg Am. 2002;84-A Suppl 2:116-122.
8. Ostlere S. How to image metal-on-metal prostheses and their complications. AJR Am J Roentgenol. 2011;197(3):558-567.
9. Long SS, Surrey D, Nazarian LN. Common sonographic findings in the painful hip after hip arthroplasty. J Ultrasound Med. 2012;31(2):301-312.
10. Wunderbaldinger P, Bremer C, Schellenberger E, Cejna M, Turetschek K, Kainberger F. Imaging features of iliopsoas bursitis. Eur Radiol. 2002;12(2):409-415.
11. Schmalzried TP, Noordin S, Amstutz HC. Update on nerve palsy associated with total hip replacement. Clin Orthop Relat Res. 1997(344):188-206.
12. Brooker AF, Bowerman JW, Robinson RA, Riley LH, Jr. Ectopic ossification following total hip replacement. Incidence and a method of classification. J Bone Joint Surg Am. 1973;55(8):1629-1632.
13. Mulcahy H, Chew FS. Current concepts of hip arthroplasty for radiologists: part 2, revisions and complications. AJR Am J Roentgenol. 2012;199(3):570-580.

# Chapter 35. Imaging After Total Knee Arthroplasty

Hyojeong Lee, MD

Radiography is the appropriate exam after knee arthroplasty. CT or MRI are often the next step if complications are suspected. The bone scan or US may be helpful in some circumstances. If infection is suspected, arthrocentesis would be appropriate.

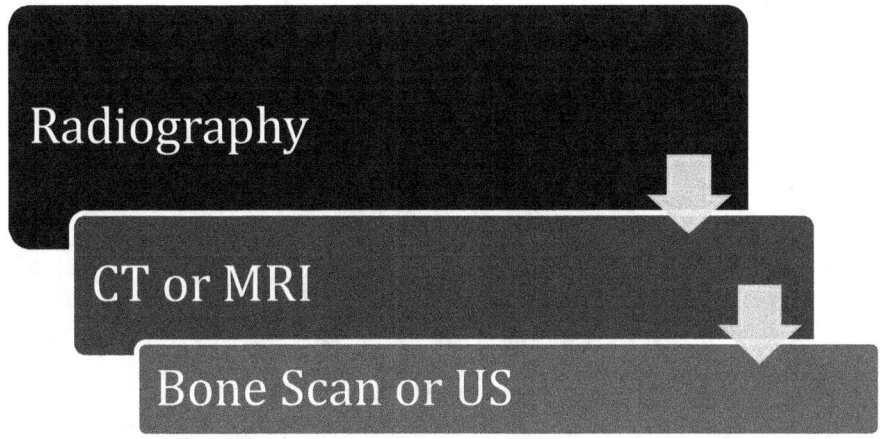

# Case 35-1

A 65-year-old woman for an annual routine check-up for her knee. She had total knee arthroplasty a year ago. What imaging test should be ordered?

This scenario concerns the routine follow-up imaging after total knee arthroplasty in an asymptomatic patient.

Sensible recommendation: XR KNEE 3 VIEW

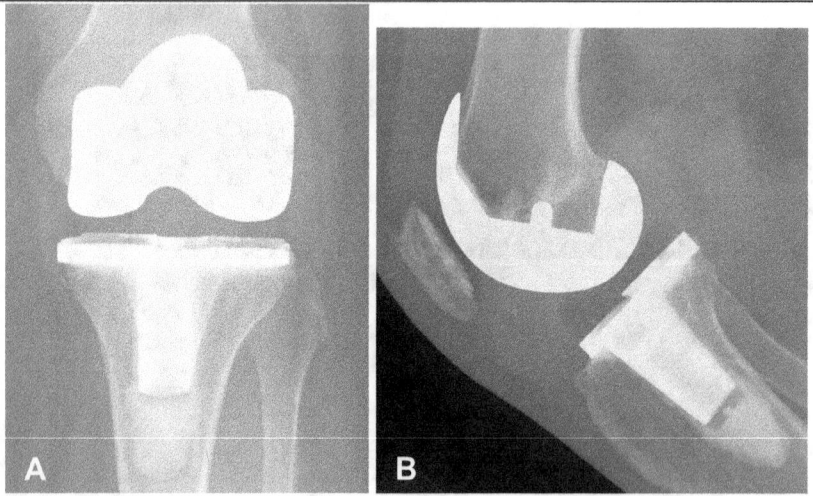

Anteroposterior (A) and lateral (B) radiographs of normal TKA. A femorotibial angle is an angle intersecting femoral anatomic axis with tibial anatomic axis. Femoral component should be placed 7° ± 3° valgus, and tibial component should be 90° ± 3° relative to anatomic axis of tibia, allowing overall 4–7° valgus angulation. Polyethylene joint space should be equivalent medially and laterally. On lateral radiograph of TKA, the horizontal portion of femoral component should be 90° relative to anatomic axis of femur. The tibial component should be horizontal or slope downward 3–7° posteriorly, and its position should be either central or posterior relative to center of tibial shaft.

Total knee arthroplasty (TKA) has become a more commonly performed procedure than total hip arthroplasty. In 2003 in the United States, 402,100 primary and 32,700 revision total knee arthroplasties were performed, and it has been estimated that by 2030, the annual demand for primary TKA will grow by 673% to 3.48 million. Patient satisfaction is greater than 90%, and there is a reported implant survival rate approaching 93% at 15 years and 83% at 20 years. Nonetheless, failures do occur, and their causes can be grouped as either extra-articular (e.g. bursitis, tendinitis, stress fracture, periprosthetic fracture) or intra-articular (including infection, instability, malalignment, aseptic loosening, prosthesis fracture, polyethylene wear, osteolysis, arthrofibrosis, soft- tissue impingement, and extensor mechanism problems such as patellar maltracking).

The timing of postoperative radiographs has been evaluated in an effort to decrease costs. Baseline radiographs are suggested at the first outpatient visit (e.g. at 6 weeks). Later follow-up is directed toward identifying any of the complications mentioned above, particularly loosening. Evaluation of serial radiographs is particularly helpful for determining subtle changes. Although follow-up radiographs are commonly performed, the frequency of assessment has not been standardized. The recommendation for follow-up every 1 or 2 years continued for the long term (>10 years).

# Case 35-2

A 69-year-old man with bilateral total knee arthroplasty presents with left knee pain. He denies any signs of infection. The clinician is concerned about polyethylene wear. What is the most appropriate first imaging test?

This scenario concerns the routine follow-up imaging after total knee arthroplasty in an asymptomatic patient.

Sensible recommendation: XR KNEE 3 VIEW

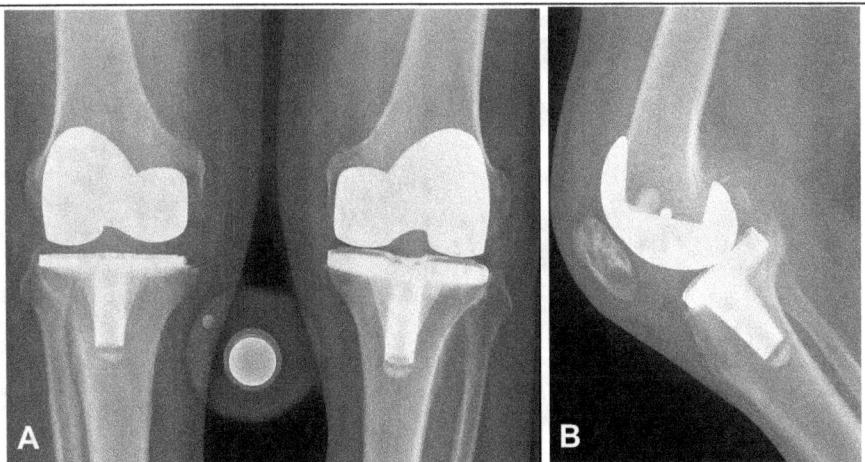

Anteroposterior radiographs of bilateral knees (A) and lateral (B) radiograph of left knee in this patient with bilateral TKA. There is joint space narrowing in left knee associated with valgus tilt (A). On lateral radiograph (B), the left knee shows metal on metal appearance in keeping with polyethylene wear.

The polyethylene articular surface of a total knee prosthesis may undergo true wear and/or deformation (sometimes termed creep), either of which can lead to a decrease in the thickness of the polyethylene. These conditions may be clinically referred to as wear. Radiographic evaluation of wear is based on weight-bearing AP and lateral radiographs and on axial radiographs. Linear wear is seen as joint space narrowing, varus or valgus deformity, or patellar tilt. An effusion may be present. Findings can be subtle and annual weight-bearing radiographs are recommended for detecting subclinical wear.

# Case 35-3

A 56-year-old man presents with ongoing left knee pain. Pain is present even at rest. He also complains of mild fever. On physical exam, he has mild fullness in the suprapatellar region. Radiograph of the knee is normal with a well-fixed and aligned prosthesis. The clinician is suspicious for infection. What imaging test should be ordered next?

This scenario concerns the initial imaging evaluation of a patient with pain after total knee arthroplasty. Periprosthetic infection not excluded. Initial imaging evaluation, including image-guided intervention.

Sensible recommendation: XR JOINT ASPIRATION KNEE

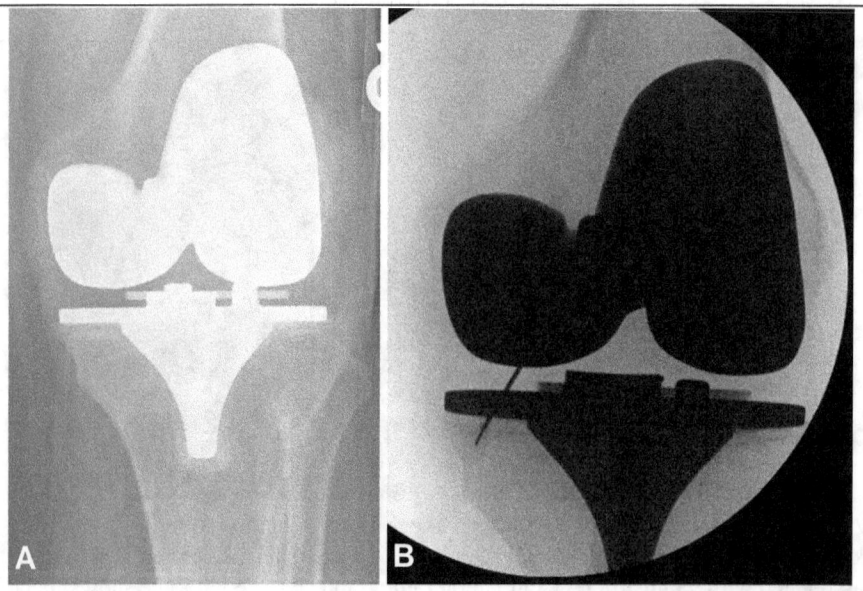

Suspected knee infection. AP radiograph of the knee (A) shows no evidence of loosening of TKA. Spot image of the knee during arthrocentesis (B). 5 ml of yellowish serous fluid was aspirated. The culture was negative for infection.

Infection is the most serious complication of joint arthroplasty and is reported in 0.8%-1.9 % of TKAs. The frequency of infection is increasing as the number of primary arthroplasties is increasing. Infection may be acute or delayed. Late infection has been defined as occurring at least 3 months after surgery. Pain is the most common presenting symptom of infection; however, it is a nonspecific finding. Night pain or pain at rest is typical of infection, whereas pain on weight bearing is more consistent with mechanical loosening. Some authors suggest that infection be excluded in all patients with persistent pain more than 6 months following joint replacement. In acute infection, findings such as pain, swelling, warmth, erythema, and fever are common, whereas chronic infections may be manifested by pain alone. Thus, a knee may be infected without the presence of fever, chills, erythema, or swelling. Loosening may result from infection.

Knee arthrocentesis has been found to be extremely useful in diagnosing joint infection after TKA. Total and differential cell count and culture should be obtained. At least 2 weeks off antibiotics is recommended before the arthrocentesis is performed (with careful clinical monitoring for sepsis). Duff *et al.* found radiographs not to be helpful since loosening, periostitis, focal osteolysis, and radiolucent lines were seen in both infected and uninfected knees. Most importantly, infection may be present with a normal radiographic appearance.

# Case 35-4

A 42-year-old woman presents with a chronic right knee pain. She has history of right distal femur osteosarcoma that was resected and reconstructed with an allograft/TKA composite, with a post-op course of multiple infections treated with debridement and several reconstructions. She denies fevers and chills but endorses fatigue. She is very tender in the popliteal fossa and has fullness in the knee. She also complains of instability with her knee while walking. C-reactive protein (CRP) was 112.8 mg/L, and erythrocyte sedimentation rate (ESR) was 60 mm/h. The knee radiograph shows joint effusion without evidence of loosening of the prosthesis. Arthrocentesis came back positive for *S. aureus*. What imaging test should be ordered next?

This scenario concerns a patient with pain after total knee arthroplasty. Joint aspiration cultures positive for infection. Additional imaging following radiographs.

Sensible recommendation: MRI KNEE WO/W CONTRAST or CT KNEE W CONTRAST

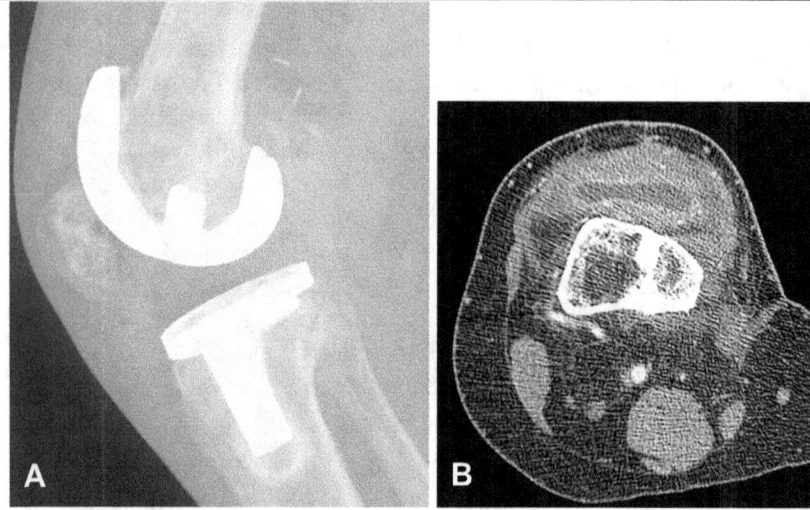

Infected knee replacement. Lateral radiograph of the knee (A) shows suprapatellar joint effusion and patellar baja. Axial CT with intravenous contrast image (B) shows suprapatellar effusion with synovial thickening and enhancement.

Infection is the most serious complication of joint arthroplasty and is reported in 0.8%-1.9 % of TKAs. Staphylococcus epidermidis and Staphylococcus aureus are the most common organisms associated with these infections. On June 18, 2010, the American Academy of Orthopedic Surgeons (AAOS) published a guideline and evidence report on The Diagnosis of Periprosthetic Joint Infections of the Hip and Knee. The work group was of the opinion that testing strategies should be planned according to whether there is a higher or lower probability that a patient has a periprosthetic infection. Patients with a high probability of infection included patients with one or more symptoms and one or more risk factors (e.g. prior knee infection, superficial surgical site infection, operative time >2.5 hours, and immunosuppression) or a physical examination finding or early implant loosening/osteolysis as detected by radiography. Laboratory findings are often nonspecific. Peripheral leukocyte counts are not elevated in most patients with infected prostheses. Sedimentation rates are abnormal in patients with infection, but this finding may also be seen in uninfected patients, limiting the value of the test. In an attempt to construct an algorithm for evaluating TKA infection, the presence of at least two positive tests for CRP (cutoff 0.93 mg/L), erythrocyte sedimentation rate (ESR) (cutoff 27 mm/h), and fibrinogen (cutoff 432 mg/dl) led to accurate results for the diagnosis of infection (sensitivity 93%, specificity 100%, and accuracy 97%).

At present, CT and MRI have a limited role in the workup of periprosthetic infection. Noncontrast CT can demonstrate the size and extent of osteolysis, periprosthetic lucencies, intraosseous or soft tissue gas, and reactive bone formation that might not be evident on radiographs. CT with IV contrast could help demonstrate periprosthetic fluid collections and fistulae. Advances in metal artifact reduction may expand the potential role of CT. In selected cases, MRI may be helpful in detecting extracapsular spread of infection and abscess formation. IV contrast may be helpful in this regard. At present, US has a limited role in the workup of periprosthetic infection, but it can be readily used to assess soft tissues and fluid collections about the knee joint in patients with TKA and can be used to guide aspiration of fluid collections about the joint.

## Case 35-5

A 62-year-old man presents with a chronic knee pain. He had a left TKA about a year ago. He did well for about 5 months, but the knee became stiffer, and warm. The patient reports the knee hurts almost all the time, sometimes even at rest. Any weight bearing is very painful. He uses crutches all the time. On exam, there is mild warmth. There is no erythema. There is synovial thickening but not a large effusion today. The knee is profoundly stiff. On laboratory exam, his CRP was 24.6 mg/L, and ESR 18 mm/h. The knee radiograph shows periprosthetic lucency around the medial femoral component and medial aspect of tibial component. The arthrocentesis was negative for infection. What imaging test should be ordered next?

This scenario concerns the imaging evaluation after total knee arthroplasty with pain. Joint aspiration culture(s) negative or inconclusive. Suspect infection. Additional imaging following radiographs, including image-guided intervention.

Sensible recommendation: In-111 WBC and SULFUR COLLOID SCAN KNEE or Tc-99m 3-PHASE BONE SCAN and In-111 WBC SCAN KNEE

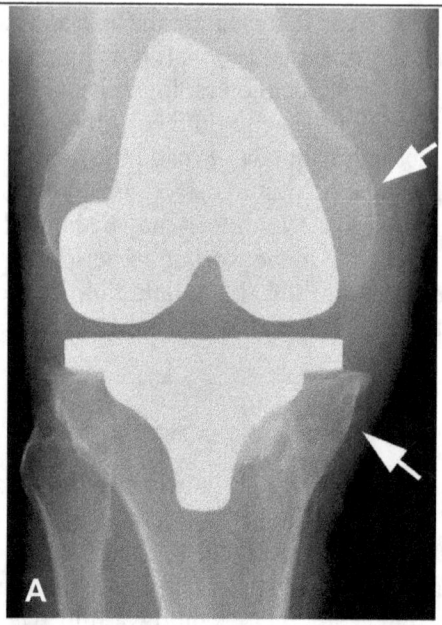

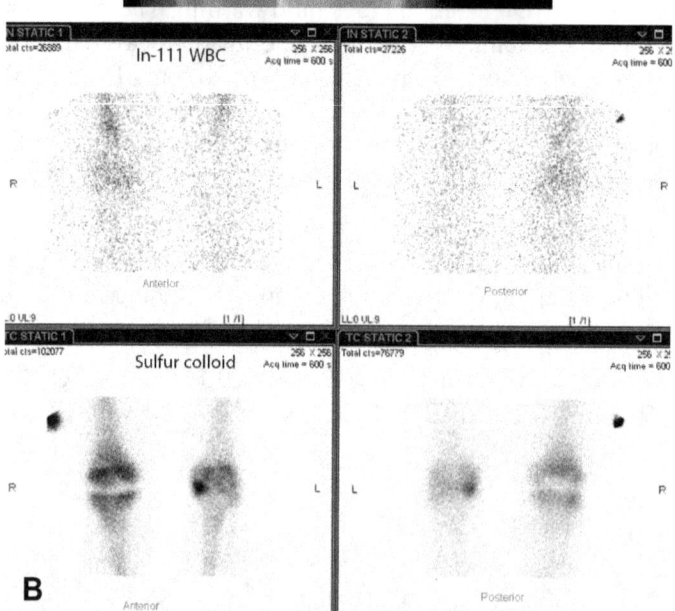

Infected knee replacement. AP radiograph of the knee (A) shows periprosthetic globular lucency around the medial aspect of the femoral and tibial components (arrows). Static images of In-111 WBC and sulfur colloid scan of the knee (B) show mismatched (incongruent) areas of pathologic leukocyte aggregation within the knee joint consistent with septic arthritis.

It is usually stated that bone scintigraphy is useful for excluding infection but of limited value in detecting it; thus specificity is higher than sensitivity. Increased uptake may persist on bone scan even at 2 years after surgery. When the equipment or expertise is not available for white blood cell (WBC) scanning, three-phase bone scanning may be valuable, even though its accuracy is lower than that of the WBC or PET scan. Infection is more likely than aseptic loosening if there is increased uptake on both blood pool and delayed images.

Gallium-67 accumulates in areas of septic or aseptic inflammation, in bone marrow, and in regions of increased bone mineral turnover. Image interpretation usually involves comparison of the isotope uptake on the gallium scan with isotope intensity and distribution on bone scan. Gallium scanning has largely been replaced by indium-labeled leukocyte imaging for diagnosing prosthetic joint infection.

Leukocyte scanning using indium-111 was introduced in the 1980s. Comparison of activity on the labeled leukocyte image to activity on the bone scan has been advocated. A positive study for infection generally requires increased activity on the labeled leukocyte study, either in a different distribution (an incongruent scan) or in greater intensity than on the bone scan. Labeled leukocyte imaging may lead to a high false positive rate because leukocytes accumulate in bone marrow as well as in infection and it is not always possible to differentiate between the two. The addition of Tc- 99m-labeled sulfur colloid bone marrow scanning has been investigated to reduce this confusion. Palestro *et al.* reported that combined leukocyte/marrow imaging was 95% accurate for diagnosing prosthetic knee infection and was superior to bone scintigraphy alone and in combination with labeled leukocyte imaging.

# Case 35-6

80-year-old man presents with right knee pain and stiffness, 6 months after revision TKA. Radiographs showed osteolysis at the tibial metal-cement interface, but arthrocentesis for possible infection was negative. What imaging test should be ordered next?

This scenario concerns the imaging evaluation after total knee arthroplasty; pain with negative studies for infection. Suspect aseptic loosening. Additional imaging following radiographs.

Sensible recommendation: CT KNEE WO CONTRAST

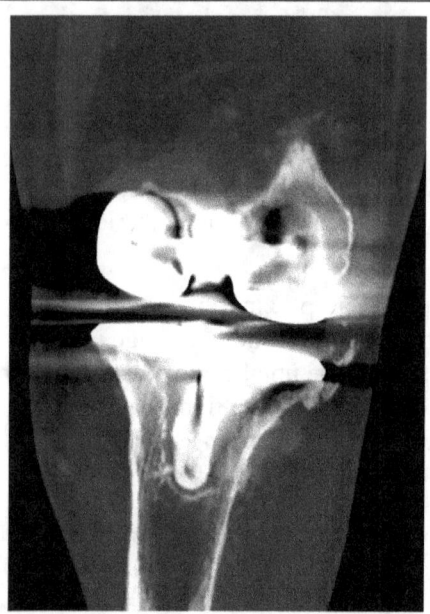

Component loosening. Coronal CT of right knee shows lucency along the metal-cement interface at the proximal tibia, along the tibial stem and medial tibial plate.

The most common cause of late TKA failure is aseptic loosening, which generally is believed to result from cumulative mechanical stresses, osteolysis secondary to particle debris, and poor bone stock. Duff *et al.* defined loosening on radiographs as the presence of prosthetic fracture, cement fracture, periprosthetic fracture, or gross component migration. Periprosthetic fractures are being encountered with increasing frequency as the number of primary TKA procedures being performed increases. Periprosthetic fractures may occur intraoperatively or postoperatively. The best treatment technique depends on whether the fracture is identified intraoperatively or postoperatively and on the fracture's location and severity. The most frequently encountered fracture occurring in juxtaposition to a TKA is a supracondylar fracture of the femur, which is often a devastating complication. Periprosthetic fractures of the tibia occur infrequently. They are classified and managed according to the anatomic location of the fracture in reference to the tibial component and whether the prosthesis is stable or unstable.

## Case 35-7

56-year-old man presents with right knee pain. He had bilateral knee replacement surgeries, right side 3 years ago, and left side 1 year ago. He started to have a sharp right knee pain 5 weeks ago. The pain is at lower aspect of knee in tibia. It is painful going up and down stairs. He denies any fever, or chills. There is no swelling on exam. Radiographs of right knee demonstrate a globular lucency about the tibial prosthesis, and particle disease is suspected. What is the most appropriate next imaging study?

This scenario concerns the next imaging evaluation of a patient with pain after total knee arthroplasty. Negative studies for infection. Suspect granulomas/osteolysis. Additional imaging following radiographs.

Sensible recommendation: CT KNEE WO CONTRAST

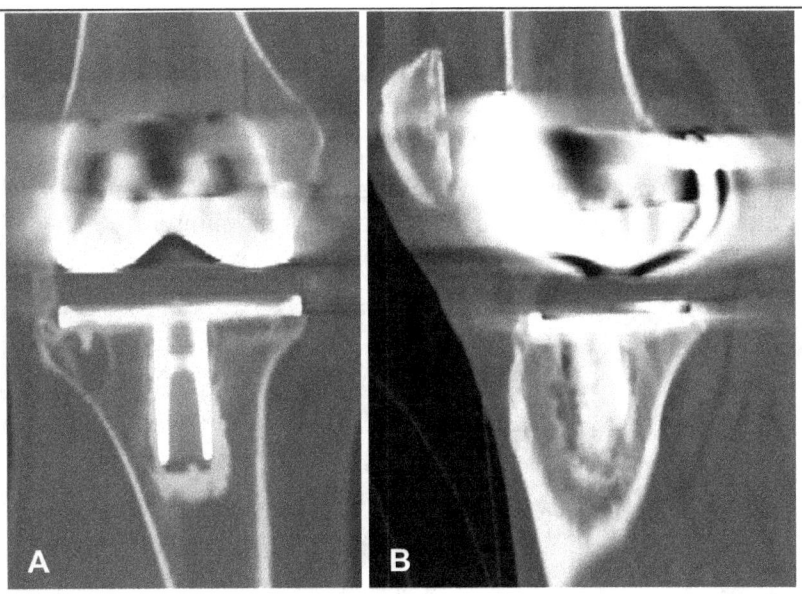

CT of knee without IV contrast. Coronal (A) and sagittal (B) reformatted images of knee. A globular lytic lesion is present at the lateral tibial plate (A). There is also periprosthetic lucency along the tibial stem with linear and lobular appearance.

Osteolysis is a leading cause of late TKA revision. Osteolysis, also known as particle disease and aggressive granulomatosis, occurs secondary to macrophage phagocytosis of particle debris. Debris from polyethylene, cement, and metal can all be causes of cell-mediated inflammatory response and osteolysis], but typically polyethylene is the most common cause. The incidence of osteolysis is higher for cementless, compared with cemented, TKAs. Osteolysis can occur anywhere but is more common in the region of the femoral condyles near the attachment of the collateral ligaments, along the periphery of the component, and along the access channels to the cancellous bone of the tibia, including screw holes. Patients with osteolysis may be asymptomatic early on but can go on to develop pain, swelling, and acute synovitis. Although small areas of osteolysis may be monitored, the presence of large areas of osteolysis suggest component loosening and may require surgery. Imaging can also help evaluate available bone stock in preparation for revision surgery. MRI and CT have both been shown to be more sensitive for detection of osteolysis than radiographs. CT can be used to detect osteolysis and to determine the total volume of osteolytic lesions, particularly when metal reduction techniques are used.

# Case 35-8

50-year-old woman presents with right knee pain. She had her right knee replacement surgery several years ago. When she walks, she feels like her knee is going out. She doesn't have any fever, or chills. There is no swelling on exam. What is the most appropriate first imaging study?

This scenario concerns the initial imaging evaluation of a patient with pain after total knee arthroplasty. Clinical concern for instability.

Sensible recommendation: XR KNEE 3 VIEW

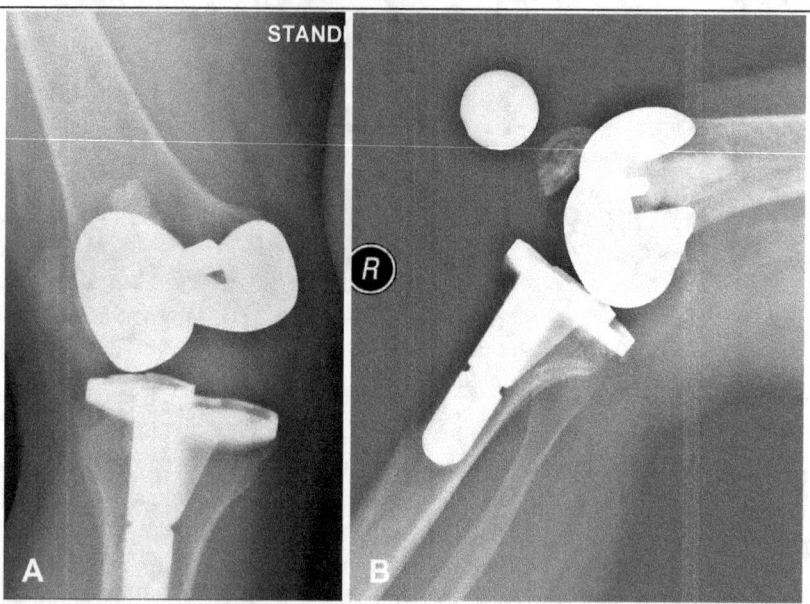

AP (A) and lateral (B) radiographs of right knee. There is marked widening of medial joint space with valgus alignment of knee on standing frontal radiograph (A). The femoral component is rotated on the lateral view (B).

Instability, one of the most common causes of early TKA failure, refers to abnormal and excessive displacement of the articular surfaces of the prosthesis. Instability usually occurs because of surgical error and poor prosthesis selection and often results in revision surgery. Severe instability can result in dislocation. Assessment of instability is based on radiographs and CT, with radiographs providing the advantage of obtaining weight-bearing and stress views.

Weight-bearing AP radiographs of the knee allow for assessment of coronal plane alignment of the knee in routine follow-up of TKA. Lateral radiographs with the knee in full extension (to assess for posterior subluxation and recurvatum and for tibial slope in a posterior cruciate–retaining prosthesis) and maximum flexion are obtained.

# Case 35-9

77-year-old woman presents with left knee pain after motor vehicle accident. On the way home after doctor's visit, she crashed her car into a pole in a parking lot. What is the most appropriate first imaging study?

This scenario concerns the initial imaging evaluation of a patient with pain after total knee arthroplasty. Clinical concern for periprosthetic fracture.

Sensible recommendation: XR KNEE 3 VIEW

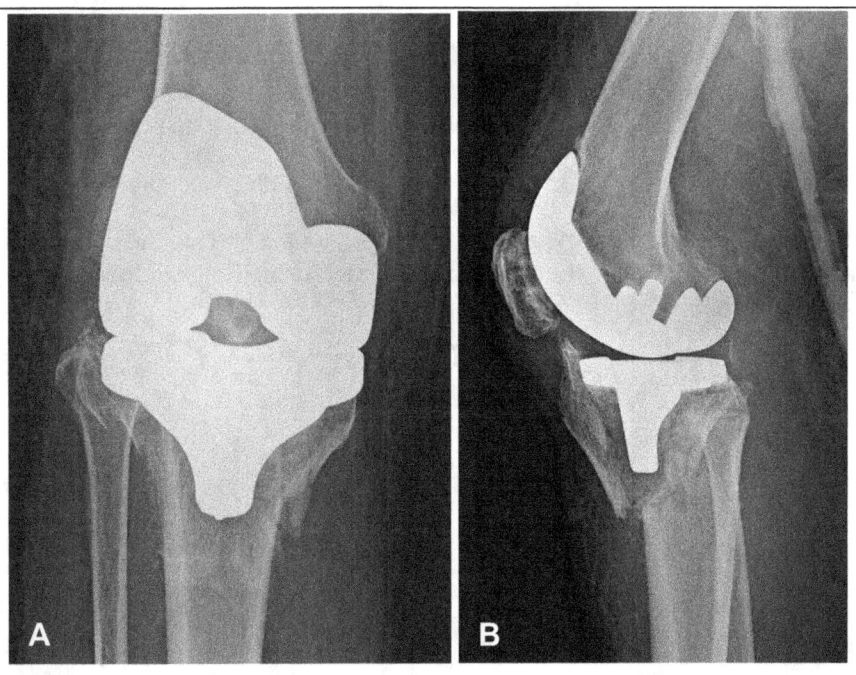

AP (A) and lateral (B) radiographs of left knee. There is a comminuted fracture in the proximal tibia. The proximal fragment containing the tibial prosthesis is displaced anteriorly.

Periprosthetic fractures may occur either during or after surgery and can involve the femur, tibia, or patella. Among periprosthetic fractures, supracondylar distal femur fractures are most common, whereas patellar fractures are rare. Supracondylar fractures occur in 0.3% to 2.5% of TKAs, usually within 2 to 4 years after surgery, and often occur in the setting of low-energy trauma. Tibial fractures are associated with loose components and malalignment. Patellar fractures are associated with rheumatoid arthritis, steroid use, osteonecrosis, and malalignment. Most patients with periprosthetic fractures are elderly, with poor bone stock. Treatment depends on fracture classification, which often includes information regarding fracture location, degree of comminution, and position and stability of the prosthesis. Radiographs are the initial examination for assessment of suspected periprosthetic fractures. Images should include the entire prosthesis as well as some surrounding bone.

# Case 35-10

80-year-old woman presents with left knee pain. She had her total knee arthroplasty eight years ago. Over the past several weeks she was having difficulty getting out of a chair. A week ago, while she was trying to get off the toilet, she heard a pop and felt severe knee pain. She is ambulating with a cane. On exam, she has a focal tenderness over her patella. What is the most appropriate first imaging study?

This scenario concerns the initial imaging evaluation of a patient with pain after total knee arthroplasty. Suspect complications related to the patella or the patellar liner (subluxation, dislocation, fracture, component loosening or wear, impingement, and osteonecrosis).

Sensible recommendation: XR KNEE 3 VIEW

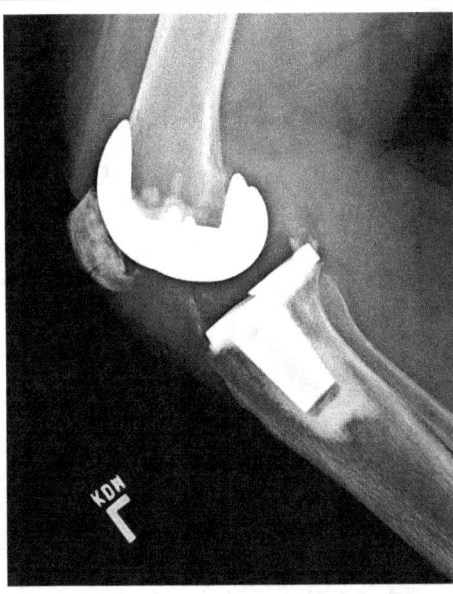

Lateral radiography of left knee shows a non-displaced fracture at the inferior pole of patella.

Patellar complications after TKA include subluxation, dislocation, fracture, component loosening or wear, impingement, and osteonecrosis. Most are not associated with prior injury, and many are asymptomatic, highlighting the importance of radiography for their identification. Transverse fractures are thought to be associated with patellar maltracking, whereas vertical fractures often occur through a fixation hole. Patellar component loosening or failure is uncommon but requires revision when it occurs. When the patella has not been resurfaced, patellar remodeling can occur and may result in anterior knee pain or fracture. Patellofemoral instability can occur from imbalance in the extensor mechanism characterized by excessive tightness of the lateral retinaculum, component malrotation, or valgus alignment of the extensor retinaculum. Radiographs are usually satisfactory for assessment of patellar complications and are helpful in guiding treatment. Axial radiographs demonstrate the degree of patellar tilt or subluxation.

## Case 35-11

70-year-old woman presents with ongoing pain, swelling, and a sense of instability. She underwent a left total knee arthroplasty a year ago. The instability seems to be the most prominent issue. She has improved substantially since her physical therapy. Clinician is concerned about her instability, and malpositioning. What is the most appropriate initial exam?

This scenario concerns the initial imaging evaluation of a patient with pain after total knee arthroplasty. Measuring component rotation.

Sensible recommendation: CT KNEE WO CONTRAST

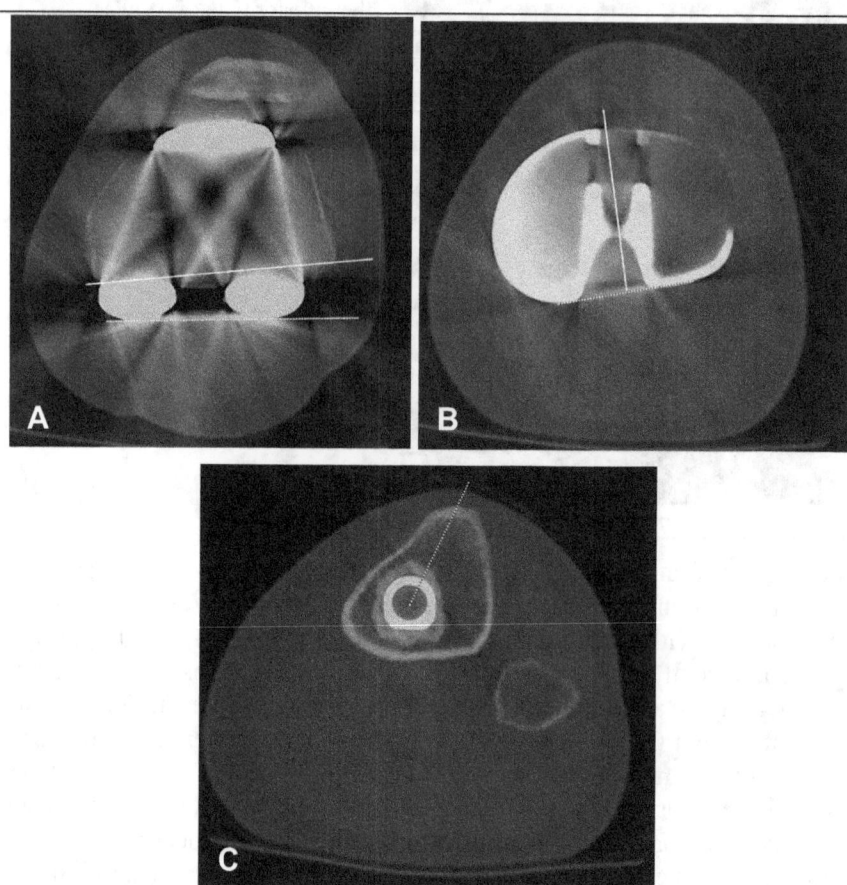

Axial CT images of knee at the level of femoral condyles (A), tibial plate (B), and tibial tubercle (C). The transepicondylar axis (TEA) is line that extends from peak of lateral epicondyle to sulcus of medial epicondyle (solid white line in A). Prosthetic posterior condylar line connects medial and lateral prosthetic posterior condylar surfaces (dotted white line in A). Rotation of femoral component is defined by angle of those two lines. At the level of polyethylene liner, perpendicular line is drawn through center point of liner (solid white line in B) to line that is parallel to posterior tibial component (dotted white line in B). At level of tibial tubercle, line bisecting tibial tubercle through center point is drawn (dotted white line in C). Tibial component rotation is defined by the angle between solid white line in B and dotted white line in C.

Malposition of femoral and tibial components may affect patellar alignment. Excessive combined internal rotation of tibial and femoral components has been shown to be associated with patellar complications. Although axial radiographs may be used to determine axial rotation of the femoral component, CT is most commonly used for this purpose. The rotation of tibial and femoral components on cross-sectional studies is most often evaluated using internal anatomic landmarks for reference. Femoral component rotation may be assessed in relation to the transepicondylar axis, or the posterior femoral condyles. The femoral component should be parallel to the transepicondylar axis, and the tibial component should be positioned in about 18° of internal rotation in relation to the tibial tubercle. Three-dimensional CT studies may also be used for assessing component rotation.

## Case 35-12

A 38-year-old man presents with pain and swelling of his right knee. He has a distant history of a right proximal tibia oncologic replacement for osteosarcoma 15 years ago. He has had multiple revisions of his implant for infection. Clinically, 2 months ago, he hit his shin on an object at home and a mass accumulated. The mass has not increased or decreased in size for the past couple weeks. He reports that he has a fluctuant swelling on the anterior aspect of his knee that has been there for quite some time and that is bothersome to him. He denies any fevers, chills, or night sweats, and he denies any lumps or bumps elsewhere. His CRP and ESR are within normal range. Radiographs of the knee demonstrate soft tissue swelling about his knee and lower leg. What imaging test should be ordered next?

This scenario concerns the imaging evaluation after total knee arthroplasty; pain but negative radiographs for loosening and low probability of infection.

Sensible recommendation: MRI KNEE WO CONTRAST

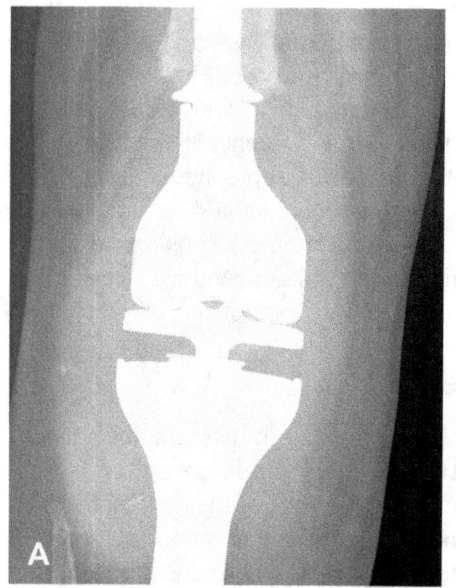

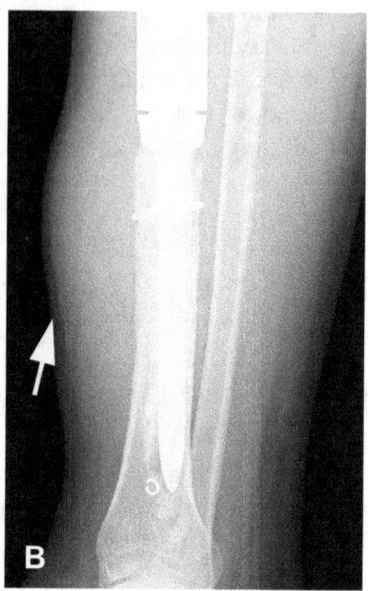

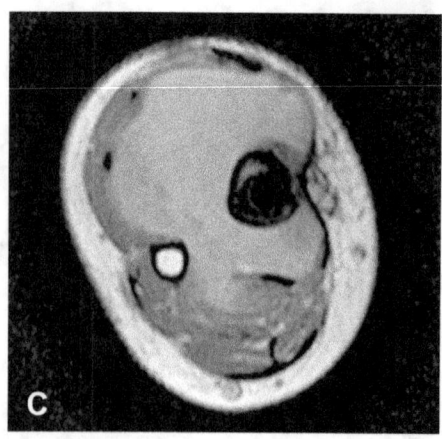

AP radiograph of the knee (A) shows an oncologic, hinged TKA. There is soft tissue density around the knee. The proximal fibular shaft is resected. The lateral radiograph of the lower leg (B) shows soft tissue swelling along the anterior calf (arrow in B). The distal tip of the tibial stem is intact. Axial T1 MRI (C) shows high signal intensity fluid collection around the tibial shaft, consistent with a subacute hematoma.

Use of modified imaging techniques may improve CT and MRI quality for evaluating the postoperative orthopedic patient. Unfortunately, radiographs have been shown to be insensitive for detecting and characterizing granulomas around total knee prostheses. CT can be used to detect osteolysis and to determine total volume of osteolytic lesions. In one study, only 17% of 48 lesions visible by CT were detected on radiographs, and detected lesions were eight times larger than radiographically occult lesions.

Similarly, MRI with techniques to decrease metal artifact can detect osteolysis even around the femoral component that is not visible on radiographs. Improved pulse sequences and techniques have facilitated the evaluation of the periprosthetic soft tissues and bone, allowing demonstration of focal osteolysis and inflammatory synovitis, as well as ligament, tendon, and nerve abnormalities. In experienced hands, US can be used to evaluate tendons, and synovitis and to guide arthrocentesis. Quadriceps or patellar tendon tears may occur, and US or MRI may be used for evaluation.

# References

1. Hochman MG, Melenevsky YV, Metter DF, Roberts CC, Bencardino JT, Cassidy RC, Fox MG, Kransdorf MJ, Mintz DN, Shah NA, Small KM, Smith SE, Tynus KM, Weissman BN. ACR Appropriateness Criteria(®) Imaging After Total Knee Arthroplasty. J Am Coll Radiol. 2017 Nov;14(11S):S421-S448. doi: 10.1016/j.jacr.2017.08.036. PMID: 29101982.
2. American College of Radiology. ACR Appropriateness Criteria: Imaging after total knee arthroplasty. American College of Radiology, revised 2017. https://acsearch.acr.org/docs/69430/Narrative/ (accessed April 24, 2021).
3. Kurtz S, Ong K, Lau E, Mowat F, Halpern M. Projections of primary and revision hip and knee arthroplasty in the United States from 2005 to 2030. J Bone Joint Surg Am. 2007 Apr;89(4):780-5. PMID: 17403800
4. American Academy of Orthopedic Surgeons. The Diagnosis of Periprosthetic Joint Infections of the Hip and Knee. Guidelines and Evidence Report. 2010; http://www.aaos.org/research/guidelines/PJIguideline.pdf. (accessed Jan 14, 2020).
5. Palestro CJ, Swyer AJ, Kim CK, Goldsmith SJ. Infected knee prosthesis: diagnosis with In-111 leukocyte, Tc-99m sulfur colloid, and Tc-99m MDP imaging. Radiology. 1991 Jun;179(3):645-8. PMID: 2027967.
6. Duff GP, Lachiewicz PF, Kelley SS. Aspiration of the knee joint before revision arthroplasty. Clin Orthop Relat Res. 1996(331):132-139.
7. Reish TG, Clarke HD, Scuderi GR, Math KR, Scott WN. Use of multi-detector computed tomography for the detection of periprosthetic osteolysis in total knee arthroplasty. J Knee Surg. 2006;19(4):259-264. PMID: 17080648.
8. Mosher TJ, Davis CM, 3rd. Magnetic resonance imaging to evaluate osteolysis around total knee arthroplasty. J Arthroplasty. 2006 Apr;21(3):460-3. PMID: 16627160.

# Chapter 36: Imaging After Shoulder Arthroplasty

Hyojeong Lee, MD.

Radiography is the appropriate exam after shoulder arthroplasty. CT or MRI are often the next step if complications are suspected. The bone scan or US may be helpful in some circumstances. If infection is suspected, arthrocentesis would be appropriate.

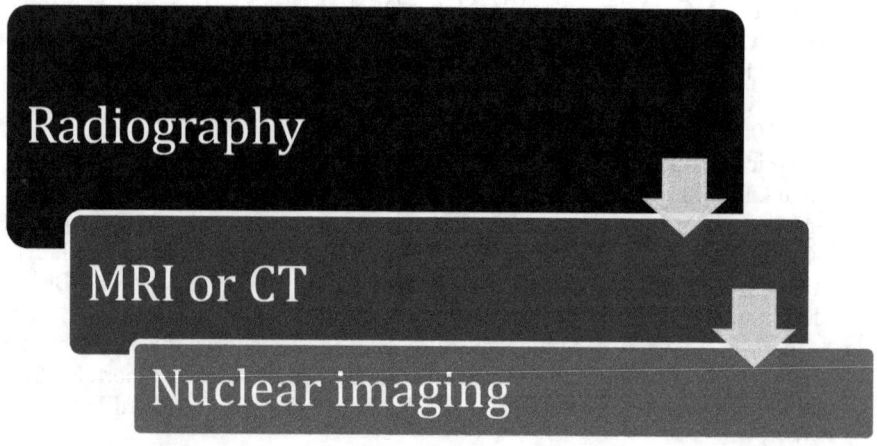

Radiography

MRI or CT

Nuclear imaging

# Case 36-1

A 55-year-old woman for an annual routine check-up for her shoulder. She had total shoulder arthroplasty two years ago. What is the most appropriate first imaging study?

This scenario concerns the routine follow-up imaging of an asymptomatic patient with a primary shoulder arthroplasty.

Sensible recommendation: XR SHOULDER 3 VIEW

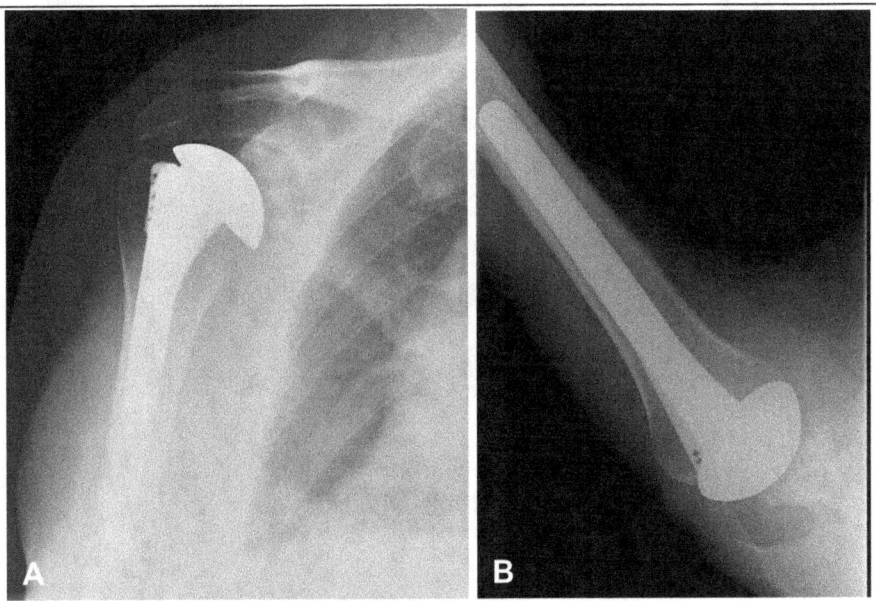

Anteroposterior (A) and axillary (B) radiographs of right total shoulder arthroplasty. On AP view, the head is superior to the greater tuberosity about 2 to 5 mm. The acromiohumeral distance is calculated by measuring the distance between an acromial line tangential to the inferior surface of the acromion and a humeral line that is tangential to the superior face of the prosthetic head. It should be more than 5 mm. On axillary view, the humeral head should be centered to the glenoid cavity.

Radiography is the first and main imaging modality utilized in the evaluation of shoulder arthroplasty. Radiographs are typically ordered within 3–6 weeks after surgery and consist of 2–4 radiographs, depending on the surgeon's preference. These may include anterior-posterior (AP), AP Grashey, scapular Y, and axillary views. Intraoperative and immediate postoperative radiographs are also ordered by some surgeons, but their value, without specific indication, has been questioned due to limitations inherent to the portable nature of the exam, patients' difficulties in cooperating with the various views, and low impact on overall patient care. n the symptomatic patient, however, radiographs are the first imaging of choice and should be performed before other more advanced cross-sectional imaging studies are performed.

# Case 36-2

A 52-year-old man presents with right shoulder pain. He underwent a resurfacing replacement of the right shoulder two years ago. He started to have pain a while ago, and now he is unable to put on a belt and has other functional deficits. He had physical therapy, but it was not that helpful. He continued to have functional deficits and pain in his shoulder. What is the most appropriate first imaging study?

This scenario concerns of a symptomatic patient with a primary shoulder arthroplasty; unknown diagnosis. Initial study.

Sensible recommendation: XR SHOULDER 3 VIEW

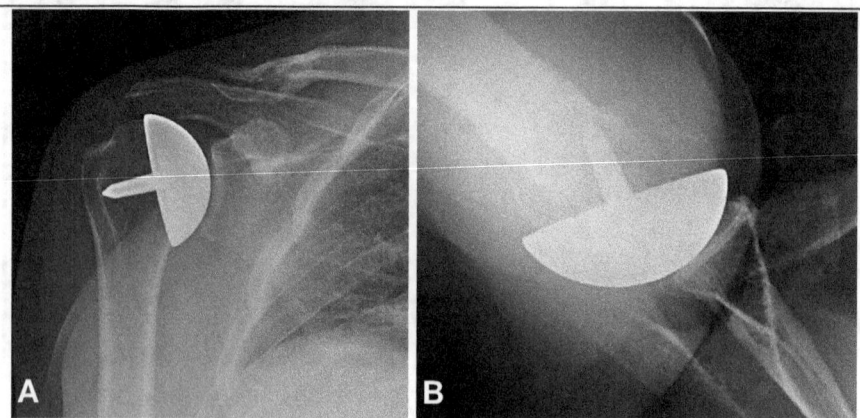

Anteroposterior (A) and axillary (B) radiographs of patient with right shoulder resurfacing hemiarthroplasty. The resurfacing stem is almost perpendicular to the long axis of humerus. On axillary view, there is surrounding globular lucency with the stem abutting to the anterior humeral cortex. The resurfacing head is posteriorly subluxated.

Radiographs should also be the first study ordered for the evaluation of the symptomatic patient with a primary shoulder arthroplasty. Humeral component loosening is less common than glenoid loosening, encompassing approximately 15% of all shoulder prosthetic complications] and more likely to occur in the setting of a noncemented component, cuff arthropathy, rheumatoid arthritis, and osteoporosis. Radiographic findings suggestive of humeral components at risk for loosening include >2 mm (width) surrounding radiolucent lines, tilt, and subsidence.

# Case 36-3

62-year-old man presents with left shoulder discomfort and dysfunction. He had his shoulder arthroplasty several years ago. He denies any signs of infection. Radiographs of his left shoulder demonstrate loosening of the glenoid component. What is the most appropriate next imaging study?

This scenario concerns a patient with a painful primary shoulder arthroplasty: suspect aseptic loosening. Additional imaging following radiographs.

Sensible recommendation: CT SHOULDER WO CONTRAST

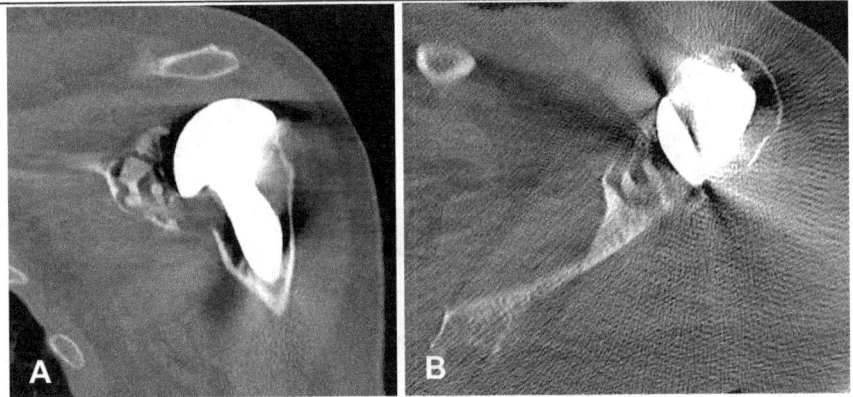

Coronal (A) and axial (B) images of left shoulder of a patient with a total shoulder arthroplasty. There is moderate amount periprosthetic lucency surrounding the glenoid component, which remodeling of the adjacent bony cortex.

Aseptic loosening, also referred to as mechanical loosening, is used to describe a hardware abnormality that results from a noninfectious etiology. Glenoid component loosening is the primary cause of failed total shoulder arthroplasties; thus the axillary view should be included in the series. Causes for glenoid component failure vary and depend on the age and sex of the patient, preoperative condition and etiology for the surgery, quality of underlying subchondral bone, type of glenoid component, and surgical technique. There is a high prevalence of radiographic radiolucencies around the glenoid component, the presence and progression of which are linked to component failure. These have been reported to become more apparent at 5 years after implantation. Evidence for glenoid loosening includes surrounding lucency >1.5–2 mm in width, migration (tilt or subsidence), or shifting of the component. Metal reduction protocols and modifications in patient positioning have greatly enhanced the ability of CT to evaluate for complications associated with shoulder arthroplasties.

## Case 36-4

49-year-old man presents with severe pain and loss of function of his left shoulder. He had his shoulder arthroplasty about six years ago. Recently he started to have pain. His shoulder radiographs were performed and demonstrated bony erosions along the glenoid. His clinician suspects infection. What is the most appropriate next imaging study?

This scenario concerns a patient with a painful primary shoulder arthroplasty: suspect infection. Additional imaging following radiographs.

Sensible recommendation: XR JOINT ASPIRATION SHOULDER

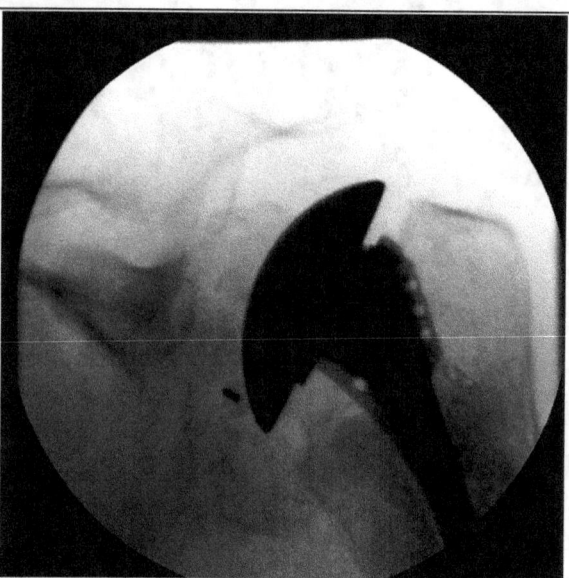

Fluoroscopic spot radiography for shoulder aspiration.

Infection, including osteomyelitis and septic arthritis, after total shoulder arthroplasty is an uncommon albeit potentially devastating complication, with a prevalence of 0.7%–2.9%, and it is more commonly seen in males and a younger age group. Predisposing underlying conditions may include rheumatoid arthritis, corticosteroid use, diabetes, repeated intra-articular steroid injections, and prior shoulder surgery. Aspiration of the shoulder should be considered when there is suspicion for an infected shoulder arthroplasty clinically, with or without radiographic evidence of infection, to avoid the destructive soft tissue and bone changes that can result from an untreated infection. Shoulder aspiration can be completed with the use of fluoroscopy, US, MRI, and CT guidance. Arthrography can be performed after the aspiration, when done under fluoroscopy or CT, if there is a clinical indication or request to evaluate for any extension of the infectious surrounding lucency >1.5–2 mm in width, migration (tilt or subsidence), or shifting of the component.

# Case 36-5

58-year -old woman with right shoulder dysfunction, and pain. She had a right shoulder total shoulder arthroplasty about three years ago. She subsequently developed shoulder stiffness on and off. She started to have pain about a month ago. Her shoulder radiographs demonstrate a minimally displaced fracture along her glenoid component. What is the most appropriate next imaging study?

This scenario concerns a patient with a painful primary shoulder arthroplasty: suspect fracture. Additional imaging following radiographs.

Sensible recommendation: CT SHOULDER WO CONTRAST

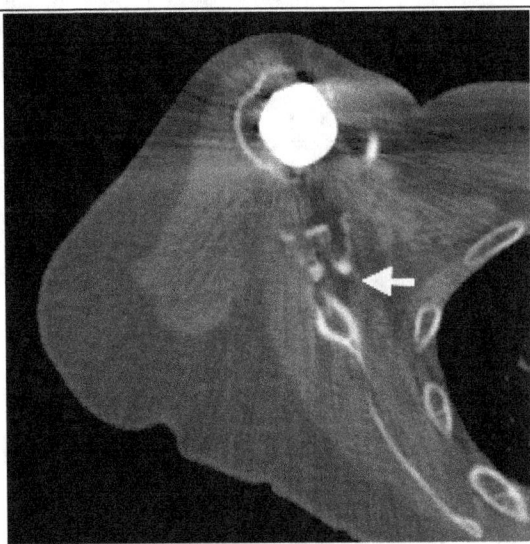

Axial CT of right shoulder of a patient with a total shoulder arthroplasty. There is a minimally displaced fracture along the glenoid stem (white arrow).

Periprosthetic fractures of the glenoid and humerus can occur intraoperatively as well as postoperatively. Complications related to surgical technique, such as excessive reaming or impaction, are the most common reasons for fractures in the intraoperative setting. In the postoperative setting, humeral fractures have been found to be more common than glenoid fractures. Fractures of the acromion and spine of the scapula are more common in the setting of reverse total shoulder arthroplasty and are thought to be related to an intraoperative complication or, more commonly, chronic stress. CT with metal reduction protocol can be used to further delineate a periprosthetic fracture seen on radiographs in terms of degree of displacement, extent, and comminution. CT can also be used when a fracture is suspected clinically but the radiographs are negative.

# Case 36-6

71-year-old woman with right shoulder pain and stiffness. She underwent a right shoulder arthroplasty about a year ago. She sustained a fracture of the greater tuberosity after a fall where she tripped on some carpet three months ago. She has had discomfort and limited range of motion. Her shoulder radiographs demonstrate no fracture or loosening. The clinician suspects rotator cuff injury. What is the most appropriate next imaging exam?

This scenario concerns a patient with a painful primary shoulder arthroplasty: patients with possible rotator cuff tear. Additional imaging following radiographs.

Sensible recommendation: US SHOULDER or CT ARTHROGRAPHY SHOULDER

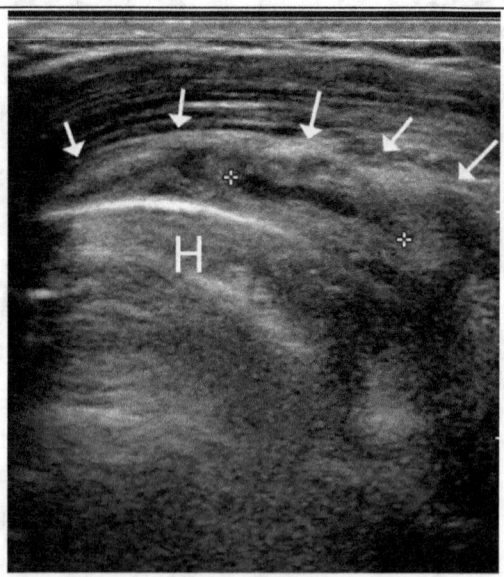

US right shoulder. Longitudinal image shows the supraspinatus (white arrows). There is linear hypoechoic area, consistent with a tear (calipers). H; humerus.

The prevalence of rotator cuff tears after arthroplasty placement has been reported to be up to 1.3%. US is a reliable option to evaluate rotator cuff tears in the setting of a shoulder arthroplasty. As opposed to evaluation on MRI, there is no prosthesis-related artifact hindering visualization of the rotator cuff on US. Tears of the supraspinatus, infraspinatus, and subscapularis tendons can all be diagnosed with US, as can long-head biceps tendon and subacromial/subdeltoid bursal pathology. US evaluation of the subscapularis tendon has been found to be more reliable than physical examination in the setting of prior tendon repair and arthroplasty placement. A limiting factor is patient body habitus. The inherent limited tissue-contrast resolution of CT detracts from its ability to detect rotator cuff tears with or without shoulder arthroplasty. CT arthrography can be used to evaluate the rotator cuff and detect any associated pathology. The technique, however, is inadequate in its ability to assess the extent of partial rotator cuff tears as well in identifying the exact location of the tear. The presence and degree of fatty muscle replacement can also be used as an indirect sign of a rotator cuff tear.

## Case 36-7

71-year-old man who presents for his right shoulder pain. He had his shoulder replaced a while ago. He also complains slowly progressing weakness. His shoulder radiographs demonstrate no loosening. He denies radicular pain. The clinician is concerned about neuropathy. What is the most appropriate next imaging study?

This scenario concerns a patient with a painful primary shoulder arthroplasty: possible nerve injury. Additional imaging following radiographs.

Sensible recommendation: MRI SHOULDER WO CONTRAST or US SHOULDER

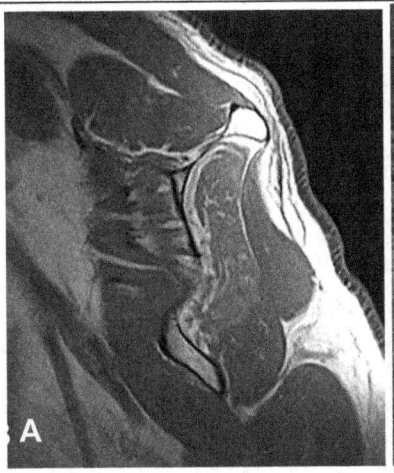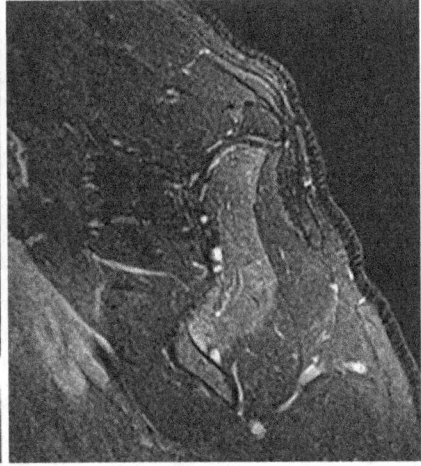

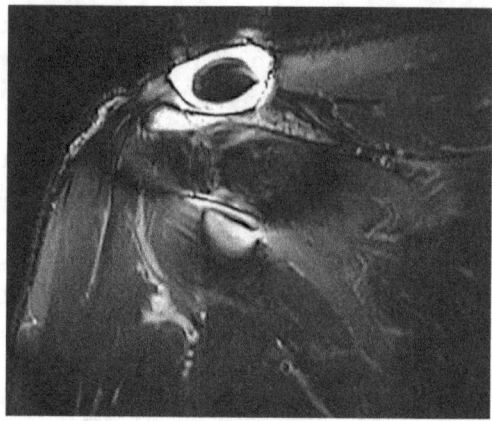

MRI of right shoulder. Sagittal T1 (A), T2 FS (B), and coronal T2FS (C) images show mild fatty atrophy (A) and edema (B, C) in the infraspinatus, in keeping with subacute denervation myopathy of suprascapular nerve.

Nerve injuries in the setting of shoulder arthroplasty are relatively common. The most common location for injury is the brachial plexus, followed by the axillary nerve and radial nerve. MRI can provide a direct evaluation of the brachial plexus as well as its branches as they course in the upper extremity. Recent advances in MRI, including high-resolution neurography, can provide greater detail in the evaluation of these nerves, allowing for an earlier diagnosis. Advanced metal reduction techniques can reduce the prosthesis-related artifact and thus improve visualization of the nerves in close proximity to the arthroplasty. Similar to CT, MRI can demonstrate the typical findings of subacute and chronic denervation in the musculature, including muscle edema, fatty infiltration, and atrophy.

# References

1. American College of Radiology. ACR Appropriateness Criteria: Imaging after shoulder arthroplasty. American College of Radiology, 2016. https://acsearch.acr.org/docs/3097049/Narrative/ (accessed April 24, 2021).

# Chapter 37: Follow-up of Musculoskeletal Lesions

Edward Derrick, MD, Kurt Scherer, MD, Laura Bancroft, MD

Radiography is the initial exam for evaluation of local tumor recurrence in the absence of comparison imaging. Follow-up at regular intervals with MRI or less often CT may be accomplished once a baseline has been established. Nuclear imaging is typically reserved for problem-solving and screening for metastases.

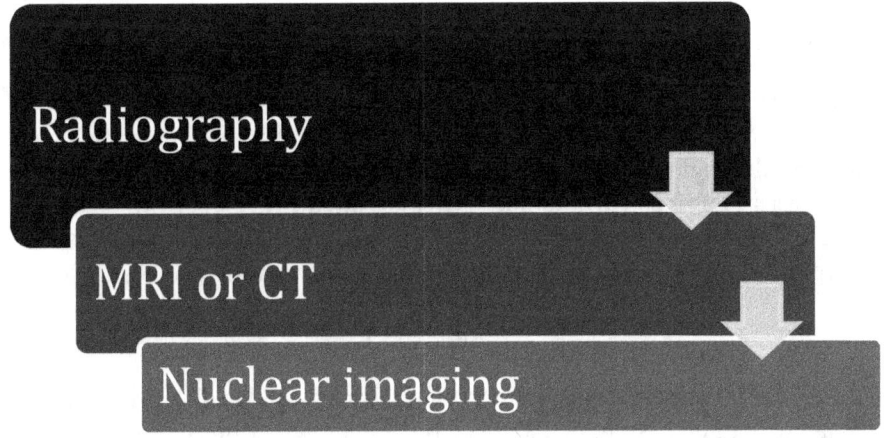

# Case 37-1

A 68-year-old patient with known primary osteosarcoma involving the left pelvis presents for follow-up. The patient is asymptomatic. What is the most appropriate study for this patient to evaluate for osseous metastatic disease at this time?

This scenario considers the evaluation for osseous metastatic disease from musculoskeletal sarcoma. Asymptomatic patient. Baseline and follow-up examination.

Sensible recommendation: NO IMAGING

In an asymptomatic patient with known musculoskeletal primary malignancy being evaluated for metastasis on follow-up, no imaging is indicated. Additional imaging should be performed if the patient is symptomatic. In most cases PET/CT or whole-body MRI has already been performed and therefore additional imaging at this time is not cost effective nor clinically appropriate and subjects the patient to unnecessary testing and cost.

# Case 37-2

A 68-year-old man presents with chest and back pain. He denies any history of trauma, but he has previously been treated known primary osteosarcoma involving the left pelvis. He has no other significant medical problems. EKG is unremarkable and laboratory values are all within normal range. What is the most appropriate study for this patient?

This scenario considers the evaluation for osseous metastatic disease from a musculoskeletal sarcoma in a symptomatic patient. Baseline and follow-up exam.

Sensible recommendation: PET/CT WHOLE BODY

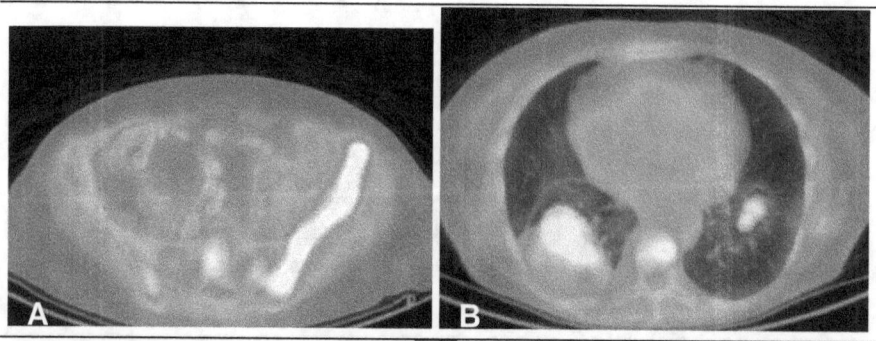

Axial PET/CT images through the pelvis (A) and chest (B). There is diffuse abnormal sclerosis involving the left iliac bone with corresponding abnormal radiotracer uptake on FDG PET/CT consistent with known osteosarcoma primary. Additionally, there are numerous hypermetabolic foci in the axial skeleton and multiple hypermetabolic nodules and masses in the bilateral lungs, consistent with metastasis.

In symptomatic patients presenting for evaluation of osseous metastasis with known primary musculoskeletal malignancy, the most appropriate baseline and follow-up imaging examination is PET/CT of the whole body. PET/CT may very accurately and sensitively detect most hypermetabolic lesions. Tc-99m bone scan can be utilized as a screening tool but it has lower spatial and anatomic resolution when compared to PET/CT. MRI whole body has been shown to have superior sensitivity and accuracy compared to PET/CT; however, this modality is not widely utilized in several institutions and requires expertise to interpret.

# Case 37-3

A 20-year-old woman presents for pain over the dorsal aspect of the left radius but has full range of motion. Two years prior patient suffered a fracture of the left distal radius and ulna after a fall, the radial fracture was found to be a pathologic fracture secondary to a low-grade chondrosarcoma. The lesion was curetted and filled with bone cement and the fractures were internally fixed. Subsequently the hardware was removed for patient comfort. MRI at that time demonstrated no residual disease. What is the most appropriate exam for this patient?

This scenario considers the imaging surveillancefor local recurrence in a patient after surgical resection of bone sarcoma, without significant hardware present.

Sensible recommendation: XR, region of interest, and MRI WO/W CONTRAST, region of interest

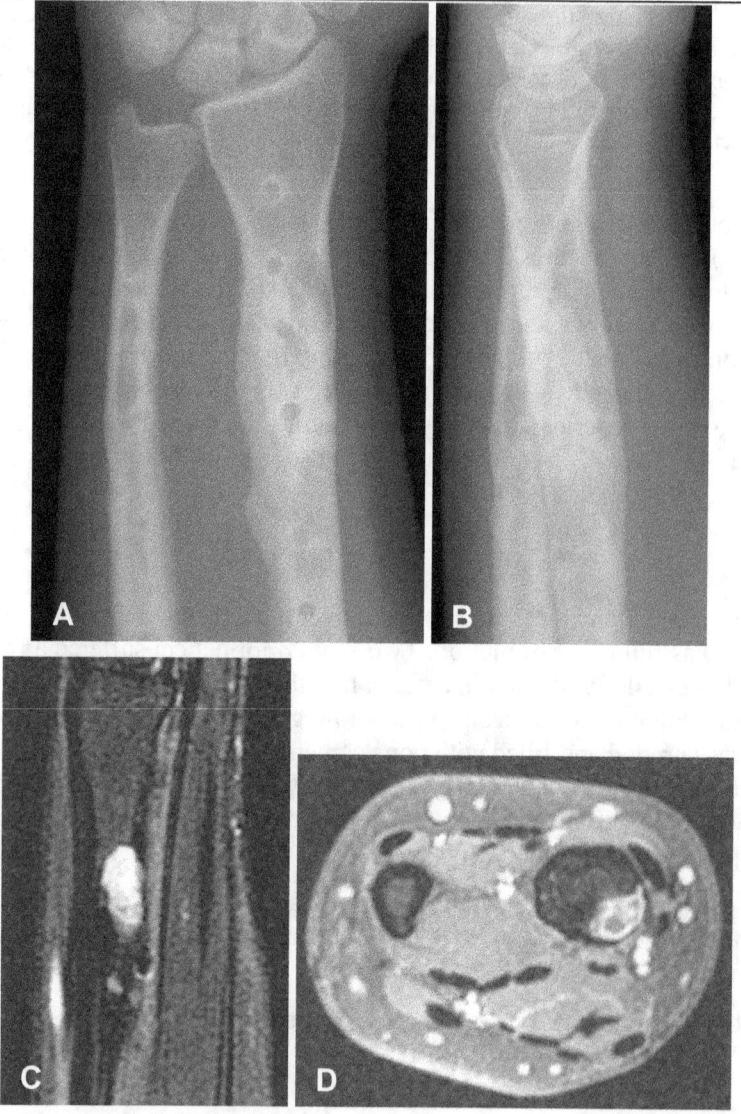

AP (A) and lateral (B) radiographs and sagittal T2 FS (C) and T1 FS Gd MRI (D) of the left distal radius. There is subtle lucency along the lateral, volar aspect of the distal radius adjacent to a region of increased sclerosis, likely representing bone cement. MRI demonstrated a lesion hyperintense on T2 with peripheral enhancement in the region of interest. Biopsy confirmed recurrent chondrosarcoma.

In a patient with a history of an osseous tumor without significant hardware with suspicion of local recurrence, the best imaging exams to perform are radiographs and MRI wo/w contrast of the region of interest. Radiography is one of the primary diagnostic tools in osseous malignancy and provides useful information by visualizing cortical structures and calcification effectively. MRI is very sensitive in detecting even subtle regions of tumor recurrence. The addition of contrast can aid in visualization of the lesion as well as facilitate the visualization of invasion, if present. PET/CT scan of the whole body may be useful in detecting distant lesions or in characterizing abnormal uptake in the region of suspected recurrence.

# Case 37-4

A 77-year-old-male with a history of sternal osteosarcoma status post resection presents with local mass in the mid-chest. Patient denies history of trauma and is otherwise reports feeling well. What is the most appropriate study for this patient?

This scenario considers the imaging surveillance for local recurrence in a patient after surgical resection of bone sarcoma, with significant hardware present.

Sensible recommendation: XR, region of interest

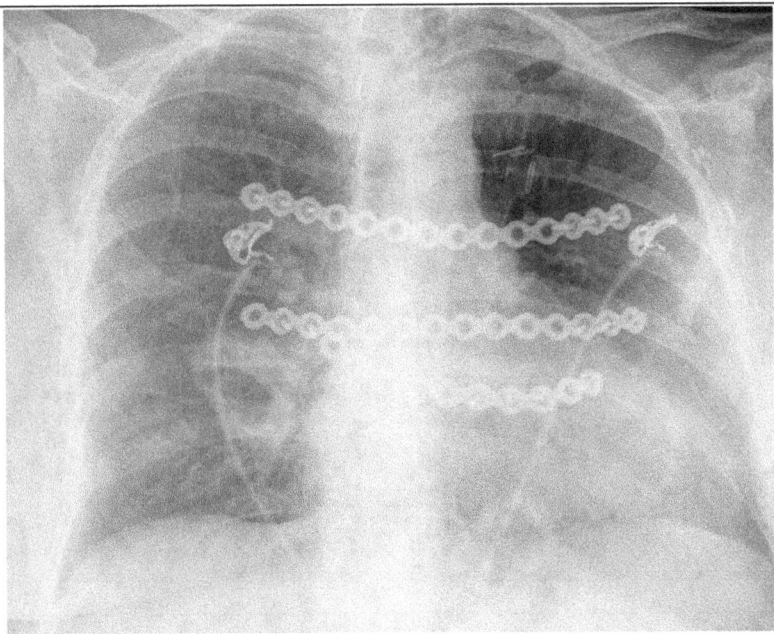

Posterior-anterior radiograph of the chest. There are post-operative sequelae consistent with prior sternal fixation. Projecting over the right infra-hilar region, there is a hyper-dense mass. Additionally, projecting over the cardiomediastinal silhouette, there is a dense region medially with a curvilinear sclerotic density periphery. This is concerning for recurrent osteosarcoma.

In a patient with a history of osseous tumor with suspicion for local recurrence with significant hardware present, the best imaging examination is radiography of the region of interest. Radiography plays a significant role in diagnosis of osseous tumors and can often detect even subtle findings. MRI of the region of interest can be used in further evaluation. Contrast can be helpful when findings are equivocal. Metal suppression techniques can be used to diminish susceptibility artifact from metal hardware. PET/CT of the whole body and CT can be utilized if MRI is not conclusive. CT technique should also be modified to decrease metal artifact.

# Case 37-5

A 46-year-old man presents for follow-up after resection of pleomorphic sarcoma of the left thigh approximately 6 months prior. Patient denies any trauma and is asymptomatic. What is the most appropriate examination?

This scenario considers the imaging surveillance for local recurrence in a patient after surgical resection of a soft tissue sarcoma tumor. Follow-up examination 3-6 months after treatment or surgery.

Sensible recommendation: MRI WO/W CONTRAST, region of interest

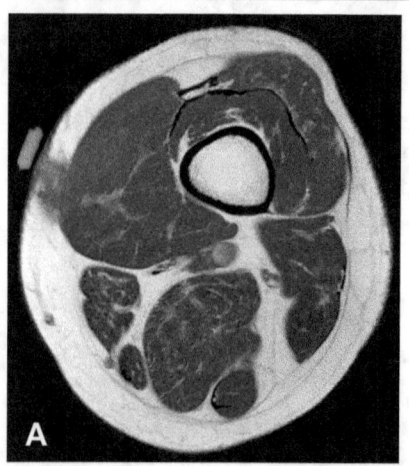 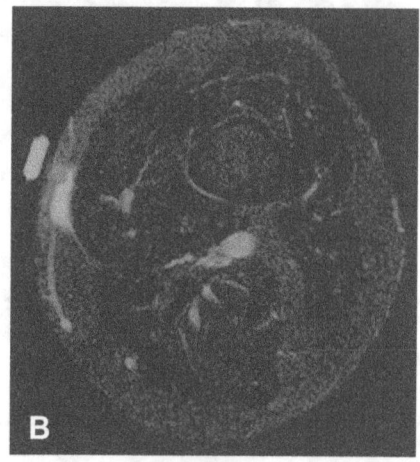

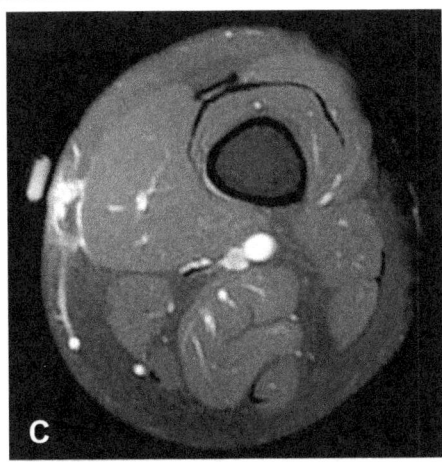

Axial T1 (A), T2 FS (B), and T1 FS Gd MRI (C) through the mid left thigh show a region of T1 hypointensity, T2 hyperintensity, and enhancement, raising the suspicion for recurrence in the subcutaneous tissues.

In patients with history of soft tissue tumor presenting for local recurrence surveillance after 3-6 months after treatment or surgery, MRI of the region of interest is the most appropriate exam. MRI is superior in evaluation of soft tissues when compared to CT. Follow-up should be performed every 3-6 months for 5 years after which the frequency can be decreased to 12 months. If a patient becomes symptomatic, it is appropriate to perform MRI earlier than these intervals. PET/CT may be helpful in equivocal cases. Ultrasound often provides sufficient penetration to visualize superficial lesions but findings are non-specific and recurrence may be difficult to distinguish from post-surgical change.

## References

1. American College of Radiology. ACR Appropriateness Criteria: Follow-up of Malignant or Aggressive Musculoskeletal Tumors. American College of Radiology, last review 2015. https://acsearch.acr.org/docs/69428/Narrative/ (accessed April 24, 2021).